AF588057

MEDIEVAL MILITARY MEDICINE

FROM THE LATE MIDDLE AGES TO THE EARLY SIXTEENTH CENTURY

For My Parents

Front Cover and Flap: Disabled veteran and battle scene (De cas des nobles hommes et femmes, 1462, Courtesy of The Huntington Library, San Marino, California HM 937, f. 1r); *Back Cover*: A soldier treats an arrow wound of a fellow warrior. (Bendicht Tschachtlan: [Berner Chronik]. Bern, [um 1470]. Courtesy of the Zentralbibliothek Zürich, Ms A 120 p. 387); *Back Inside Flap*: Tools for trepanation, (1564 – *Instrumenta chyrurgiae et icones anathomicae* / [Ambroise Paré], p. 245. Courtesy of the Wellcome Collection)

MEDIEVAL MILITARY MEDICINE

FROM THE LATE MIDDLE AGES TO THE EARLY SIXTEENTH CENTURY

BRIAN BURFIELD

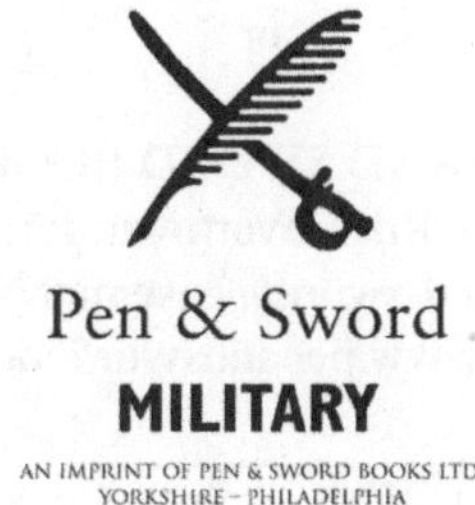

Pen & Sword
MILITARY
AN IMPRINT OF PEN & SWORD BOOKS LTD.
YORKSHIRE – PHILADELPHIA

First published in Great Britain in 2026 by
PEN AND SWORD MILITARY
An imprint of
Pen & Sword Books Limited
Yorkshire – Philadelphia

Copyright © Brian Burfield, 2026

ISBN 978 1 39904 093 8

The right of Brian Burfield to be identified as Author of this work has been asserted by him in accordance with the Copyright, Designs and Patents Act 1988.

A CIP catalogue record for this book is available from the British Library.

All rights reserved. No part of this book may be reproduced, transmitted, downloaded, decompiled or reverse engineered in any form or by any means, electronic or mechanical including photocopying, recording or by any information storage and retrieval system, without permission from the Publisher in writing. NO AI TRAINING: Without in any way limiting the Author's and Publisher's exclusive rights under copyright, any use of this publication to "train" generative artificial intelligence (AI) technologies to generate text is expressly prohibited. The Author and Publisher reserve all rights to license uses of this work for generative AI training and development of machine learning language models.

Typeset in Times New Roman 11/14.5 by
SJmagic DESIGN SERVICES, India.
Printed and bound in the UK by CPI Group (UK) Ltd.

The Publisher's authorised representative in the EU for product safety is Authorised Rep Compliance Ltd., Ground Floor, 71 Lower Baggot Street, Dublin D02 P593, Ireland.
www.arccompliance.com

For a complete list of Pen & Sword titles please contact
PEN & SWORD BOOKS LIMITED
George House, Units 12 & 13, Beevor Street, Off Pontefract Road,
Barnsley, South Yorkshire, S71 1HN, England
E-mail: enquiries@pen-and-sword.co.uk
Website: www.pen-and-sword.co.uk

or

PEN AND SWORD BOOKS
1950 Lawrence Rd, Havertown, PA 19083, USA
E-mail: uspen-and-sword@casematepublishers.com
Website: www.penandswordbooks.com

CONTENTS

LIST OF PLATES

Colour

Black and White

8. An apothecary publicly preparing the drug theriac, under the supervision of a physician. It was used to treat both wounds and diseases, including the bubonic plague. (From Hieronymus Brunschwig, Woodcut – 1500–99, Reference: 16050i. Courtesy of the Wellcome Collection)
9. An image called *Der Tod als Kriegsknecht umarmt ein Mädchen,* or *Death as a soldier embraces a girl.* (Artist: Niklaus Manuel Deutsch, mixed media on fir, 1517, Courtesy of Kunstmuseum Basel, AmerbachKabinett (Photo Credit: Martin P. Bühler)
10. Two mercenary soldiers approach a seated sex worker while Death sits in a tree pointing to an hourglass indicating that syphilis will soon take its toll. (Etching after Urs Graf, 1524, Reference: 33730i. Courtesy of the Wellcome Collection)

PREFACE

> How many have I seen, who, wounded and thrust through the bodie with swords, arrows, pikes, bullets, have had a portion of the brain cut off by a wound of the head, an arm or leg taken awaie by a cannon-bullet, yet recovered? And how manie on the contrarie, have died of light and small wounds, not worth speaking of?[1]
>
> Ambroise Paré

These observations by the prominent sixteenth-century surgeon Ambroise Paré capture the essence of military medicine in Europe from the late medieval period through the early decades of the sixteenth century and form the foundation of this volume. While gunpowder weapons were beginning to appear on battlefields, traditional arms such as swords, arrows and pikes continued to be widely used. Disease and infected wounds still posed a constant threat to soldiers' lives. Yet this period also witnessed significant medical progress and a revival of knowledge, much of it driven by the experiences and innovations of battlefield surgeons treating the wounded.

ACKNOWLEDGEMENTS

It gives me tremendous pleasure to be able to acknowledge my appreciation for the many people and institutions who helped to make this second volume a reality. Their knowledge and counsel have been indispensable.

To begin, my parents, to whom this book is dedicated, deserve a great deal of recognition for their enthusiasm and love. I will be forever thankful for their immeasurable support. There are many others who deserve to be mentioned for everything they have done for me along the way: Steph, Ruth, Steve, Andrew, Tyler, Alison, Emma-Rae, Grace, Lauren, Harri, Moira, Norm, Kelly, Erica, Quinn, and Emma. I extend my heartfelt thanks to each of them. Their love and encouragement have been limitless.

This book would certainly not have been possible without the assistance and knowledge of institutions such as the British Library, the Wellcome Collection, The National Archives and Internet Archive. It is essential that they are able to thrive and inspire without interruption. Supporting them ensures that their invaluable contributions to knowledge and culture continue to flourish.

The assistance of D. Goldring was once again instrumental in the production of this book. He reviewed ideas and initial drafts of chapters with honesty, thoughtfulness and necessary hard-heartedness. I am incredibly grateful for his tireless contributions to this volume. I am also deeply indebted to both Nancy C. D. Costa and Teresa Costa for their tremendous assistance with the translation and understanding of several historical Portuguese texts.

I am forever grateful to Pen & Sword Publishing, especially commissioning editor Amy Jordan, for allowing me the opportunity to take the review of military medicine into the late Middle Ages and the decades that followed. Stephen Chumbley, the copy editor for this book, did a tremendous amount of meticulous work to prepare this text for publication and I am very grateful for his professional assistance.

Finally, there is no one to whom I owe more than Catarina. Maintaining that she missed the piles of books and papers that surrounded my desk during the production of the first volume, she was insistent that I begin work on this second book. It was her belief and encouragement throughout the process that enabled me to finally complete it. Her translation skills in several languages also proved to be incredibly important along the way. She will always have my inestimable love and gratitude.

Chapter 1

MEDICINE FROM THE LATE MIDDLE AGES TO THE EARLY SIXTEENTH CENTURY

> For a short space of time they had fought so viciously against one another, that you could see one of them lying there with his brains showing, over there another with his arm cut off, a third with his throat sliced open, there a fourth with his chest pierced, and along the whole street it was filled with the corpses of the slain.
>
> *Chronicle of the Monastery of St Albans*[1]

This eyewitness account of the First Battle of St Albans in 1455, taken from the *Chronicle of the Monastery of St Albans* and authored by John Whethamstede, serves as a bleak reminder of the brutal nature of warfare in Europe from the late Middle Ages into the early sixteenth century.[2] It is certainly not unique; throughout the period, chroniclers strove to capture the horrors of war. Yet even an anonymous witness who attempted to document what they saw at the Battle of Crécy in 1346 in a *rijmkroniek*, or *rhyming chronicle* acknowledged how distressing this task could be, 'Of the bitter battle we cannot describe, for it was so horrible and so ghastly'.[3] It is perhaps understandable that such gruesome scenes proved difficult to portray since this was a time when the art of killing and wounding was advancing with cruel efficiency. Traditional weapons were still in use and many of them had increased in both range and lethality.[4] The introduction of gunpowder weaponry was a significant turning point in military technology that over time only became more prevalent on battlefields across Europe. These advancements enabled warriors to inflict greater damage on one another.[5] Furthermore, many of the wars of the late medieval period and early sixteenth century were marked by a general increase in size and devastation over what had come before, among them the Hundred Years War (1337–1453) and the Italian Wars (1494–1559). Compounding the misery, these conflicts took place during a period of rampant disease, further intensifying the hardships endured by both soldiers and civilians.[6]

Finding The Evidence

> Many say, and especially men of battle that prayer miraculously heals all curable wounds.
>
> John Mirfield[7]

The chief objective of the previous volume was to explore how soldiers of Europe's early and high Middle Ages survived their wounds and illnesses. This time, it is the turn of those who fought during the late medieval period and the decades that followed. Indeed, it is the hope that this edition can continue to try and answer the challenge set by the eminent surgeon and professor George E. Gask a century ago:

> . . . the old chroniclers, delighting in the narratives of which they were the actors or witnesses, have failed to tell us the fate of those who fell in battle, how they were nursed, or how their wounds were tended . . . It is only by diligent search of contemporary documents and by inference that we can hope to repair this omission.[8]

While it may be true that most chroniclers did stop short of explaining how the wounded were treated, their works do provide valuable information in this quest, including details of names, locations, battles and tournaments.[9] Still, as Gask aptly points out, a thorough investigation of a variety of other sources and materials is necessary to reveal much more about the treatment of soldiers who were wounded or became ill. These records include medical texts, poetry and literature, miracle collections and modern scientific studies in areas such as archaeology. Medical practitioners, knights, soldiers and others whose names and lives are recorded in such documents remain of particular interest since they offer a tangible link to the subject matter addressed in this edition. One such individual from the late medieval period is the cleric John Mirfield (d. 1407), an acquaintance of Adam Rous, who was himself surgeon to King Edward III of England (1312–77).[10] While not a practitioner himself, Mirfield had a significant interest in the subject of medicine.[11] Written towards the end of the fourteenth century, his text summarises the medical procedures that were common in England at the time, which included many of the therapies that had been recommended by well-known surgeons like William of Saliceto (c.1210–77) and Lanfranchi of Milan (c. 1250–1315) nearly a century earlier.[12]

The preceding book focused on five significant medical texts spanning the 500-year period between 800 and 1300 to explore the injuries and illnesses suffered by the warriors of the time: *Bald's Leechbook* and *Leechbook III* from the tenth century, Roger Frugard's influential twelfth-century work, and two surgeries from the thirteenth century, specifically those of Theodoric and William of Saliceto.[13] This volume examines the military medicine of the 250 years from 1300 to 1550, centring on the contributions of five individuals: Henri de Mondeville, Jehan Yperman, Guy de Chauliac, Heinrich von Pfolspeundt and Ambroise Paré. All of them, with the exception of de Chauliac, spent much of their careers as combat surgeons.[14] Additional details about their lives, work and texts are examined in the following chapter.

Contemporary stories and poems, ranging from *The Canterbury Tales* in the fourteenth century to *The Seven Merchants of Naples* (*Les sept marchans de Naples*) in the early sixteenth century are featured throughout this book. Literary works like these contain worthwhile information about the battles, soldiers, medicine and culture from this period. The fifteenth century carol called *The Rose of Ryse*, or *The Rose, which is the fairest flower*, offers an example. Composed originally in Middle English, it not only commemorates the victory of King Henry V of England (1387–1422) over the French at the Battle of Agincourt in 1415, but it also includes a verse that extolls the virtues of the rose, specifically its healing properties:

> The rose is the fairest flower
> The rose is the sweetest in odour
> The rose in care it is comforter
> The rose in sickness is healer
> The rose so bright
> In medicines it is most of might.[15]

Rose oil, rose honey and rose syrup were included in many of the healing salves and ointments used during this time, including those that would have been employed to treat the wounded at Agincourt.[16]

A poem by Colins de Beaumont, entitled *On the Crécy Dead*, written not long after the eponymous battle in 1346, is another work of interest, since it expresses the value of poetry over prose when reporting what occurred:

> It would be good that this affair
> Be set in rhyme, and not in prose,
> For in rhyme is it perceived to be more truthful
> And is stamped longer in the memory.[17]

This concept of truth in poetry is one that continues to have some merit when it comes to warfare. The real horrors of the First World War were often more honestly depicted in the poems of writers like Osbert Sitwell and Siegfried Sassoon than in the news reports of the time.[18] Verses by such twentieth-century war poets are occasionally included alongside works from the period under review in this volume. As shown above, they help highlight the many parallels between soldiers of these different times, creating another connection to the past.

Miracle accounts that feature sick and wounded soldiers continue to be examined, albeit there are fewer of them than in the first volume. This reduction reflects the significant decline in the documentation and collection of miracle claims of all types that took place during the late Middle Ages.[19] The inclusion of these records remains focused on the associated details they contain, rather than the miracles themselves.[20] An example can be found in the *Miracles of King Henry VI*, which contains the particulars of a man named Henry Walter de Guildford who was injured by cannon shot during fierce fighting at sea in the late spring of 1484, while he was a sailor under the command of Sir Thomas Everingham in the fleet of Richard III of England (1452–85).[21] As the men patrolled the waters around England, they met with what the report calls 'Some enemies, or it may be pirates . . .', and fighting broke out between the two sides.[22] Guildford sustained a severe injury when a small cannonball struck him in the abdomen during the skirmish.[23] It was decided that his injuries were too serious to be treated aboard the ship. When he finally reached shore, the account notes he was taken to a hospital, but his requests for a doctor went unanswered as none wished to come to treat him for fear he would soon expire, and they might be apportioned some of the blame.[24] Eventually, a surgeon was found who agreed to operate on him. He cut away the gangrenous tissue around the injury and treated it with soothing ointments before bandaging the area. Despite the intervention of the surgeon, each time the dressings were changed, it was discovered that undigested food was oozing from his belly, the entry noting, 'What could be more desperate for one who still fought for his life?'.[25] It is here that the details surrounding his treatment stop. The record picks up sometime around August 1484, when de Guildford was sent home so that he might convalesce in more comfort.[26] It was also the same time the body of King Henry VI of England (1421–71) was transferred to St George's Chapel at Windsor Castle, and miracles began being attributed to the deceased monarch. Despite being back home, it is clear that de Guildford was not fully recovered from his injuries. He summoned his sister, asking her to take a votive offering in the form of a wax image of himself to Henry VI's shrine in Windsor in the hope that he too might benefit from a healing miracle.[27] The account then states, '. . . from that time on he was more comforted each day in body and mind . . .'.[28] Later, de Guildford made the obligatory visit to the shrine at Windsor, where he told the story of his miracle to an assembly of magistrates and others, bringing with him some of his neighbours to bear witness to the details.[29] He was more than happy to show off his scar, a clear indication that his wound had eventually healed.[30]

The names and dates found in this miracle story provide proof that Henry Walter de Guildford was a real person who existed during the late fifteenth century. Several of the other details are not only evidential but also informative, including the fact that initially no doctor wanted to treat his wounds. It speaks to the reluctance of many medieval practitioners to treat those whose injuries were so serious that they might die anyway, despite intervention. When it came to wounds involving the heart, lungs and stomach, the seminal twelfth-century surgeon Roger Frugard stated: 'Wounds of those organs and of the diaphragm are beyond our abilities. Therefore, to avoid accusations that your interventions caused the death, decline to undertake treatment.'[31]

The surgeon who was eventually found partially treated de Guildford's injuries but either neglected or was unable to fix his leaking intestines. Undoubtedly, there was a recognized method for treating perforated bowels during this period, although the circumstances of de Guildford's eventual recovery remain unclear.[32] As is often the case in miracle accounts, the work of surgeons and physicians was frequently minimized by the scribes who recorded them. It helped to enhance the perception that something wondrous had taken place during the individual's recuperation.[33]

The advances in science-based disciplines, including archaeology and bioarchaeology, have been incredibly significant over the past few decades, enabling a much greater understanding of how people lived, fought, and were healed many centuries ago. For instance, an individual's approximate date and place of birth, sex, what they ate, estimated age at death, and whether any injuries were sustained prior to or at the moment they died can often be determined by examining their teeth and bones.[34] A recent study of mass graves related to the Siege of Rennes in 1491, during the French-Breton War (1487–91), has uncovered the bones of several individuals from both sides of the conflict who display healed injuries from previous bouts of violence.[35] Studies of a skeleton belonging to a Breton soldier, designated as 20183, suggest that he was likely a professional soldier and nobleman. His bones show several healed stab wounds incurred in the years leading up to the siege during which he was killed.[36] This kind of information lends credence to the idea that the therapies for such injuries, as outlined in the military surgeons' textbooks, could indeed be effective.

Evidence drawn from sources such as those above, and many more beyond, is used throughout this book to explore a range of topics related to the health and welfare of the warriors of this time. These include discussions of injuries inflicted by gunpowder and early firearms, along with the impact of diseases such as the bubonic plague and syphilis. Other chapters in this book cover broken and dislocated bones, disability, and the mental health of soldiers and civilians who were affected by war. This chapter, however, concludes by examining medicine in the late Middle Ages and early sixteenth century, as well as its evolving relationship with warfare.

The Moon and Good Humours

> He knew the cause of every ailment, were it of hot humour or cold, moist or dry, and where it was engendered, and of what humour.
>
> *The Canterbury Tales – The Prologue*[37]

Just as it had done for many centuries, the ancient Greek doctrine of the four humours continued to guide all facets of medicine during this time. This fundamental concept proposed that the body contained four vital fluids, referred to as humours: black bile, yellow bile, blood and phlegm. It was believed that everyone had a different balance of these humours, with the most dominant of the four determining their disposition. If black bile was believed to be the primary humour in an individual, they were considered Melancholic, meaning they had a thoughtful and sad disposition. A prevalence of yellow bile in a person indicated they were Choleric, someone with a fiery and irritable personality. A Sanguine temperament, one that was optimistic and sociable, belonged to those whose overriding humour was blood. Rather aptly, the primary humour in a Phlegmatic person was phlegm. Those in this category were thought to be both calm and stable.[38] There were also other factors linked to this theory, such as the four elements of air, water, earth and fire, as well as the qualities of dry, hot, wet and cold.[39] When an individual became unwell through injury or illness it was believed that their humours had been knocked out of balance. Proper treatment relied on the medical practitioner's knowledge that each patient was different and required bespoke care based on several factors.[40] As described by the prominent surgeon Lanfranchi of Milan, it was up to the medical practitioner to ensure that the combination of therapies they used properly rebalanced the patient's humours: 'The surgeon should know how to rid the patient of evil humours and to restore depleted humours and how to maintain the patient in a temperate mood, thereby to further the healing process.'[41] Bloodletting, cupping and evacuation of the bowels were among the practices employed by surgeons, alongside sutures, splints and bandages, to help restore the balance of the patient's humours and health to their natural state.[42]

When it came to healing, astrology was another important consideration for practitioners of medicine during this period.[43] In Geoffrey Chaucer's *Canterbury Tales*, the physician, who was among the group of pilgrims on their way to Canterbury, was said to be very knowledgeable about the subject, '. . . for he was well grounded in astrology. He watched well times and seasons for his patient . . .'.[44] It was something that was approached with great conviction, constituting an essential part of the medical curriculum at Europe's universities, such as Padua, Bologna and Paris.[45] During the early fifteenth century, at the university in Bologna, the coursework that formed part of the four years of study included such lectures as the 'Theory of the Planets'.[46]

The phases of the moon were believed to play a crucial role in determining the optimal time for doctors to treat a particular area of a patient's body. The basic theory was described by the fourteenth-century English army surgeon, John Arderne (1307–c.1380):

> A cyrurgien ow noȝt for to kutte or brenne in any member of a mannes body, ne do fleobotomye whiles þe mone is in a signe gouernyng or tokenyng þat membre.[47]
>
> A surgeon should not cut or cauterize any part of a man's body, nor do any bloodletting while the moon is in a sign governing or signifying that part of the body.

In medical texts of the era, it was usual to see a human figure known as a 'Zodiac Man' with the signs of the zodiac around or on the area of the body to which they applied.[48] For instance, Aries was linked to the head, Taurus to the neck and shoulders, Gemini to the hands and arms, and so on.[49] The image was typically accompanied by complex charts and instructions to assist practitioners in determining when treatment was suitable. The Flemish surgeon Jehan Yperman provides a useful example for Aries, stating, 'A head-wound during the month of Aries is influenced by the moon during two days of its fullness and for three days before and after'.[50] This meant that the surgeon should not operate on a patient's head during those eight days.

The Medical Hierarchy

> Then leeches had envy, and letters they sent him
> To dress as a doctor, and dwell with them ever.
>
> *Piers Plowman*[51]

During this time, the medical profession was primarily divided into four key groups: physicians, surgeons, barber-surgeons and apothecaries.[52] Across Europe, each was regulated and promoted by a craft guild that was dedicated to its interests.[53] Although rivalry existed between them, cooperation was not uncommon, particularly when it served the welfare of both the practitioners and the wider community.[54] In 1493, the Barbers' Company of London and the Surgeons' Guild put aside their differences to try to stop quack doctors from operating in the city.[55] In another example, the Germanic surgeon Hieronymus Brunschwig, who saw a few outbreaks of the bubonic plague during his lifetime, published a treatise on the malady in 1500. He acknowledged that it was the responsibility of physicians to treat the disease; nevertheless, he suggested that collaboration with surgeons could enhance efforts to alleviate the suffering that was caused by the plague.[56]

In addition to the four main groups, there were various other less qualified specialists, including midwives, tooth-pullers, bonesetters and rural practitioners.[57] They often filled the gaps in healthcare by taking on tasks that the professionals considered outside of their remit or unworthy of their attention.[58] While battlefield medicine was usually the domain of surgeons and barber-surgeons, in times of war medical practitioners of most types might find themselves treating the injured. During the mid-1360s, when the city-state of Florence was at war with Pisa, a state-employed bonesetter and a local wound doctor were called into service to help look after the wounded.[59]

Physicians were unquestionably the highest-ranking group among the medical experts. They were university-trained and educated individuals and, as such, usually represented the category with the smallest number of professionals.[60] Records indicate that England's two universities, Cambridge and Oxford, generated fewer than seventy-five physicians over the course of the fifteenth century. Although the numbers were bolstered by practitioners from abroad, less than 100 identifiable physicians from that century can be found working in England, which meant that the bulk of the medical work was handled by others of a lesser standing.[61]

They were often regarded as a rather self-important lot. In the 1530s in Paris, for instance, physicians from the Faculty of Medicine believed themselves to be in control of all aspects of the medical field. Despite lacking any genuine authority, they took it upon themselves to check and oversee the work being done by other practitioners.[62] Returning once again to the prologue of Chaucer's *Canterbury Tales*, a further sense of this pomposity can be seen in the physical description of the well-dressed physician who was going on pilgrimage:

> He was clad all in sanguine and blue, lined with taffeta
> And sarcenet; and yet he was but moderate in expenditure;
> he kept what he won in time of pestilence; for gold in physic
> is a cordial; wherefore he loved gold especially.[63]

Physicians were focused mainly on the internal problems of their patients.[64] Establishing what was wrong with an individual first involved classifying them according to the doctrine of the four humours. They also conducted various tests on the patient, such as checking their pulse and examining their urine for irregularities. The information the physician gained from this analysis enabled them to recommend assorted therapies and medicines to then treat the patient.[65] While they could usually be found looking after wealthy patients in Europe's towns and cities, occasionally they turn up in the records among those who treated the sick and wounded on the battlefields of Europe.[66] Marcello Cumano was one such physician. He was present at the Battle of Fornovo on 6 July 1495, administering medicine to soldiers in the Venetian army.[67]

Surgeons, whether they were university-educated or the product of the apprentice system, were at a level below the prestige that physicians enjoyed.[68] Their focus was a more hands-on approach to medicine, which primarily involved surgical procedures and treating injuries.[69] An existing record from 2 February 1369 in London, describes the swearing in of three of the city's master surgeons in which their responsibilities are outlined:

> . . . that they would well and faithfully serve the people, in undertaking their cures, would take reasonably from them . . . would faithfully follow their calling, and would present to the said Mayor and Aldermen the defaults of others undertaking cures, so often as should be necessary; and that they would be ready, at all times when they should be warned, to attend the maimed or wounded, and other persons . . .[70]

The surgeons' skill set made them particularly suited for the demands of the battlefield.[71] As some of their predecessors had done, several army surgeons from this period wrote medical texts referred to as 'surgeries'. As noted earlier, these serve as sources for much of this book and encompass a variety of techniques and remedies, including those employed by their forerunners. The tried and tested 'red powder' found in Roger Frugard's twelfth-century surgery is one such treatment. When applied to wounds, this mixture was effective in stopping the flow of blood and facilitating the healing process. It was composed of iron oxide-rich clay, known as bol d'armenie or Armenian bole, blended with frankincense, greek tar, sangdragon, mastic and one or two other ingredients, that could differ depending on the surgeon.[72]

When they were not looking after injured soldiers, numerous surgeons dedicated their time to providing medical care to individuals across all levels of society. Occasionally, this work involved participating in charitable initiatives aimed at assisting those who were unable to afford healthcare.[73]

The barber-surgeon is described in a short sixteenth-century verse by the Nuremberg-born poet Hans Sachs (1494–1576), which accompanies an image by Jost Ammann showing the practitioner at work:

> I am called everywhere.
> I can make many healing ointments
> To heal fresh wounds with grace,
> As well as broken legs and old injuries,
> To heal syphilis and treat cataracts,
> To get rid of gangrene and pull teeth.
> I also wash, shave and cut hair
> And I gladly perform bloodletting.[74]

The profession of barber-surgeon originated in the public baths of Europe, where these individuals shaved and cut the hair of their customers. They also offered basic healthcare services, such as bloodletting and tooth extraction.[75] As the barber-surgeons' popularity increased, the role evolved to include more advanced surgical procedures.[76] Guilds were established, and more control was gained over their education, which took place over several years as an apprentice.[77] Most barber-surgeons and even some surgeons lacked the ability to read Greek and Latin, which at the time were the languages of medical literature. To address this issue, initiatives were undertaken to render important medical texts into more accessible languages. The faculty at the Université de Montpellier, a prominent European centre for the study of medicine, translated the ancient works of Hippocrates, Galen and various others into French.[78] Similarly, in England, significant medical texts, such as the surgery of Lanfranchi of Milan, were successfully converted into English.[79] The education and practical skills of the barber-surgeons made them ideal practitioners to accompany Europe's armies into battle during the late medieval period and early sixteenth century. The fact that they were more numerous than surgeons was another factor that made them appealing to military forces.[80]

Apothecaries and herbalists were commonly the most accessible of the medical professionals during much of this period, offering advice to the average person. Certain apothecaries were even established to provide free medical services to disadvantaged members of the public. In Valencia during the mid-fourteenth century, an apothecary run by a man called Guillelmus Caner catered to the needs of those who could not otherwise afford it.[81] At Orléans, in 1407, Henry le Vistre donated funding for an apothecary's shop to be established within the city to provide drugs and medical attention for the poor free of charge.[82]

Apothecaries were usually literate and could rely on a wealth of experience gained through constant contact with their customers.[83] They kept their own medical texts and compendiums which they could use for reference and the preparation of medicines.[84] Their shops offered a diverse range of drugs, spices and groceries, similar those described by the sixteenth-century scholar and physician François Rabelais (d. 1553) in *Gargantua and Pantagruel*. The story depicts the experiences of two giants of the same name who are father and son, respectively. During the early stages of the story, Gargantua and his teacher would often abandon their studies on rainy days to wander through Paris, visiting various tradespeople. They especially enjoyed investigating the apothecaries, where the two '. . . diligently considered the fruits, roots, leaves, gums, seeds, the grease and ointments of some foreign parts . . .'.[85] As Rabelais suggests, these establishments offered exotic goods from far-off lands. It would not be unusual to find an elephant's tusk or a desiccated baby crocodile on display in an apothecary's window, drawing curious customers inside.[86]

Not only did they support the public at large, but apothecaries also worked closely with many surgeons and physicians. The medical texts of the army surgeons discussed in this book often refer to apothecaries as sources for the various medicines and ointments they needed for their patients.[87] In places such as Florence and Venice, between the fourteenth and sixteenth centuries, physicians and apothecaries entered into agreements that stipulated that the doctor would treat members of the public at a particular apothecary, provided they prescribed drugs and ointments offered by the shop.[88]

***

Remarkably, King David II of Scotland (1324–71) stands as a rare example of someone whose war wounds were treated by practitioners from all four tiers of the medical hierarchy during his eleven years of captivity. In October 1346, while fighting at the Battle of Neville's Cross, the king was struck in the face by two arrows.[89] He was captured by the English and held at Bamburgh Castle.[90] His treatment began when two barber-surgeons, Hugo de Kilvington and William de Bolton, were summoned from York to remove the arrows from his face. The men were paid the quite considerable sum of £6 for their services.[91] Following this initial treatment, it would be ten weeks before the king was well enough to make the trip to the Tower of London, where next he would be seen by the English royal surgeon, Roger de Heyton (also Eyton).[92] It appears that his wounds may have continued to trouble him for many years, as near the end of his confinement he is known to have required expensive herbal medications and a poultice, which were purchased from the London apothecary of John Adam. Around the time of his release, the king was examined not only by the English royal physician, Master Jordan of Canterbury, but also by his own physician, Hector le Leche, perhaps as a result of the king reaggravating his injuries.[93] Clearly, the fact that David II was the King of Scotland speaks to why he was treated by so many of the top practitioners of the time. Of course, for the average soldier, this sort of extended expert care would have been well beyond their financial means and station in life.

Quacks

> Witches, Conjurers, Diviners, Soothsayers, Magicians, and such like, boast of curing many diseases . . .
>
> Ambroise Paré[94]

As alluded to previously, quacks and fraudsters posed a significant obstacle to the medical community. These charlatans, who continued to flourish during this era, exploited the sick and injured, cheating them out of their health and money.[95] A case from London in 1382 illustrates some of the ridiculous schemes that certain imposters tried to execute, highlighting the lengths to which they would go to deceive others. A quack named Roger Clerk tried to pass himself off as a genuine man of medicine, claiming to another with the same first name, Roger atte Hacche, that he could cure his wife Johanna of her fever and infirmity. Hacche provided the quack with a partial payment of his fees in advance. In return, he received a fragment of parchment torn from an old book, which Clerk claimed contained a charm for fevers. The little parchment parcel had been wrapped in gold cloth, with Clerk suggesting it be placed around Johanna's neck so she would be healed of her ailments. When Hacche discovered that he and his wife had been deceived, the matter was taken to court. It emerged during the proceedings that there was no charm inscribed on the parchment, as it was revealed that Clerk was in fact illiterate.[96] He was found guilty of being, '. . . altogether ignorant of the art of physic or of surgery . . .'.[97] Clerk's punishment involved being paraded through the streets of London on horseback while trumpets and pipes played loudly. Throughout this ordeal, he was forced to wear the piece of parchment and a whetstone around his neck, with a physician's urine flask placed both in front and behind him.[98]

These frauds also feature in the literature of these centuries, where they are frequently the subject of ridicule. *The Fenyeit Freir of Tungland*, also known as *The False Friar of Tungland*, is a late medieval Scottish poem written by William Dunbar (c. 1460 – died before 1530) that provides an example. The tale focuses on a cleric named John Damian, a charlatan who travelled to Scotland from Lombardy. While much of the story is true, Dunbar is not above embellishing it for the benefit of the reader. It begins with the cleric visiting France, where he tries to pass himself off as a medical professional.[99] After being exposed as a fraud, Damian travels to Scotland and succeeds in convincing King James IV (1473–1513) that he is both an alchemist and a doctor. He is soon appointed abbot of Tongland Abbey in the south-west of Scotland. However, after three years, he is unable to produce any gold by alchemy and his medical falsehoods ultimately catch up with him.[100] Trying to save face, Damian claims that he can fly from Stirling Castle to France. With feathered wings attached to his arms, he perches himself on the walls of Stirling Castle and leaps off the stone ramparts only to plunge straight to the ground below, breaking his femur.[101]

The difficulties caused by quack practitioners impacted all aspects of the medical community, including those who were involved in military medicine. Henri de Mondeville, a distinguished surgeon in the French army and one of the subjects of this volume, highlights the challenges faced by military surgeons due to their presence. These charlatans dismissed the medical qualifications of those who treated soldiers, claiming that their own healing powers were superior thanks to divine intervention.[102] The absurdity of their beliefs is underlined by de Mondeville in an anecdote from the early fourteenth century involving a surgeon friend of his who was treating a patient suffering from a fistula, a condition known as St Eloi's disease. As he was grinding the medicines necessary for healing his patient, the mortar broke. The quacks and superstitious public interpreted his broken mortar as clear evidence that de Mondeville's learned friend should not be meddling in areas that were meant for God's chosen practitioners:

> . . . this was a divine miracle and revenge, for his wanting to cure a disease attributed to a saint, the treatment of which should really be reserved for divine surgeons alone.[103]

In a section of his work entitled '*Of certain juggling and deceitfull wayes of curing*', the sixteenth-century surgeon, Ambroise Paré, who is also featured in this text, discusses a number of dishonest practices that were prevalent across Europe at the time.[104] Unscrupulous practitioners attempted to persuade victims of gunshot wounds, broken or dislocated limbs and other injuries that they could heal them through various means that offered little or no actual benefit. Paré describes one of the treatments as a new trend that had appeared in an area of what is now Germany:

> . . . they beat into fine powder a stone which in their mother tongue they call Bembruch, and give it in drink to any who have a bone broken, or dislocated, and affirm that it is sufficient to cure them.[105]

Paré held a strong contempt for these healers who had been shown to be fraudulent, observing that they 'pollute, pervert and defame' the noble art of healing.[106] Despite his strong feelings, Paré was open to exploring the treatments employed by most untrained healers. He recognized that their seemingly strange approaches might offer valuable insights that could enrich his own understanding of medicine.[107]

Female Practitioners of Medicine

> For in suche cas she was a prudent leche
>
> *An Epistle to Sibille*[108]

During this time, female medical practitioners faced many obstacles, including the church, exclusion from some forms of higher education, controls on licensing and continued prejudice, all of which meant that their names and work were seldom recorded.[109] In fact, the documented names of female healers from the thirteenth to the fifteenth centuries account for less than 2 per cent of all known practitioners from that period, despite many more having clearly been involved in this field.[110] It makes trying to establish the identities of women who looked after the wounds of battle even more difficult, although they certainly do exist. During the fourteenth century, there was a female surgeon living in Frankfurt, the daughter of a physician called Hans der Wolff. Having been taught by her father, she was decorated several times for her ability to successfully treat wounded soldiers.[111] Similarly, in Hildesheim, there were two women who were known to have looked after the casualties of war and been compensated for their services.[112] Queen Isabella I of Castile (1451–1504) had a great interest in medicine, especially the positive impact it could have on the battlefield. During the fight to retake the Kingdom of Granada, she directed the construction of four large tents that served as field hospitals for her soldiers, providing them with more comfortable care when they were sick or injured. The queen ensured that the men were well looked after by professional physicians, surgeons, and apothecaries, whose assistants were generally women.[113] Similarly, in the sixteenth century, the Holy Roman Emperor, Charles V, employed female nurses to care for his soldiers.[114]

Despite the gradual decrease in the number of female characters in the literature of this period, it remained the one place where healers who were women could repeatedly be found treating the wounded.[115] The fourteenth-century story by an unknown Iberian author titled *Amadís of Gaul* contains a female surgeon who successfully treats two formerly estranged brother knights, '. . . Corisanda, being skilful in chirurgery, looked to their wounds herself with great care . . .'.[116] Elsewhere, the late fifteenth-century poem *The Story of Grey-Steel* contains a female healer, the aptly named *Loosepaine*, and according to the tale, there was '. . . no better leech in all the world!'[117] Francisco de Moraes Cabral's epic romance, *Palmerin of England*, written in the first half of the sixteenth century, features several scenes in which women treat the story's wounded, including a scene in which a badly-injured knight is cared for by two sisters:

> . . . they came speedily unto him, and taking off his armour, were careful to stanch the bleeding of his wound. Orianda, the eldest of the sisters, who had greater experience in medicine than the other twain, attended to him with such care as he deserved at her hands; supplying herself with things needful from a dispensary . . .[118]

There are many more stories beyond these where women with superior skills in medicine can be found, including the epic Valencian chivalric romance of the late fifteenth-century *Tirant Lo Blanc* or *Tirant the White*.[119] While the talents of most female practitioners who cared for the warriors of this time may have been overlooked by the medical profession, there is no doubt that the poets and storytellers of the era continued to acknowledge their invaluable contributions, much like their predecessors had done.[120]

Echoes of Metalsmiths and Medicine

> . . . there are many sorts of trepans invented . . . you shall find none more safe, than that I invented and have here delineated.
>
> Ambroise Paré[121]

London's Wellcome Collection holds a fifteenth-century manuscript of medical and alchemical works with the shelf number MS.117, which is a text that was originally transcribed from a book belonging to a medieval Florentine physician and goldsmith called Bisticius.[122] This man from Florence is representative of the notable relationship between medicine and metalsmithing during the timeframe being examined in this volume.

In earlier centuries, metalsmiths were often seen as both healers and metalworkers. They were regularly sought out to treat all sorts of medical issues, everything from injuries and illnesses to difficult pregnancies. To cure some problems, the patient was positioned over the smith's anvil, and the metalworker, with hammer in hand, pretended to strike the body part that was thought to be afflicted.[123] By the late medieval period, treatments involving anvils and large hammers had waned, and a much more practical connection existed between practitioners of medicine and metalworking.[124] While it often involved surgeons, there are many examples of others in the medical community who were also linked to metalworking, like the fourteenth-century French doctor called Master Jean Fusoris. At first, he pursued a career as a coppersmith, just as his father had done, before deciding to study medicine at the University of Paris.[125] His breadth of knowledge, which also included other subjects like mathematics and astrology, soon brought him to the attention of the court of King Charles V of France (1338–80), where he would become a member of the French embassy.[126] Another was John Hexham, an English apothecary living and working in London in 1415. He decided to use his metalworking skills for a much more nefarious purpose: counterfeiting coins, a crime he would eventually pay for with his life.[127]

The knowledge of metalworking enabled many surgeons to design and create their own medical instruments and tools.[128] During times of conflict, the ability to produce such implements for the care of the wounded was particularly beneficial. As will be seen in Chapter 3, the English surgeon, John Bradmore, managed to save the life of the young Prince Henry by extracting an arrow from his face. A specialized metal instrument had to be devised by Bradmore for the procedure to be a success.[129] In preparation for renewed hostilities with France, an entry found in the *Calendar of the Patent Rolls* of Henry V of England, dated 14 June 1416, gives licence to the king's two surgeons, Thomas Morestede (also Morstead), a member of the goldsmith's guild, and William Bredewardyn (also Bradwardyn), to begin making the surgical instruments that would be necessary for the treatment of the wounded:

> Commission to Thomas Morestede and William Bredewardyn, the king's surgeons, to take surgeons and other artificers for

> making certain instruments necessary to their mistery for the king's present voyage at sea.[130]

Ambroise Paré developed a vast array of surgical tools, instruments and prosthetics in the sixteenth century, designed to treat and assist both soldiers and citizens who had suffered injuries and the effects of disease. His contributions were significant not only in his own time but also for centuries to come.[131]

Chapter 2

SURGEONS, CONFLICTS AND TOURNAMENTS

> Five things are proper to the duty of a Chirurgeon; to take away that which is superfluous; to restore to their places such things as are displaced; to separate those things which are joyned together; to joyn those which are separated; and to supply the defects of nature.
>
> Ambroise Paré[1]

As noted in the previous chapter, much of the focus of this book is on five practitioners of medicine. Four of these men – Henri de Mondeville, Jehan Yperman, Heinrich von Pfolspeundt and Ambroise Paré – spent many years as battlefield surgeons, while the other, Guy de Chauliac, became one of the most influential figures of medieval medicine. Each authored at least one surgical text during their lifetime that brings to light the methods and treatments used to care for sick or wounded soldiers during this period. Given this context, it is worth devoting a few pages to a brief exploration of their lives and some of the challenges each faced.

Born in Normandy around 1260, very little is known about the early life of Henri de Mondeville. He would later become a cleric and study medicine in France, likely in Paris and Montpellier. After leaving France, he journeyed to Bologna, where he was mentored by the renowned surgeon Theodoric.[2] Mondeville learnt and adopted Theodoric's innovative 'dry healing' method, which sought to inhibit pus formation in wounds by avoiding the application of things such as ointments. Instead, wine was used to cleanse the injury before clean and dry bandages were applied. It was then left for a few days so that the body could start to heal naturally. This approach contradicted the prevailing theory of the time, which assumed that the formation of white pus, known as 'laudable pus', was essential for proper wound healing.[3]

Upon his return to France, de Mondeville served King Philip IV (1268–1314) and his armies until the ruler's death. He carried on in the same capacity under Philip's successor, Louis X (1289–1316).[4] Mondeville continued using the 'dry healing' technique in his day-to-day work and even tried to improve upon its effectiveness.[5] Despite his success with it, particularly in treating soldiers' injuries, he found it difficult to convince other medical professionals to adopt this novel approach, as he makes abundantly evident in his surgical text:

> This is how it was with the treatment of wounds according to Theodoric's method. Master Jean Pitard and I, were the first to bring this new technique to France, using it in Paris and in several battles to treat the wounded. We did this against the advice and will of everyone, particularly the medical community. We have had to endure abuse, threats, and even violence from others, including our own colleagues, and other surgeons . . . But the Most Serene Prince Charles, Count of Valois, came to our aid, as did a few others, who had previously seen us in the military camps successfully using this method of healing to treat the wounded.[6]

In the early fourteenth century, only a few surgeons, such as de Mondeville and Pitard (1228–1315), had the courage and willingness to practice the 'dry healing' method. The fact that so few practitioners were prepared to champion this approach led to its decline and eventual disappearance.[7] By the time of Guy de Chauliac, later in the century, the technique had faded into obscurity and would not return for many centuries.[8]

Mondeville's extensive military service and education shaped him into an accomplished man of medicine. He held a position at the Université de Montpellier, where he taught anatomy, medicine and surgery in the very early years of the fourteenth century. He stayed there until 1306, when he moved to Paris to teach in a similar capacity.[9] It was around this time that he also began work on his voluminous surgical text. The death of Louis X in 1316 marked the beginning of de Mondeville's own failing health, which forced him to retire from military service. Stating, 'I am not destined to live long, being asthmatic, coughing, and suffering from consumption . . .', it seems likely that he was suffering from pulmonary tuberculosis.[10] He continued to compose his book during the final years of his life but sadly never finished it. Still considered one of France's greatest surgeons, Henri de Mondeville died in 1320, around the age of 60.[11]

Long considered the father of Flemish surgery, Jehan Yperman was both a soldier and a surgeon who served in the Ypres militia during the first part of the fourteenth century, eventually becoming the leader of its surgical staff.[12] Born around 1260, he studied medicine in Paris in the late thirteenth century under the master surgeon Lanfranchi of Milan.[13] Afterwards, he returned home to Ypres, where he lived next to the Belle Hospital when he was not away with the military.[14] Although there is some discrepancy about the date, it seems likely that Yperman wrote his surgical text around 1328.[15] Unusually, he composed the volume in his mother tongue, which is to say, not Latin but rather a dialect of medieval Flemish called Thiois.[16] According to Yperman, he chose to write it in this language so that his son, who apparently neither read nor spoke Latin, could understand it.[17] His surgery is full of references to his famous mentor, with statements such as '. . . what Lanfranchi taught me . . .' and 'Lanfranchi of Milan said this was the best treatment'.[18] Yperman also included the teachings of ancient physicians like Galen (129–216), as well as those of other medieval surgeons, such as Bruno da Longoburgo and Theodoric, whose works were only a few decades old by that time.[19] As well, he made sure to include his own observations and experiences in the text, along with several sketches of medical instruments, something that was unusual among similar works of the period.[20]

From time to time, Yperman's work offers unexpected opportunities to discover some of the views and superstitions of the medical community and society at large during the early fourteenth century. His section on facial wounds, for example, takes a sudden turn as he discusses contemporary beliefs about children born with congenital anomalies. One theory about such conditions was that they were the result of a mother's fantasies during the conception of her child.[21] It was an idea that was still alive 250 years after Yperman penned his text. Ambroise Paré, the last of our military surgeons, included an entire chapter on the notion that anomalies present at birth were the result of the mother's imaginings during intercourse.[22] Yperman did address and dispel one superstition here: the belief that a cleft lip, then commonly referred to as a 'harelip', was the result of the mother consuming hare or red mullet during pregnancy. He deemed these ideas to be utter nonsense.[23] Yperman would continue to practice medicine until his death around the year 1331.

As stated, Guy de Chauliac is the one individual among this group of five practitioners who was not an army surgeon. However, he remains arguably late medieval Europe's most significant man of medicine. Born in the Auvergne, France around 1300, de Chauliac pursued his studies at universities in Toulouse, Paris and Montpellier.[24] He continued his education under a master surgeon in the city of Bologna, where there was another well-regarded school of medical science.[25] From there he journeyed around Europe, honing his surgical abilities and acquiring new techniques along the way.[26] Remarkably, he qualified as both a physician and a surgeon, which was somewhat unusual for the time. In addition to being accredited in these two branches of medicine, he also took holy orders, becoming chaplain and doctor to Popes Clement VI, Innocent VI and Urban V.[27]

As well as his vast education and experience, Chauliac owned a huge library of both Western and Islamic medical books, including several rare texts that are only cited by him.[28] Among the volumes he collected were a few military surgical tomes written by the Teutonic Knights.[29] Chauliac composed his *Chirurgia Magna*, or *Great Surgery*, in 1363, not long after some of the bloodiest battles of the Hundred Years War had been fought. The significance of his writing stems not only from the immense knowledge he acquired but also from its clarity. Designed as an instructional text, the book contains a huge number of treatments and therapies that would remain relevant until the eighteenth century.[30]

One area of de Chauliac's work that is particularly noteworthy surrounds the bubonic plague, known at the time as the Black Death, which arrived in Europe during the middle of the fourteenth century. Unlike most physicians who fled the disease, de Chauliac remained with his patients, treating them as best he could. During this time, he also became afflicted with the plague and was sick for some six weeks, but unlike so many others, he managed to recover.[31] Guy de Chauliac lived to be 68 years of age before his death at Avignon in 1368.

The least well-known and understood member of the group under review here is no doubt Heinrich von Pfolspeundt (also Pfolsprundt), a fifteenth-century soldier and barber-surgeon who flourished around 1460. A member of the Teutonic Order of Knights, it appears likely that he originally came from Thuringia, in what is now central Germany. As with de Mondeville, almost nothing is known about von Pfolspeundt's early life.[32] He does not appear to have had much of a formal education, but he would become exposed to medicine as an apprentice barber-surgeon, learning under a few now-obscure master surgeons, such as Johann von Birer (also Birris).[33] As a part of the Teutonic Order of Knights, von Pfolspeundt travelled throughout Germany and France. During the Thirteen Years War (1454–66), he managed to develop his medical skills further by treating many combat-related injuries.[34] Von Pfolspeundt wrote his surgical text following the Siege of Marienburg in 1460, but it would eventually become lost to history. It was only rediscovered during the second half of the nineteenth century when a manuscript copy was found amongst a box of papers in what was then Breslau, now Wrocław, Poland.[35] Von Pfolspeundt's work is certainly a worthwhile volume, not least because it is the earliest known text written by a battle surgeon from what is now Germany. It was composed decades before more widely known works by Hieronymus Brunschwig (c.1450–c.1512) and Hans von Gersdorff (c. 1455–1529), which were not published until 1497 and 1517, respectively.[36]

Von Pfolspeundt's book is quite unusual for the time in that it does not mention any of the well-known ancient, Islamic or European medical practitioners, like Galen, Avicenna (980–1037) and de Chauliac, as was common in other surgeries. It only gives the occasional nod to men such as von Birer.[37] As much as anything, this likely points to von Pfolspeundt's lack of a proper education in the science of medicine, as does his limited of knowledge of human anatomy.[38] Like most medieval surgeries, his text contains several seemingly strange ideas that challenge the twenty-first-century mind. In one passage, von Pfolspeundt advises surgeons not to eat onions or engage in 'suspicious sex' before treating patients, for fear of poisoning the injuries with their breath.[39] However, none of these aspects diminish the value of his work, which offers a realistic glimpse into the care of the sick and wounded on mid-fifteenth-century battlefields; rather, they add to it.[40] Von Pfolspeundt was a devout man who proposed that surgeons hear Mass before treating difficult cases, although this must surely have delayed the treatment of many unfortunate patients waiting to be looked after. He also possessed wisdom and humility, passing cases that went beyond his level of skill as a surgeon to a more experienced practitioner.[41]

While his surgery may seem to be the least erudite of those under review in this book, it contains procedures that are not found in most of the others, including the treatment of gunshot wounds and the reconstruction of a nose lost to violence or disease.

The last of these military surgeons, Ambroise Paré, was born around 1510 in Bourg-Hersent, a small village that is now part of the town of Laval in France. His early life and education are something of a mystery, as is his time as an apprentice barber-surgeon, although he certainly read the celebrated medical texts of men like Guy de Chauliac and the Genoese surgeon Giovanni de Vigo (1450–1525).[42] He had an older brother named Jean, a master barber-surgeon practising in Brittany, and a sister named Catherine, who was married to a barber-surgeon called Gaspard Martin, based in Paris. Given the family's strong involvement in the medical field, it appears probable that at least one of them contributed to his education.[43] He eventually moved into the Hôtel Dieu, a hospital in Paris, where he became *compagnon chirurgien*, a position not far removed from that of a modern hospital intern. At that time, this was the only true public hospital in all of Paris, a place where Paré must have gained a wide range of practical experience that would later serve him well.[44] After just three or four years of training and not yet qualifying as a barber-surgeon, Paré left the Hôtel Dieu in 1536. Despite his lack of credentials, he joined the French army, where he was soon able to make use of his medical skills while on campaign to Turin in 1537. After Paré's return to Paris, he qualified as a barber-surgeon in 1541. He eventually advanced to the rank of surgeon and ultimately became chief surgeon to the Kings of France. As with the campaign to Turin, Paré continued to accompany the French army to numerous areas of conflict between the 1530s and the 1560s, treating the sick and wounded. Much of this work would go on to inform his medical and surgical writing. His first book, published in 1545, focused on the treatment of wounds caused by gunpowder weapons and other projectiles.[45] He would then go on to write several more volumes about other aspects of surgery and medicine. When not on the battlefield, he spent much of his time treating the poor and sick of Paris. Paré's many experiences developed him into a highly skilled battlefield surgeon, inventor, and philanthropist. He was never too proud to offer up his well-worn phrase when describing his medical successes, 'I dressed him, and God healed him'.[46] In 1590, he died in Paris at the age of 80.

In addition to these five men of medicine, this volume features several other physicians, surgeons, barber-surgeons, apothecaries and clerics whose lives and work are also connected to the soldiers of these centuries. Among them is the previously mentioned Englishman John Arderne, who was no stranger to the battlefield and whose medical speciality became the treatment of anal fistulas, haemorrhoids, and other matters of this delicate area of the body. The works of the notable Giovanni de Vigo are also examined in later chapters. His insights regarding gunshot wounds and syphilis provide an understanding of the medical landscape during the late fifteenth and early sixteenth centuries. Despite practitioners such as these being acknowledged only briefly in this text, their contributions to the history of military medicine are not insignificant. As before, the lack of detail surrounding their lives and work merely reflects the constraints of space available for each of the topics under discussion in this book.

The Assistant

> If the assistants are not careful and conscientious . . . it creates many problems for the surgical work.
>
> Henri de Mondeville[47]

Assistant, fellow of the leech and surgeon's mate were just a few of the terms used to describe those who worked alongside the surgeons and barber-surgeons during these two and a half centuries. These individuals provided the professionals with vital support during medical procedures, cared for the patients as they healed, and managed several of the administrative responsibilities within the surgeon's practice.[48] It was a demanding role that could at times be exceptionally stressful, especially during times of conflict. This was the case in the early fourteenth century, when the Ypres' militia fought at Groningen. Led by Jehan Yperman, the small but busy team of surgeons and assistants is described as treating the wounded soldiers from Ypres during a very 'bloody affair'.[49]

Assistants were not unique to surgeons and barber-surgeons; they could also be found working alongside the physicians and apothecaries during this period.[50] Occasionally a name of one of these aides can be found, such as Claude Viart (also Viard), the long-time assistant and student of

Ambroise Paré. However, more often than not, their names were omitted from the texts and treatises of their masters.[51]

The guidelines and expectations of an effective subordinate continued to be included in the surgeries of this period, just as they had been in earlier medical texts.[52] Several times in his work, Henri de Mondeville mentions the traits that a useful assistant should possess. In their interactions with the surgeon, they were expected to be sharp, attentive and capable of following commands. When in the presence of a patient, they were expected to be pleasant, obliging and able to maintain confidentiality.[53] These guidelines were summed up in just four words by the Catalan physician Arnald of Villanova (c.1240–c.1311): kindness, agreeability, loyalty and discretion.[54]

Throughout the period, the merit of the assistant can be found in many of the procedures that involved fractured or dislocated bones, where more than one pair of hands were required to fix or realign a patient's damaged limbs. The thirteenth-century surgeon Theodoric suggested two assistants for these operations and used descriptions such as 'trained' or 'who knows well' when noting the sort of competent subordinates necessary for more complex situations.[55] In Jehan Yperman's fourteenth-century surgical text, his method for treating a broken leg suggests the help of two aides to provide the countertraction necessary for such a procedure. One was to hold the patient's thigh, while the other pulled from the foot, enabling the surgeon to carefully manipulate the bones back into their proper alignment.[56]

While the treatment of dislocations and fractures formed some of the less gruesome parts of the surgeon's work, there were many other operations that required a tolerance for the sight of blood and gore.[57] It was understood that some assistants might lose consciousness during one of these gorier procedures. Henri de Mondeville included a few sets of recommendations for dealing with such an eventuality. The initial approach involved more passive measures, such as removing the aide from the room when it became evident that they were struggling. However, the proposed measures for reviving a subordinate who collapsed and could not be revived relied much more on violence:

> . . . he (the surgeon) will pull hard on the assistant's hair from the temples, yell loudly at him as if he were quarrelling with him, call his name several times and strike him with whatever

> is at hand, give him a slap, rub his extremities, induce sneezing or vomiting with a feather or finger, dry or soaked in oil . . .[58]

If these methods were not successful, smelling salts or spices could be used to bring the poor helper back into the land of the living.[59]

Assistants were often responsible for other tasks, such as collecting payment on their master's behalf for certain services rendered. This could be particularly challenging, as some individuals from the nobility and wealthier classes, including judges, lawyers and bailiffs, were rather unwilling to settle their bills. They often attempted to avoid paying the surgeon for his work by dressing in 'habit de pauvre' or 'pauper's clothing' so as not to appear like someone of wealth and position.[60] If the patient was a friend or relative of the surgeon or someone truly unable to pay, their bill could be settled with a food parcel or homemade gift for the doctor. It was the assistant's job to make sure that these gifts in lieu of payment were items the surgeon actually wanted or needed by saying things such as:

> No! The master would not want that! However, you could make him some nice pottery or something like that, however, I know he does not really expect anything.[61]

By practicing such diplomacy, de Mondeville noted that a shrewd assistant could manage to earn their keep by bringing in a significant income for the surgeon's practice in the form of food and goods.[62]

Medicine in Times of War

> The wounded he caused to lie in secret hiding, and had surgeons brought to them till they were whole.
>
> *The Bruce*[63]

In the earlier centuries of the medieval period, it was less common for European armies to include dedicated surgical or medical support among their troops, but they were not unknown. The tenth-century law code of Welsh king Hywel Dha, or Howel the Good, provides evidence, stipulating that the royal physician was to be a part of the army whenever it went into battle. Amid periods of conflict in thirteenth-century Bologna, the city's surgeon became part of the Bolognese army, attending to the wounded during campaigns like the Fifth Crusade.[64] By the late Middle Ages, things began to change, and more military leaders incorporated small but professional medical corps into their armies.[65] During the Flemish revolt (1323–8), the Yprois militia joined those from Bruges in their fight against the Count of Flanders, Louis de Crécy. It was here that the surgeon Jehan Yperman was appointed 'chargé du service chirurgical', or the 'head of the surgical service'.[66] Another medical practitioner responsible for an army's medical needs was Stephen of Paris, surgeon to King Edward II of England (1284–1327).[67] In 1322, he took charge of the medical services and supplies necessary for Edward's campaign against Scotland.[68] Europe's land armies were not the only ones employing medical professionals during the fourteenth century. Many of the republics that now make up Italy included surgeons on their ships in times of both war and peace. A manuscript from 1337 contains an agreement between Philip VI of France (1293–1350) and Anton d'Oria of Genoa providing the French with 40 Genoese galleys, each with 210 men, which included a surgeon and his assistant.[69]

One of the better-known medical units of the fifteenth century was that organized by Henry V of England as he prepared for his campaign against the French in 1415. He took his own physician, Nicholas Colnet, along with two surgeons, the previously mentioned Thomas Morestede and William Bredewardyn. Each of these men of medicine was provided with three archers, whose purpose appears to have been for the doctors' protection.[70] As well, Henry's two lead surgeons each had a small group of nine surgeons reporting to them.[71] The wartime laws that go back to Henry V's reign, or possibly even earlier, acknowledge the value of such medical professionals to an army.[72] Within these ordinances are two items that stipulate that no leech, surgeon or barber-surgeon was to be harmed by anyone in any manner under the pain of death.[73]

There are other examples that come from this century, including Edward IV of England (1442–83). On his military expedition to France in 1475, he chose to take with him his physician, Master Jacobus Fryle, plus physician and surgeon Master William Hobbis (also Hobbes), and a staff of a dozen more surgeons.[74] Charles the Bold, Duke of Burgundy (1433–77), was another who understood the need for medical professionals amongst his forces, employing one surgeon for every one hundred of his spearmen.[75] At the end of the century, during the Italian Wars, Alessandro Benedetti (c. 1450–1512) was a physician to the Venetian army where he composed an important diary of his experiences, known as *Diaria de bello Carolino*, or *Diary of the Caroline War*.[76]

In the first part of the sixteenth century, Henry VII of England (1457–1509) was known to have employed surgeons in his navy, but it was his successor Henry VIII (1491–1547) who brought structure to the medical corps that formed part of the English fleet. He would introduce several reforms to the medical community, helping to increase the number of surgeons he needed to supply his armies and Navy Royal.[77] Charles V, Holy Roman Emperor (1500–58) gathered physicians and surgeons from far and wide to be a part of his campaigns, creating field hospitals for the wounded, just as his grandmother, Isabella I of Castile, had done.[78]

The value of such professional medical support to Europe's armies and navies was undeniably significant, enabling many of the sick and wounded to live and even fight another day. The fifteenth-century tale *Le Morte d'Arthur*, which has traditionally been attributed to Sir Thomas Malory of Newbold Revell, describes their usefulness. After King Arthur and his army had defeated the emperor Lucius and his men, the former made certain that his own wounded were well looked after, 'And them that were hurt he let the surgeons do search their hurts and wounds, and commanded to spare no salves nor medicines till they were whole'.[79] While surgeons and physicians such as these typically served the nobility and knightly classes, there is evidence that common soldiers, sailors and even prisoners occasionally received professional medical care. The *Diaria de bello Carolino* of Benedetti provides a first-hand account of the dire condition of the wounded brought into the Venetian camp after the Battle of Fornovo in July 1495. It underscores the critical role that medical practitioners played in saving lives, at times on both sides:

> Very many wounded were found naked among the corpses, some begging aid, some half-dead. They were weakened by hunger and loss of blood . . . In this affair no form of cruelty seemed to be lacking. There were 115 of these; some Frenchmen were mingled among them, begrimed with mud and blood and

> looking like slaves, and these without distinction were brought into the Venetian camp and attended by the surgeons at public expense. Some still breathed after hands and feet had been amputated, intestines collapsed, brains laid bare, so unyielding of life is nature.[80]

Some among the knightly classes had personal surgeons and physicians to treat their wounds from battle or tournament. Others, however, were more than capable of tending to some of their own injuries and those of their comrades.[81] Such lifesaving skills would have been invaluable to any fighting force during this time.[82] In Paris, during the early decades of the 1300s, a knight called John of Padua is mentioned as being, '. . . a soldier, a surgeon, the dean of distinguished men'.[83] In 1445, a young Spanish knight called Ferrandus of Córdoba was already a very accomplished soldier by the age of 20, before he attended the Collège de Navarre, part of the University of Paris, to become a Doctor of Medicine.[84] Returning to Malory's *Le Morte d'Arthur*, it too features knights like these, men that could not only fight, but look after injuries as well, including Sir Baudewin of Brittany, '. . . a full noble surgeon, and a good leech'.[85] Sir Mador is another in the story who uses his skills of medicine to treat and heal Lancelot's wounds.[86]

Although professional treatment was sometimes available, most soldiers continued to care for their own wounds and those of their comrades, as they had in earlier times.[87] This self-treatment is also referenced by Benedetti, when he describes a brief respite during the Battle of Fornovo in which, '. . . the soldiers were caring for their bodies'.[88] How soldiers acquired medical skills remains something of a mystery. They may have learnt them through first-hand experience, or perhaps the knowledge was passed down to them informally.[89] One of the few references to the medicine of the common soldier comes from the late fourteenth-century text of the English cleric and medical enthusiast, John Mirfield. He gives the impression that they were not overly sophisticated in their methods but were trusted none the less, explaining that some used 'their local medicines' beyond the battlefield to assist the poor.[90] When soldiers were not successful with these unschooled cures, they often turned to what Mirfield refers to as charms and oaths.[91] The cleric included one such charm that was apparently used to stop the flow of blood from a wound. Adding the patient's name, the following incantation was to be repeated over them nine times once the first few verses from the Gospel of John and a prayer had been recited:

> Cease, blood, in the name of Father and the Son. Stay blood, in the name of the Holy Spirit. Christ Jesus put to flight the pains and haemorrhage of thy servant (name), in the name of the Father and the Son and the Holy Spirit. Amen[92]

Next, the paternoster and Ave Maria were recited nine times. This practice of repeating a charm nine times, frequently alongside Christian prayers, evokes the remedies found in much earlier medical texts, such as the tenth-century *Bald's Leechbook*.[93] Although Mirfield was not opposed to the use of such incantations, he stopped short of fully endorsing them, claiming he included them for any potential benefit they might offer.[94]

The Tournament

> Be it in tournament, or in combat,
> In joust, or in battle.
>
> *Poem of the Eight Coats-of-Arms*[95]

Over the course of the 250 years covered by this book, warriors continued to face peril not only on Europe's battlefields but also at the many tournaments that were held, which makes them relevant to this study.[96] Despite the potential for injury or even death, men-at-arms sought glory and an opportunity to enhance their skills by participating in these popular events, sometimes resorting to borrowing money to cover the costs involved.[97] The fourteenth-century text *The Book of Chivalry* describes the tournament as a place that could '. . . earn men praise and esteem . . .'.[98] While this book has long been attributed to the French knight Geoffroi de Charny (1306–56), recent studies suggest that it was more likely authored by his son, Geoffroi II de Charny (d. 1398), perhaps as a tribute to his father's legacy.[99] In any case, the work also confirms the risks that went with the glory of the tournament, as there was always the potential for '. . . physical hardship, crushing and wounding, and sometimes danger of death'.[100]

During the fifteenth century, these events evolved into even more extravagant displays of grandeur, and yet, for the combatants, the dangers continued to be very real.[101] The late fourteenth- or early fifteenth-century English romance *Sir Degrevant* contains a useful description of the blend of pageantry and chaos that made up the tournaments of this time:

> In the clear sunshine, five hundred knights with their banners assembled, featly armed, and their servants as well. And all the broad countryside came thither that day to see the sport . . . With trumpet and drum and clear-sounding shawm they rushed together, and when they met, many a bold knight was thrown by the way and lay stunned and fouled under the horses' feet. They smote mightily with their swords, and soon many of these fierce fellows in their armour had no longer any joy of life. Barons were sitting on the bent, shamefully hacked about the shoulders, and with bleeding brows; and many a man was hurt . . .[102]

These events continued to be held into the sixteenth century, with enormous contests being organized by Europe's heads of state, including Henry VIII of England, Francis I of France (1494–1547) and James IV of Scotland. Battles and sieges were reenacted in front of the crowds and were made more monumental by the elaborate structures that were erected as backdrops to the fighting.[103]

The violent nature of tournaments throughout this period can be illustrated with examples of the types of casualties that were a common occurrence. According to the *Chronica Johannis de Reading*, during an event at Windsor in 1358 that honoured the feast of St George, Henry, Duke of Lancaster, was severely injured by a blow from a lance.[104] His leg was badly damaged, leaving him disabled.[105] The fifteenth-century manuscript, known sometimes as the *Warwick Pageant*, describes the life of Earl Richard Beauchamp and includes images of tournament battles where the combatants fought on horseback, as well as on foot. The potential dangers of such competitions are depicted and explained throughout, with notations such as, 'Here shews howe a myghty Duke chalenged Erle Richard for his lady sake/ And he Justyng slewe the Duke/'.[106]

Much like the medical teams at Premier League football matches who provide assistance to injured players, practitioners were typically on hand to care for the wounded during these contests. In 1390, during the reign of Charles VI of France (1368–1422), a large tournament was held at Saint-

Inglevert, near Calais. As described by the Monk of Saint-Denys, Michel Pintoin (c.1350–c.1421), knights wounded during the contest were treated by the king's own doctors:

> They dealt Sir Boucicault and Renaud de Roye severe blows which left them lying in bed for nine days; but thanks to the expert care of the doctors whom the king had sent and placed at their disposal as well as other servants of his court, the two completely recovered.[107]

The chronicler Enguerrand de Monstrelet (1400–53) recalls a five-day event held by the Duke of Burgundy at Arras in February 1429. It was fought between five Burgundian knights and an equal number of French men-at-arms.[108] During the combat, two of the French knights received serious wounds when their visors were knocked off by opposing lances that also struck them in the face.[109] Monstrelet explains that their injuries were such that neither was well enough to leave once the tournament was finished. Instead, they stayed behind at Arras, where they were cared for by the duke's personal surgeon, who eventually healed them.[110] The literary works of the time also feature doctors who were at the ready during these tournaments, as exemplified by the chivalric romance *Tirant Lo Blanc*. In one passage, Tirant is wounded in the neck during a joust but is quickly seen by surgeons who are called in to treat his injuries.[111]

During the summer of 1559, a remarkable tournament was held as part of the festivities organized by King Henry II of France (1519–59) to celebrate the end of the Italian Wars and the marriages of his sister and daughter. Jousting represented a large part of the revelries, and the king himself rode against Gabriel de Montgomery, the captain of his Scots Guard. As the two clashed, Henry suffered a blow to the face from fragments of de Montgomery's lance or perhaps the lance itself. Despite the efforts of many physicians and surgeons to save him, they ultimately could not prevent his demise, prompting an autopsy to be carried out.[112] Among the many doctors present was Ambroise Paré, who managed to record the details:

> His skull being opened after his death, there was a great deal of blood found between the *Dura*, and *Pia Mater*, poured forth in the part opposite to the blow, at the middle of the suture

> of the hind part of the head; & there appeared signs by the native colour turned yellow, that the substance of the brain was corrupted, as much as one might cover with ones thumb. Which things caused the death of the most Christian King, and not only the wounding of the eye, as many have falsly thought. For we have seen many others, who have not dyed of farre more grievous wounds in the eye.[113]

Drawing on the accounts of Paré and others who were there at the time, including the Brussels-born physician Andreas Vesalius (1514–64), modern investigations into the cause of Henry II's death have been unable to positively identify the cause of his demise. One of the more prominent theories under consideration is that the king likely died due to inflammation of the brain and the surrounding membranes.[114] While the level of medical detail and investigation surrounding the death of Henry II is unusual, his case is indicative of the genuine danger of death that existed at these contests, irrespective of social status.[115]

Accounts of injuries, both minor and severe, suffered by men-at-arms at the tournaments during the period examined here are interspersed throughout this edition, adding to our understanding of contemporary medical practice.

Chapter 3

DISCOVERY AND REDISCOVERY

The leches seide that they him hele wolde;
With goddis helpe they it doo sholde.

The Romance of Guy of Warwick[1]

From the latter part of the Middle Ages through the decades that followed, the improvement of traditional weapons and the development of firearms were the catalysts that drove many of innovations, discoveries and rediscoveries in medicine.[2] As the French surgeon Henri de Mondeville noted in his text, '. . . what is new requires a new opinion and the surgeon needs to have a ready and natural genius'.[3] To turn these new opinions into something useful regularly involved perseverance and repetition on the part of the practitioner. The English surgeon John Arderne used the image of a closed door to symbolize the persistence he believed practitioners needed to solve difficult medical problems, stating, 'It is not opened to them that knock as they pass by, but to those who stand and knock'.[4]

Experimentation was another important part of the discovery process for these surgeons, both for wounds and disease.[5] As difficult as it may be to comprehend from a 21st-century perspective, this could include testing on cadavers, animals, condemned criminals, soldiers and the poor.[6] One such operation took place in 1474 and involved an archer from Meudon, near Paris, who was sentenced to death for robbery.[7] Importantly, the soldier had also been afflicted by an unknown illness that was affecting many others in the area, raising concern among local doctors. Described as '. . . stone colic, passion and malady of the flank', the condition led surgeons to operate on the archer while he was still alive to study the condition in a living person:[8]

> Whereupon an opening and incision was made in the body of the said archer, and therein they searched and sought the place of the said maladies, and after it had been seen, was sewed up with his entrails replaced within.[9]

Having received the best post-surgical care available, the archer survived and soon began feeling well again.[10] His crimes were pardoned, and he was even rewarded for all he had been through. Just what this affliction was, however, remains a mystery.[11]

Time and again, resolving difficult medical issues relied on doctors' knowledge of metalsmithing to produce new tools for treating patients, though not always to the best effect, as will be seen. Combined with expertise, persistence, and experimentation, often in the context of treating wounded soldiers, this practical knowledge enabled surgeons such as Henri de Mondeville, Heinrich von Pfolspeundt and Ambroise Paré to arrive at a number of discoveries and rediscoveries, some small and others more significant. A few of these devices and procedures are highlighted in this chapter, with more being found throughout the rest of this volume.

Spider Silk

> . . . apply spider's web soaked in common oil and vinegar.
>
> John of Mirfield[12]

Cuts and lacerations were naturally very common among medieval soldiers. There were any number of sharp-edged weapons that were capable of causing such harm to the warriors of the age. Provided infection did not decide to play too significant a role in the injury, repairing the damage was usually well within the capability of those who treated their wounds. The female leech named Loosepaine, for instance, who appears in *The Story of Grey-Steel*, is frequently depicted treating such injuries, using an assortment of sutures, salves and expensive spices.[13]

One of the more unusual-sounding elements that was employed to heal lacerations is spider silk, sometimes known as *toile d'araignée*. It is something that would not have been out of place among the treatments of someone like Loosepaine. It was a substance used by Greek and Roman physicians and later by Islamic doctors, such as Abulcasis (936–1013).[14] It appears less frequently in the texts of European surgeons during the high Middle Ages, before enjoying something of a resurgence with practitioners in the period examined here.[15] In the early fourteenth century, de Mondeville suggested using spider silk to strengthen topical salves and medicines, while the Flemish surgeon Jehan Yperman recommended it as part of a mixture to help control bleeding in wounds.[16] Later in the century, Guy de Chauliac described a medicine containing spiders' webs, which he noted would help stop bleeding and promote healing.[17] John Mirfield, too, endorsed its use in his late fourteenth-century collection of cures and treatments but warned against the dangers of leaving foreign matter in the silk, which could cause contamination in the wound:

> Or if a spider's web cleansed of dust may be put on, it cures the wound because it cleanses and consolidates, but take care that neither the foot nor any part of the spider stays in it which could easily infect the whole body.[18]

Ambroise Paré included spiders' webs among his large list of medicines derived from animals, plants and minerals, believing them to be useful in the treatment of diseases.[19]

The value of spider silk in wound healing remains a topic of debate, with modern scientific studies yielding mixed results. While some research highlights its antimicrobial properties and suggests improved rates of healing and tissue growth, other studies indicate that the substance may have little medical value.[20] What is not disputed is the strength, durability and biodegradability of spider silk, which makes it very useful for wound dressings. These qualities allow, among other things, the capacity for such dressings to better cradle antiseptic and healing agents.[21] John Mirfield prescribed spiders' webs specifically for this very purpose, noting that they could be soaked in vinegar or oil and then applied to simple injuries.[22]

One of the drawbacks of using spider silk may have been sourcing enough of it to satisfy all who required it. Spiders tend to be extremely territorial and prone to cannibalism, making them difficult to farm on a large-enough scale to produce viable quantities of silk. Just as it is today, one suspects that there may have only been limited quantities of spider silk available to medieval practitioners wishing to use this natural material.[23] Perhaps this explains why, unlike other resources, it was only used for very specific applications.

A Strong Man with a Hammer

:. . . it was necessary to invent a new machine.

Henri de Mondeville[24]

Despite the advent of gunpowder weapons in the late Middle Ages, throughout most of the period arrows and crossbow bolts remained the most common types of projectiles used on the battlefield.[25] Large and small, barbed and smooth, socketed and solid, poisoned and not, there was almost no end to the different types of iron heads or points being used by this time.[26] Any of them could be lethal, especially those that struck the major organs of the body or that resulted in serious infections.[27] Still, many of the injuries caused by these weapons could be successfully treated by military surgeons. Mondeville wrote extensively about these types of wounds in his large, early fourteenth-century surgical text. He was a proponent of removing arrows from soldiers as quickly as possible, quoting the prominent Islamic physician Avicenna: 'If we remove the arrow, then maybe the wounded will be saved.'[28] This was not common practice among all surgeons at the time, nor would it become so in the centuries to come. Many chose to leave the projectile in the wound for several days before attempting to remove it.[29] The barber-surgeon von Pfolspeundt provides an example of this practice. In the fifteenth century, he advocated cutting the wooden shaft of the arrow at skin level and leaving the metal arrowhead within the body for 12 to 14 days. As the tissues surrounding the arrow began to putrefy and soften, it could then be removed.[30]

In his surgery, de Mondeville incorporated several specialized extraction techniques for projectiles, including one for a partially-exposed arrow in an arm or leg that was difficult to remove. First, the patient's limb was tied to something secure before a length of strong cord was fixed to the head of the arrow. The other end of the cord was attached to the taut string of an empty crossbow which was in the 'ready to shoot' position. When the trigger on the crossbow was pulled, the force acting on the cord would be strong enough to withdraw the stubborn arrow from the patient. Mondeville noted that he had never seen this procedure fail.[31] Another of his techniques was designed around warriors who wore mail. Many of the arrows of the day could pierce the protective metal rings, pulling some of the mail into the wound. Mondeville suggested that a surgeon be prepared for such situations by having an armourer on hand to assist with the procedure. First, the shaft of the arrow was severed to prevent it from obstructing the operation. Subsequently, the armourer and surgeon worked together, with the armourer removing the mail from in and around the wound so that the surgeon could extract the arrow safely.[32]

Occasionally, soldiers found themselves in unusual situations that required even more specialized help. Mondeville describes a case that he observed, noting, 'It is sometimes necessary for the surgeon to invent his own equipment that is different from that which already exists . . .'.[33] The situation involved an unnamed man whose knee had been pierced by a piece of iron. The object measured several centimetres in length, being slender in the middle, while the ends were thicker than the central section. There is some debate as to what it was, with Nicaise's late nineteenth-century translation of de Mondeville's work referring to it as a crossbow bolt.[34] In his modern version of the text, Dr. Rosenman suggests that this piece of metal was part of the equipment used for pulling taut the string of an arbalest, a type of powerful crossbow. It may have come loose under high tension and impaled the poor user as he was attempting to load the weapon.[35] Whatever it was, it had clearly required considerable force to drive the unusual shape through the victim's knee, so that a portion of its length stuck out on each side.

A piece of equipment was devised that would allow the metal bar to be removed, while protecting the victim's knee from further harm. It consisted of a column of some sort, likely a log, which was sufficiently hollowed out to a depth and width that could comfortably hold the patient's leg, along with some protective padding. Channels were cut into the sides of the column to accommodate the metal ends jutting out from the man's knee, before it was partially buried in the ground to provide stability. With care for his knee, the victim's leg was then guided into the proper position within the column. Cloth pads were used to secure and protect his leg while it was inside the device. A metal lid was fashioned with corresponding grooves cut into it to for the protruding ends of the piece of iron. It was then fitted into place.[36] With the man's limb now steady, cushioned and protected, Nicaise's translation picks up de Mondeville's story:

> Alors un homme fort frappa vigoureusement sur la pointe du garrot avec un marteau de fer, et le garrot jaillit de l'autre côté de la colonne.[37]

> Then a strong man forcefully struck the end of the piece of metal with an iron hammer, and it shot out from the other side of the column.

It must have been an incredibly intense few minutes for all involved as they anticipated the swing of the hammer, to say nothing of the patient who awaited the strike. It seems that the column did its job of protecting his knee from the hammer blow, but we will likely never know for certain, as de Mondeville's anecdote ends without any further information on the health or welfare of the individual once the operation was done.

Soporific Sponge

> . . . such remedies did he apply that the pain presently abated, so that he fell asleep.
>
> *Amadís of Gaul*[38]

Procedures like the one described by Henri de Mondeville above, as well as other more dangerous surgical operations carried out in the period examined in this volume, raise questions about the sedation of patients during them. Clearly, a narcotic mixture that allowed medieval practitioners to perform surgery while the patient remained unconscious or at least heavily sedated would have been extremely useful, and there is considerable evidence to show that one existed. To be sure, it was not anaesthesia in the modern sense but rather a type of sedation that could cause drowsiness or unconsciousness in the patient, enabling the surgeon to treat them more easily.[39]

Avicenna included a type of powerful sedative in his eleventh-century medical text, which featured opium, henbane and mandrake among its ingredients. It could be given to a patient by the surgeon when a deep level of sedation was required for a painful operation.[40] The military surgeon Master Hugo and his son Theodoric helped to bring to light a similar narcotic concoction during the second half of the thirteenth century.[41]

This soporific, or sleep-inducing drug, was another powerful mixture of narcotic ingredients, like opium, henbane and hemlock, combined with other substances.[42] The concoction was absorbed with a sponge, which was left to dry in the hot sun.[43] Later, a surgeon could soak the sponge for an hour in hot water and then place it under a patient's nose until they fell asleep.[44] Once the surgical procedure was finished, the patient could be reawakened by waving a vinegar-soaked sponge under their nose.[45]

The acceptance and use of such a strong sedative for surgical purposes reached its peak of popularity during the fourteenth and fifteenth centuries, with varying ingredients and methods for delivering the drugs being used. The reputation of such a technique even went beyond the medical community, being included in the tale of *Amadís of Gaul*. The story's learned physician, Master Helisabad, uses something similar to assist the badly wounded Amadís, here disguised as the Knight of the Green Sword, after his battle with the great beast Endriago, '. . . then he took a sponge that was steeped in a confection good against the poison, and placed it at his nostrils whereby he greatly recovered'.[46]

The physician Arnald of Villanova chose to apply his formula to the foreheads and noses of his patients using a rag instead of a sponge.[47] John Arderne deployed his in a different manner, binding the ingredients together with lard rather than a sponge.[48] The surgeon then rubbed the soporific ointment onto the patient's forehead, temples, pulse points, armpits, palms and soles of their feet until they, '. . . schal slepe so þat he schal fele no kuttyng'.[49] The Frenchman Guy de Chauliac borrowed Theodoric's anaesthetic sponge method almost verbatim, placing it appropriately in his section on amputations.[50] He also noted that some surgeons foolishly chose to give their patients opium to drink instead of applying an external concoction. Chauliac considered this to be very dangerous, as it could potentially lead to the patient's demise.[51]

During the fifteenth century, in what is now Germany, the barber-surgeon Heinrich von Pfolspeundt also recommended a nearly identical sedative mixture and method of delivery to that of Theodoric.[52] Its inclusion in his surgery is interesting, predominantly since von Pfolspeundt appears to have had no comprehension of practitioners like Theodoric or de Chauliac. It suggests that this knowledge of a strong sedative may have had an even wider circulation across Europe by means of less-established channels. In the late fifteenth century, Hieronymus Brunschwig used a formula not unlike the others, while in the early sixteenth century, Hans von Gersdorff says he performed nearly 200 amputations using a soporific sponge.[53] Finally, Ambroise Paré suggested a modified use for the sedative, helping a patient to sleep so they could recuperate from their injuries.[54]

By the time of von Gersdorff and Paré, the use of soporific medicines was beginning to fall out of favour among surgeons.[55] This was probably due to the inherent risks associated with them, something already noted by de Chauliac. The dosing of these mixtures was difficult enough to estimate, and the fact that few surgical texts contained any recommended measures for the ingredients meant that tragic accidents were bound to happen.[56] Through Theodoric's text, we get an understanding of the types of challenges surgeons faced. He advised that some practitioners were using too much of the sedative in head trauma cases, causing the deaths of their patients. The injuries had already altered the levels of consciousness in these individuals, making it challenging for a surgeon to determine the appropriate amount of the mixture required, which led to numerous cases of overdose.[57] Despite his boasts, von Gersdorff also stated, in no uncertain terms, that these concoctions were causing the deaths of patients.[58]

The fact that so many practitioners of medicine included one of these anaesthetic techniques in their texts gives weight to the idea that surgery during this period was possible while the patient was drowsy or even unconscious. Grimly, even deaths of patients noted by Theodoric, de Chauliac and von Gersdorff offer further proof that such methods of sedation were genuinely being used. However, some of the best evidence comes from the modern discovery of several caches containing the seeds of black henbane, opium poppy and hemlock found in the 'medical waste' at Soutra Aisle, an Augustinian monastery in the Scottish Borders where quite advanced surgical practices were taking place during the medieval period.[59] It is noteworthy that modern pharmacologists have proposed that ingesting a cocktail of drugs similar to those found at Soutra Aisle would have grave repercussions. This appears to support the argument for using an external delivery system, such as a sponge or lard, to administer the drugs.[60] Modern tests done on laboratory rats using the soporific sponge technique have certainly had some success.[61] Understandably, there have been few modern experiments done on human subjects using these ingredients, but in the nineteenth century, the soporific sponge method was apparently applied successfully to five individuals requiring surgery.[62]

Fistula-In-Ano

> I sawe a man of Northampton þat had þre holes in þe lefte buttok, and þre in þe testicles.
>
> John Arderne[63]

While serving with the English army in France under Sir Henry Plantagenet, the fourteenth-century knight Adam Everyngham suffered from a delicate but relatively common medical problem, an anal fistula, also known as a fistula-in-ano. He sought the help of leeches and surgeons from across Gascony, but none could assist him.[64] It was only when Everyngham returned home to England, sometime before 1358, that he finally found relief, apparently becoming the first person to benefit from an innovative surgical procedure established by the army surgeon, John Arderne.[65]

During this period, people from all walks of life could be impacted by anal fistulas, just as they are now.[66] Even so, they do seem to have been quite common among the knightly classes. The list of Arderne's patients who were treated for this condition includes other warriors, like Sir Reynald Grey de Wilton and Sir Henry Blakborne, men who had also fought in France.[67] Perhaps this was due in part to the long hours spent in the saddle in cold, wet weather, further exacerbated by the additional weight of their armour, as noted by Sir D'Arcy Power in his edition of Arderne's work.[68]

There are several ways anal fistulas can start, but most commonly, they begin as an anorectal abscess. The ulceration creates a small channel that eventually connects the anal canal to the exterior skin around the anus, groin, or buttocks. In addition to the relentless, throbbing pain they can cause, these small openings can release faecal matter, gas and a foul-smelling, fishy odour, which can make life terribly difficult and potentially embarrassing for the sufferer.[69] It is quite usual for more than one of these channels to occur, as Arderne noted in his treatise on the subject, '. . . Thomas Broune, that had 15 holes by whiche went out wynde with egestious odour'.[70]

Remarkably, mid-thirteenth-century practitioners like Bruno da Longoburgo and Theodoric appear to have understood what was required to treat anal fistulas by following the earlier work of the brilliant Islamic doctor Abulcasis.[71] However, by the last quarter of the thirteenth century, things had changed, and strangely, these therapies were no longer trusted. In his medical text of 1275, the well-respected surgeon, William of Saliceto, noted that the problem, '. . . is difficult to cure, in fact, it would be better and more honourable for the surgeon to abandon it altogether'.[72] Despite the caution, William did provide details of an operation to treat an anal fistula, but it came with a further warning that he had seen this method end poorly on many occasions.[73] So, for about 100 years, things remained the same, with medical practitioners seeming to have lost their way when it came to remedying the problem.[74]

Arderne devised his method of treating anal fistulas by reintroducing two of Abulcasis' surgical procedures and combining them with his own gentle post-operative care.[75] In 1376, he would detail his solution in a treatise, which includes full-scale illustrations of the metal instruments that he himself designed for the procedure.[76] Unfortunately, in this case, the awkward nature of his tools only served to make the operation more difficult than it needed to be.[77]

The procedure began in a well-lit room, with the patient lying on their back, legs flexed, spread, and secured.[78] Using a probe, threads were pushed through the entire length of the fistula until the rectum was reached. The surgeon then brought the ends of the threads down through the anal orifice and joined them with the other ends hanging from the fistula. They were tied together and slowly drawn taut. This provided an accurate guide that the surgeon could follow with a curved scalpel to cut cleanly through the entire length of the fistula, right to the rectum. A metal shield, placed inside the rectum and likely held secure by the practitioner's assistant, enabled the surgeon to know when to stop cutting so that no unnecessary damage was caused. As the incision was completed, the shield and threads were withdrawn. If other fistulas existed, they might also be repaired at the same time, depending on the patient's level of tolerance.[79]

The incision was then allowed to heal naturally. The biggest advancement in the operation was Arderne's post-operative care, which avoided the use of cauterization and corrosive substances so commonly employed by other surgeons.[80] Instead, he chose just to wash the incision with warm water and a sponge, apply gentle salves made from things like egg whites and rose oil and change the dressing as infrequently as possible. Arderne also used a simple enema of salt and water to keep things moving smoothly and easily through the patient while they recovered.[81]

For obvious reasons, modern-day surgical procedures to fix anal fistulas are done under general anaesthesia.[82] By contrast, Arderne's patients seem to have been awake for the procedure, with the instructions that they remain brave and cooperative, staying as still as possible so as not to risk further damage from the surgeon's knife.[83] Oddly contradictory are Arderne's general instructions for his soporific lard, which state that using it would allow the patient to, '. . . suffre kuttyng in any place of þe body without felyng or akyng'.[84] One could almost underline the words 'any place' in consideration of this difficult procedure on one of the most delicate areas on the body.

The Royal Treatment

> And in this Bataylle was the Prince Herry shotte into the heede with an Arowe.
>
> *Chronicles of London*[85]

An entry in the letters patent from the reign of King Henry IV of England (1367–1413), dated at Shrewsbury on 23 July 1403, provides the names of those who were to provide protection against a Welsh attack:

> Appointment of Richard, earl of Arundel, Thomas Berkele of Berkele, Edward de Cherlton, Hugh Burnell and John Tuchet of Audelee to govern the marches of England towards Wales and resist the invasions of Owin de Gleyndourdy and other rebels there, as the king's son the prince of Wales cannot attend to this.[86]

The reason the teenaged Prince of Wales, the future king Henry V of England, could not look after such a matter of importance was that just two days earlier, while leading the left side of his father's forces at the Battle of Shrewsbury, he had been '. . . smetyn in the face be syd the nose on the lefte syd with an arow'.[87] According to some accounts, like that of the chronicler Titus Livius, Henry continued fighting after receiving the wound, even asking to be taken forward so that he could lead his men.[88] Whatever the truth of it might be, at some point Henry was removed from the field of battle and taken to the 'castell of kelyngworth' for treatment.[89] First, local physicians attempted to help the prince but were unsuccessful. They did little more than remove the shaft of the arrow, leaving the small, barbless, bodkin-type iron arrowhead buried several inches deep inside Henry's face.[90] He may well have perished from the injury were it not for the skill and ingenuity of the king's own surgeon, John Bradmore, who managed to succeed where other medical professionals had failed. Two fifteenth-century manuscripts found in the British Library, known by shelf numbers Sloane MS 2272 and Harley MS 1736, contain versions of Bradmore's procedure. The first is an early fifteenth-century Latin edition authored by Bradmore himself, taken from a folio titled *Philomena*.[91] The second, composed in Middle English in 1446, draws heavily on Bradmore's version, providing a more concise account of the surgery with some small variations in detail.[92]

According to the manuscripts, Bradmore fashioned graduated probes, referred to as *tents*, by wrapping sticks of dried elder in clean linen cloth and dipping them in rose honey. These were used to prevent the wound from closing.[93] He made the tents increasingly thicker and longer, gradually inserting them into the wound one after another until he had created a path that was sufficiently wide and deep within Henry's flesh to accommodate an instrument capable of reaching the arrowhead. The specialized surgical tool that could extract the weapon had to be designed and made by Bradmore. It is illustrated in each of the manuscripts, with the version in Harley MS 1746 being the more elaborate of the two images.[94] It is quite a clever instrument, as described by Bradmore in *Philomena*:

> . . . tunc reparaui de nouo tenaculas paruas et concauas ad quantitatem unius sagitte et in medio tenacule intrauit quoddam vyse . . .[95]

> . . . then I made small hollow clamps, the width of an arrow and through the middle of the clamps ran a type of screw . . .

The sides of the clamps were smooth and curved so that they met at the bottom. As Bradmore guided the device through the expanded wound, he could feel it reaching and entering the empty socket of the arrowhead, where the wooden shaft had once been. He then turned the central screw at the top of the instrument, causing the sides of the clamps to spread apart and press against the inner walls of the socket. When he felt that he had a tight enough grip on the arrowhead, he began withdrawing the instrument slowly and carefully. As the weapon finally emerged from the wound, all those who stood watching were said to have excitedly given thanks to God.

Next, Bradmore cleansed the injury with white wine.[96] The alcohol would have acted as an antiseptic, although the surgeon would not have understood the science behind it. He made an ointment by taking white breadcrumbs and boiling them in water, then squeezing the liquid out through a cloth. He added barley flour and honey to the soaked breadcrumbs, boiling them together over a slow fire and eventually adding turpentine to the mixture. Over the next twenty days, he used the graduated probes to push the ointment into the wound to promote healing. Bradmore applied another antibacterial substance made of various resins and gums, which he referred to as his 'brown ointment'.[97] The surgeon continued to care for the prince in this way until he was once again well.

Bradmore does not specify whether a sedative was administered during the operation. Certainly, the existence of soporific recipes in England is supported by Arderne's treatise on the matter. There is no doubt that it would have been extremely useful, especially in the performance of such a tricky and potentially lethal surgery. Also, given the nature of the operation, it may have been unrealistic to expect the young prince to endure it without any form of pain control. On the other hand, Bradmore may have considered the available mixtures too risky to use on the king's son. In the end, it seems we may never know for certain whether the young prince was sedated for this groundbreaking surgical procedure.

As noted earlier, contemporary sources indicate that the arrow struck the young Henry on the left side of his face. Yet, there are still questions about which side of his countenance was hit by the projectile. One of the most famous portraits of Henry V hangs in London's National Portrait Gallery (NPG 545). It depicts the left side of his face but shows no sign of a scar whatsoever. The problem with the artwork is that the unknown artist who painted it did so nearly 200 years after Henry had died. If they painted this detail incorrectly, it would be completely understandable.[98] However, could it be that the painter was right all along? Some have questioned whether Bradmore could have mixed up right with left when he recorded his procedure.[99] It does seem unlikely that such a competent man of medicine would get this simple detail wrong, but then again, these sorts of things happen in modern medicine with a fair degree of regularity.[100] Whichever side of his face it was, there is little doubt that Henry was extremely fortunate in so many aspects of his injury. The small, barbless arrow that struck him somehow managed to miss his spine and brain by the smallest of margins. Even with the benefit of these things, Henry's wound was still extremely serious. He would have almost certainly lost his life had it not been for John Bradmore, a man whose ingenuity and familiarity with medicine and metalsmithing, along with the weapons of the time, made him the ideal surgeon for the job.[101]

Rhinoplasty

> . . . they cut their noses so that they would be recognized by others.
>
> *Chronicle of the Este Family*[102]

At the time of the Wars of the Roses, a Hanseatic merchant named Gerhard von Wesel was living in London. In a letter dated 17 April 1471, to authorities back home in Cologne, he did his best to update them on the current situation in England. This included a description of the events that had occurred just three days earlier at the Battle of Barnet. In it, he described the terrible injuries suffered by some of those who had fought in the conflict:

> Those who had set out with good horses and sound bodies returned home with sorry nags and bandaged faces, some without noses . . .[103]

This passage from von Wesel's newsletter underlines a common type of facial wound during this time, one that left survivors terribly disfigured and with little hope of a return to normal life. However, in fifteenth-century Sicily, there was a glimmer of optimism for anyone who had suffered the loss of their nose. A form of rhinoplasty was being practiced by a secretive Sicilian surgical family called Branc. The procedure used skin from another area of the body to help create a replacement. Just where and how they rediscovered this operation remains a mystery.[104] A few decades later, von Pfolspeundt learned the technique from an unknown Italian practitioner and included a description in his medical text.[105] The procedure itself can be traced as far back as the middle of the first millennium BC to an Indian physician called Sushruta.[106] It was also recorded by Abulcasis, some 500 years before von Pfolspeundt included it in his surgical text.[107] One of the biggest distinctions between von Pfolspeundt's procedure and the operation described by Sushruta and Abulcasis is the area of donor skin used to construct the new nose. Von Pfolspeundt suggested that the skin should come from the upper arm, while Sushruta and Abulcasis proposed that it come from the cheek.[108]

The procedure in von Pfolspeundt's surgery calls for a template to be made of the patient's missing nose using leather or parchment. Great consideration was to be given to its size, shape and placement on the face.[109] The guide was then to be laid sideways and flat across the biceps of the patient's arm and traced with ink. A scalpel was then used to cut and expose the skin along both sides of the outline, right up to the top where they met, with the bottom line of the marked area remaining uncut for the time being. Haeser and Middeldorpf, who edited von Pfolspeundt's manuscript in the nineteenth century, rightly noted that this portion of the operation does, unfortunately, suffer somewhat from a lack of detail.[110] The practitioner was also required to create freshly cut edges around the nasal cavity to ensure an adequate blood supply for the skin graft taken from the arm.[111] The patient's arm was then folded across their face so that the donor tissue of the upper arm lined up exactly with the nasal cavity. Towels and bandages were used to keep the patient's arm immobilized so that the donor tissue could be shaped and sutured onto the face. This uncomfortable set-up had to remain in place for a period of eight to ten days, after which the final cut could be made to free the skin from the arm. This portion was then sutured above the patient's lip, with allowances made for the two nostrils, which were created using hollow quills wrapped in flax. These were left inside the cavities, and bags were laid externally on either side of the nose to help keep its structure in place while it healed.[112]

It appears highly probable that von Pfolspeundt employed his soporific recipe to sedate patients during this and other procedures. His prescription, along with the instructions for its application, occupies a dedicated section in the earlier part of his text under the heading, 'The first thing you will learn is how to make a patient's body sleep'. It begins by saying, 'How to make a person unresponsive so that you may cut them open or give sleep to a sick person suffering from insomnia'.[113]

Helping to give von Pfolspeundt's operation a greater air of plausibility is the work of Ambroise Paré in the following century. Concurring with von Pfolspeundt, Paré also describes '. . . a surgeon of Italie of late years . . .', who had performed a very similar-sounding operation.[114] Paré even reported a case he knew of where this method of rhinoplasty had been successful:

> A younger brother of the familie of St Thoan, beeing wearie of a silver-nose, which beeing artificially made, hee had worn in the place of his nose that was cut off, went to this Chirurgian into Italie, and by the mean fore-named practice hee recovered a nose of flesh again, to the great admiration of all those that knew him before.[115]

One of the crucial differences between Paré's technique and the method suggested by von Pfolspeundt was the length of time the patient's arm was to be kept in position above their face before the final line of skin was cut away. Instead of the eight or ten days suggested by von Pfolspeundt, Paré advocated 40 days. During this time, the French surgeon also recommended that the patient be fed easily digestible foods and liquids like soup and jelly.[116] Paré did warn both the patient and the surgeon regarding the operation:

> This thing truly is possible to bee don, but it is verie difficult both to the patient suffering, and also to the Chirurgian working. For that the flesh that is taken out of the arm is not of the like temperature as the flesh of the nose is; also the holes of the restored nose cannot bee made as the were before.[117]

Chapter 4

FIRE AND GUNPOWDER

> There came to my gate the last summer . . . a very miserable man, and much deformed, as burnt in the face . . .
>
> *A Caveat or Warning for Common Cursitors*[1]

Long before the emergence of gunpowder and gunpowder weapons on European battlefields in the fourteenth century, fire was already regarded as one of the most feared instruments of war, making it effective for both attacking and defending. Unpredictable and sometimes uncontrollable in its various forms, fire inflicted appalling injuries and caused the deaths of many, not to mention the extensive damage to property it could produce. The literary works of the military commander, Oswald von Wolkenstein (c. 1377–1445), include a poem titled *'Nu huss!' sprach der Michel von Wolkenstein*, or *'Attack!' Spoke Sir Michael von Wolkenstein*. It commemorates the successful defence of Greifenstein Castle in 1418 and illustrates the devastation that fire can cause when used as a weapon:

> And then a rain of fire began to fall
> down on the heads beneath the castle wall
> and burned on armour, helmets, bows and all;
> they left these as they ran, which caused us no dismay.
>
> Their heavy weapons, tents and fire shield
> were burned to ashes in the upper field;
> I hear an evil loan will evil yield
> and thus we're glad to give Duke Friedrich all his pay.[2]

Throughout the period, weapons that made use of fire and heat came in many different types. The fourteenth-century poem by John Barbour, called *The*

Bruce, describes how fire was intended to be used by Scottish forces in the defence of Berwick in 1319. When the English began their assault on the town, they spent the first several days constructing large wooden siege engines that could be used to breach the walls. Among them was a heavily protected and wheeled shelter known as a sow. It could be manoeuvred into place against the town's wall so that soldiers inside could work to make an opening in the fortifications in relative safety.[3] The poem details how the Scots arranged to deal with the sow using a crane that had been constructed inside the town:

> They also took pitch and tar, with lint and hards and brimstone, and dry sticks that would burn easily . . . They planned to use them in a blazing bundle by means of their crane, and if the sow came to the wall, to let them fall burning upon her, and with a strong chain keep her there till all were burnt who were within.[4]

In the end, this method was not required as the Scots were able to smash the sow using a catapult.[5] However, being constructed of wood, there were many times when such devices were set ablaze by city and castle defenders, causing terrible injuries and deaths to those inside. At the Siege of Breteuil in 1356, for instance, a huge French siege tower was set on fire, trapping and killing many of the soldiers inside.[6]

All manner of projectiles, doused in flammable materials like pitch or resin, could be shot or hurled at enemy soldiers. Boiling liquids, especially water, could be poured onto unsuspecting adversaries through specially designed shafts or spouts set in castle or city defences.[7] Those who defended the town of Harfleur against the English in the late summer of 1415 employed several of these methods:

> . . . flinging fire-hot torches from the battlements, pouring hot water or boiling oil and fat from the brattice, or shooting mallets distaffs and tow-trenders, i.e. flaming arrows rolled round with tow dipped in resin or pitch . . .[8]

Such weapons were not just used on land. In *Tirant Lo Blanc*, the author describes a moment when Tirant's galleon is attacked by Muslim ships. One of his experienced sailors, the wonderfully named *Look-what-you-do*, organizes huge cauldrons of pitch and oil to be boiled, which Tirant's men then fling at their enemies as they come alongside them in their ships. It created such chaos among the Muslim sailors that they were forced to abandon their attack.[9]

Greek fire continued to be used during the first part of this period. Likely originating in the Byzantine Empire many centuries earlier, the exact nature of this highly flammable liquid remains a mystery.[10] Pumped through syphons or thrown using catapults and clay grenades, Greek fire burnt ferociously and proved to be very difficult to extinguish.[11] The Battle of St Omer in 1340, and the sieges of Algeciras in 1343 and Breteuil in 1356 all saw Greek fire employed as a weapon.[12] At times, it was used alongside gunpowder weapons, as was the case at the ill-fated Siege of Ypres in the summer of 1383, when forces led by the Bishop of Norwich, Henry le Despenser, were repelled by the townspeople:

> . . . villani occurant totis animis, et cum lapidibus, lanceis, et sagittis, igne Græco, et missilibus quæ 'gunna' vocantur, nostros ubique repellunt.[13]

> . . . the villagers attacked us wholeheartedly, and with stones, lances, and arrows, with Greek fire, and with the missiles which are called 'gunna', drove away our men everywhere.

Despite these examples, the use of Greek fire did remain somewhat limited throughout fourteenth-century Europe.[14] It was not especially easy to obtain and appears to have required some specialist knowledge to be used safely and effectively. Military engineers are regularly mentioned in connection with Greek fire; their knowledge and experience seem to have qualified them on both counts.[15] Returning to John Barbour's poem *The Bruce*, the author explains that the defending Scottish forces had a Flemish engineer called John Crab in their employ, and it was he who had '. . . procured Greek fire . . .' for the Scots.[16] Its use dwindled even further in the fifteenth century, with writers like Christine de Pizan (1364–c.1430) stating that Greek fire was a weapon not befitting a Christian warrior.[17] In the mid-1460s, the French soldier and author Jean de Bueil recounted much of de Pizan's work in his text called *Le Jouvencel*. He reiterated the fact that Christians should not be permitted to use something so barbaric as Greek fire, even in times of war.[18]

The terrible injuries suffered by soldiers and sailors who were caught on the wrong side of a siege tower engulfed in flames, a clay grenade filled with Greek fire, or cauldrons of boiling pitch are truly unthinkable.

It is uncommon to find references to soldiers with healed burn injuries; however, one such instance can be found in *Áns saga bogsveigis*, or *The Saga of Án Bow-Bender*, which is an Icelandic outlaw tale dating from the late fourteenth or early fifteenth century. The passage describes a wrestling match that takes place inside a hall between two rival warriors: the story's namesake and Björn 'The Strong'. During the fight, Án lifts Björn and hurls him into the fire. Björn's retainers rush to his aid and pull him from the flames, but he is badly harmed.[19] The narrative uses dark humour to describe the incident and the subsequent injuries sustained by Björn:

> It occurred during the encounter,
> I added some wood to the blaze;
> Denied him distinction;
> Damned ever be that man.[20]

While the methods used to treat Björn's burns are not described in *The Saga of Án Bow-Bender*, there are many salves and remedies found among the medical texts explored in this volume that were meant for that purpose. Yperman listed the instructions for fourteen different treatments, which were drawn from several sources, including Galen and a now-lost thirteenth-century treatise called *Experimentator*.[21] One of them simply involved placing a thin sheet of lead over the wound.[22] Many of the salves suggested by Yperman were to be applied with a feather or feather brush to prevent causing the patient more discomfort. One such preparation, borrowed from Galen, was made up of the chopped rinds of fresh limes that were boiled in water for a considerable period. Once the soggy lumps had been removed, the resulting liquid could be applied to the area of the burn with a feather brush.[23]

Mondeville and de Chauliac outlined actual treatment strategies for patients with burn injuries, rather than merely listing ointments and remedies. They focused on preventing the formation of blisters, managing those that did occur and facilitating the healing process. The initial step involved the repeated application of cooling treatments, such as cold cloths soaked in a mixture of rose honey and water, to the burnt areas of skin.[24] These cooling therapies likely worked not only to prevent blisters but also provided analgesic benefits for the patient. Regarding pain control, only de Chauliac suggested the topical use of opium at any point during this stage.[25] When it came to removing the blisters, de Mondeville followed a four-step approach: regulating the patient's diet, clearing their bowels to rebalance their humours, applying healing ointments and surgically excising the blisters.[26] Guy de Chauliac, though, used just a few words for this part, stating, 'The second step is accomplished by removing the blisters with scissors or a blade'.[27] He suggested the use of healing ointments as a separate step, proposing such things as cooked garlic or burnt dove-droppings mixed with rose honey, which could be applied to the burns.[28]

Ambroise Paré's sixteenth-century text contains several remedies for burn injuries, including one that provides further evidence of the active role that women played in healing during this period.[29] It came from an elderly woman he encountered in an apothecary, where he had gone to obtain supplies to treat the injuries of a kitchen boy in the service of the Marshal of Montejan, who was also Paré's employer. The boy had suffered severe burns after falling into a cauldron of hot oil:

> . . . by chance a certain old countrey woman, who hearing that I desired medicins for a burn, perswaded me at the first dressing, that I should lay two raw Onions beaten with a little salt; for so I should hinder the breaking out of blisters or pustules, as she had found by certain and frequent experience.[30]

Paré applied this technique solely to the boy's face, while for the remaining burns, he used his standard cooling treatments.[31] The process recommended by the woman worked just as she had suggested, but the other areas where Paré had not used it ended up completely blistered.[32] This treatment highlights Paré's willingness to experiment with techniques he was unfamiliar with, even if it did come at the expense of the poor kitchen boy who ended up as a guinea pig in the French surgeon's trials with salt and onions.[33]

Missing Evidence

> . . . powder for that devilish instrument of war colloquially termed gunne.
>
> John Mirfield[34]

In her volume *Le livre des fais d'armes et de chevalerie*, or *The Book of Deeds of Arms and of Chivalry*, Christine de Pizan included a section entitled

Provisions Needed for a Castle or Town in Time of War, in which she advises defenders to have on hand '. . . a very good supply of gunpowder . . .'.[35] When she wrote these words in the early fifteenth century, gunpowder, one of the most significant innovations in the history of warfare, had already been used in Europe's battles and sieges since around the 1320s.[36] From the early decades of the fourteenth century to around 1460, numerous other writers and chroniclers documented the use of gunpowder, its weapons, and the injuries they caused.[37] Yet, despite this, there is a striking absence of substantial references to them in the medical texts of the period.[38] There is a passing mention in the surgery of Jehan Yperman, which was penned around 1328. In his section on wounds to the oesophagus, he wrote, 'You must examine minutely all wounds [caused] by cutting weapons or by firearms that enter the neck or throat until you are certain about their severity'.[39] Guy de Chauliac did not comment on gunpowder, or the weapons associated with it, but it is perhaps worth remembering that, unlike Yperman, de Chauliac was not a battlefield surgeon.[40] Other works, like those belonging to John Arderne and John Mirfield, include recipes for making gunpowder but little else on the subject.[41] As the epigraph for this section portrays, Mirfield had an obvious dislike for gunpowder. It is puzzling that he would provide details on creating such a cruel instrument of war in conjunction with his medical writings yet fail to address how to treat the injuries it might inflict.[42] The first known instructions for treating gunpowder and gunshot wounds do not appear until von Pfolspeundt's surgical text of 1460.[43] Although there may be other yet-undiscovered or lost-to-history medical texts that describe such therapies, von Pfolspeundt's remains the earliest example of its kind, the details of which are discussed later in this chapter.

Gunpowder and Gunpowder Burns

> . . . great negligence set on fire a great bag of gun-powder; wherewith hee was burned together with ten or twelv souldiers.
>
> Ambroise Paré[44]

Gunpowder is made from a combination of charcoal, sulphur and potassium nitrate, more commonly known as saltpetre.[45] When mixed in the correct ratios and ignited, it burns rapidly and produces the gases necessary to force projectiles from the barrels of cannons and guns. These same properties were later found to be useful in an almost endless list of weapons, such as fire arrows, fire pots and mines.[46] In the first part of the fourteenth century, gunpowder was still fairly new to Europe, although it had existed in China for centuries.[47] Initially, it suffered from a few problems, including the fact that the force it could create was fairly weak. Saltpetre was also in short supply, and what did exist was expensive.[48] However, as the fifteenth century drew closer, saltpetre started to become easier to obtain in larger quantities, which caused prices to drop and made gunpowder more readily available.[49] Improvements in the mixing method also contributed to the increased potency of gunpowder.[50] Greater quantities of a more effective product meant that accidents and misuse by soldiers became regular occurrences, causing some of the most shocking burn injuries and deaths. At times, it must have seemed like this new weapon could cause almost as many problems for those who used it as it did for those for whom it was intended.[51] During the Battle of Gavere in the summer of 1453, a gunner on the rebel Ghent side accidentally set fire to several barrels of gunpowder. The resulting explosions led the gunner's comrades to believe they were under attack and caused them to flee the battlefield. It was this action that signalled the beginning of the end for the insurgents in their fight against Philip the Good of Burgundy during the Revolt of Ghent (1449–53).[52]

An account of Charles the Bold, Duke of Burgundy, from the mid-1470s describes the awful injuries suffered by many of his own troops during training exercises:

> . . . le duc est prince chevaleureux, et de tel exercise de guerre, que par blessure de coup à main, de trait de pouldre ou aultrement, il a bien souvent tant de gens blessez en sa maison et en ses ordonnances, que aultre part en divers lieux blessez, que cincquante chirurgiens diligens auroyent assez à besoigner, à faire leur devoir des cures qui surviennent.[53]

> . . . the Duke is a chivalrous prince and during war exercises there are just as many of his contingent who are wounded by guns or burned by gunpowder and other such things as are injured in other places, so that as many as fifty diligent surgeons have sufficient work to do treating these cases.

The treatment of gunpowder burns is briefly mentioned in von Pfolspeundt's surgical text; however, this reference primarily concerns the localized area around a bullet wound, rather than addressing any significant burn injuries.[54] In contrast, Ambroise Paré witnessed, treated and recorded some truly horrific injuries caused by gunpowder during his campaigns as a surgeon with the French army. Among them is an incident involving a soldier whose, '. . . flasque full of Gunpouder set on fire, whereby his hands and face were grievously burnt'.[55] At the time this soldier was injured, Paré was still experimenting with the mixture of salt and onions he had learnt from the woman he met at the apothecary. He applied this remedy to the middle part of the soldier's face, while on the rest of the burns, Paré employed his usual therapies. Once again, the surgeon found the new method to be far superior to his own.[56] Despite his initial success with the treatment, it took further experimentation before he felt confident enough in the salt and onions remedy to endorse its use.[57]

Paré warned of the risks that serious burns such as these could pose to certain parts of the body, including the eyelids and the sides of the fingers. If left alone, these areas could become affixed to one another by scar tissue. He therefore recommended placing linen cloths between them to help prevent it from occurring during the healing process.[58]

Generally, when it came to the burns caused by gunpowder, Paré acknowledged that they were particularly difficult to care for and always left a scar, no matter what types of treatments were applied.[59] A lack of understanding of bacteria meant that burns, whether resulting from gunpowder or other factors, were highly susceptible to infection during this period, which could ultimately lead to death. Furthermore, significant burns were beyond the scope of available treatments.[60] Indeed, it has been less than a century since therapies such as topical antibiotics, burn resuscitation and successful skin graft techniques have been employed in the treatment of patients with severe burn injuries. The lack of effective therapies during this period is illustrated by Paré in an excerpt from his text. He recounts a distressing scene from the early days of his medical career with the French army, where he encounters several soldiers who have suffered terrible harm:

> . . . their faces wholly disfigured, and neither saw nor heard, nor spoke: and their clothes did yet flame with gun-powder

> which had burnt them. Beholding them with pittie, there happened to com an old Souldier, who asked mee if there were anie possible means to cure them, I told him no . . .[61]

Gunpowder Weapons

> The canonys, the bumbard, and the gunne.
>
> *Of Knyghthode and Bataile*[62]

Constructed using iron or bronze, early European gunpowder weapons were small cannons that looked like a vase or bulbous flask laid sideways, with combustion occurring in the bulb-shaped base.[63] An English manuscript, attributed to Walter of Milemete and dating from 1326–7, *De Nobilitatibus Sapientii et Prudentiis Regum*, or *Of the Nobility, Wisdom, and Prudence of Kings*, includes one of the earliest European images of such a weapon.[64] Sticking out from the barrel of this cannon is a large dart-shaped weapon with a metal point and wooden shaft that went by many names, including *quarrel* and *garrock*.[65] Weighing around seven ounces, nearly three times the weight of a regular crossbow bolt, these early projectiles were stabilized for flight using brass or iron feathers and protected at the base with an iron cap.[66] To fire one of these cannons, gunpowder would be set inside the base, and a leather-wrapped dart pushed down the barrel. The leather helped provide a tight fit and seal to ensure that as little pressure as possible escaped past the dart when the cannon was fired. The gunpowder was ignited by placing a red-hot priming iron at the touchhole located at the base of the cannon. The rapid combustion of the gunpowder produced the gases necessary to propel the projectile back up through the cannon's barrel and out of the opening at the top.[67]

The dart-shaped projectiles were soon replaced by balls made from stone, lead, or, in rare cases, even iron and brass.[68] With other modest improvements being made during the last few decades of the fourteenth century, artillery began to be used a little more regularly on the battlefield.[69] During the Revolt of Ghent (1379–85), at the Battle of Beverhoutsveld near Bruges in 1382, the attacking Ghent army deployed artillery against a much larger force from Bruges. By firing their weapons and charging at the enemy soldiers, the men from Ghent managed to frighten them into retreating toward the town gates, where they overran them and captured the town. A few months later, however, during the same uprising, this time at the Battle of Roosebeke, troops were far less frightened by artillery, which greatly diminished its impact.[70] Elsewhere, cannons were used in 1385 at the Battle of Aljubarrota in Portugal and in 1387 at the Battle of Castagnaro in what is today northern Italy.[71] Despite the improvements to these weapons, issues with size and mobility meant that their value on the battlefield remained inconsistent at best. Rain-soaked gunpowder was another problem that could quickly render an army's artillery completely useless.[72] These problems would remain throughout most of the fifteenth century. Agincourt in 1415 and Towton in 1461 offer examples of battles that were won in large part because of factors such as archers and the weather, rather than the gunpowder weapons that were present. It would still be many decades before artillery began to properly replace more traditional weapons such as bows and crossbows on Europe's battlefields.[73]

However, the one area of warfare where gunpowder weapons proved to be very useful, both for attackers and defenders, was the siege.[74] Gunpowder supplies could be more easily protected, and these confrontations did not require the mobility of a pitched battle, making larger, more devastating guns more practical. By the fifteenth century, siege cannons were capable of launching enormous projectiles.[75] At the Siege of Maastricht, between 1407 and 1408, some thirty large stone balls were fired at the town each day by troops from Liège, totalling more than 1,500 by the time all was said and done.[76] During the Siege of Harfleur, Henry V of England commanded fewer than a dozen cannons, yet they were remarkably large. Some of these formidable weapons weighed nearly two tonnes and were capable of firing massive stone projectiles ranging from 400 to 500lbs. The process of firing them was slow, but the impact these weapons had on Harfleur was extremely detrimental.[77] Naturally, cannons of this size could cause catastrophic injuries. The significant human cost of weapons like these is described in the *Major Chronicle of Thomas Walsingham*:

> . . . per gunnas regias (nam ab ipsis evolantia saxa ingenti verberis ictu, obvia fregere quaeque ruentes, nec tantum corpora pressa necabant, sed totos cum sanguine dissipant artus, et singula cesserunt ictibus arms)[78]

> . . . by the royal guns (the rocks flying from them struck huge blows smashing every obstacle in their way including bodies that were crushed and killed under their weight, while also dismembering and scattering bloody limbs everywhere)

Such devastating casualties could come from either side of the walls during these conflicts, as underscored by the English siege of the French town of Meaux in 1421. Among the English losses was the 17-year-old son of the Lord of Cornwall, who was killed by a French cannonball. He had been a brave and well-liked young man, and his death caused deep sadness among many of the English nobles, not least his poor father, who had witnessed the horrific event.[79] On the French side, a 25-year-old captain called Michiel Bouyer was taken captive after one of his legs was smashed by a cannonball. He became terribly ill due to his injury, but neither he nor his wife had the means to buy his release from captivity.[80]

As with gunpowder itself, these new weapons were susceptible to dreadful accidents, misuse and failures. Poor construction, substandard materials or too much gunpowder could cause a piece of ordnance to burst apart, frequently with deadly consequences. The city of London produced a large siege cannon, called 'London', for Henry V of England, which he used at the Siege of Melun in 1420. The large quantity of gunpowder required to fire the huge stone balls eventually took its toll on the weapon, so that '. . . the explosions split the gun itself and finally broke it utterly into pieces'.[81] King James II of Scotland was present at the Siege of Roxburgh Castle in the summer of 1460, trying to take back the fortress from the English. As he stood near his cannons, one of them suddenly exploded, killing the Scottish ruler.[82] The illuminated German manuscript called *War Technology* illustrates the moment when such an explosion occurred. Two gunners turn away in horror just as jagged pieces of iron begin breaking apart from the cannon and flying in every direction.[83] The force of these blasts, combined with the irregularly shaped metal fragments they produced, frequently resulted in fatal injuries for anyone nearby.[84] The wounds they caused were likely not dissimilar to the devastating shrapnel injuries seen during the First World War; wounds that challenged early twentieth-century surgeons, let alone those practicing in the late medieval period and early sixteenth century.[85]

Treating Gunshot Wounds

> Wounds made by Gunshot are known by their figure . . .
>
> Ambroise Paré[86]

By the early part of the fifteenth century, soldiers began to use smaller, handheld guns on the battlefield. Early design problems took some time to overcome, but as the century moved forward, the use of these weapons became increasingly widespread.[87] Accounts of injuries can be found in various records, including the miracles of Katherine of Fierbois. In the summer of 1444, an esquire called Jehan Prevost was struck in the leg by a stone ball fired from a type of handgun called a culverin. The account says that he, '. . . could find no cure nor no remedy, for the stone of the culverin abode fast in his leg'.[88] As is routinely the case in miracle accounts, there is very little detail about the cures and remedies used to try and remove the stone bullet from Prevost's leg. According to the record, he vowed to God, the Virgin Mary and St Katherine that if he recovered from his injury, he would visit the saint's church to give thanks. Shortly afterwards, while out riding his horse, the ball suddenly came loose and fell from his leg.[89] As promised, he later attended the church in gratitude for the miracle.[90]

A very similar injury comes from the 1451 Siege of Bayonne, when a nobleman called Bernard de Béarn was also struck by a ball from a culverin. He was hit in the lower leg, and the bullet became lodged between the tibia and fibula bones.[91] The *Chronique de Charles VII, Roi de France* explains that unnamed surgeons were able to remove it immediately without much difficulty and with no need to cauterize the wound.[92]

The above incident predates von Pfolspeundt's entry on gunshot wounds by a few years, providing proof that practitioners were successfully treating soldiers injured by gunpowder weapons well before the barber-surgeon's text of 1460. When it came to removing bullets, as described by von Pflospeundt, the process began with the use of a metal probe:

> You can do such a search for the bullet that had been shot into the body from the gun using a piece of iron . . . then you can remove it, along with whatever else went inside the wound.[93]

His suggestion to use an iron probe to search for the bullet by sound would have made it much easier to find a metal or stone projectile buried in a patient's flesh. It was an age-old method that had been used to find iron arrowheads lodged inside individuals. The twelfth-century surgeon Roger Frugard was one of many who proposed using a probe to establish the location of an arrowhead deep within a patient's face so that it could then be removed.[94] An example of this technique of finding a bullet comes from September 1495, when a lead ball struck the Count of Pitigliano, Niccolò Orsini, near his right kidney and travelled all the way up to his left scapula. Physicians were able to locate the bullet by using a long bronze probe.[95]

Elsewhere in his text, von Pfolspeundt discusses the treatment for gunshot wounds once the projectile had been extracted. It involved rinsing the affected area with 'frawenn milch' or 'women's milk' to treat the powder burns and eliminate any gunpowder residue. A bandage soaked in turpentine and either rose oil or linseed oil could then be applied.[96] Neither von Pfolspeundt's surgery nor other early recorded examples of gunshot injuries seem to indicate that these wounds were believed to be poisoned in some way.[97] The Venetian army physician, Alessandro Benedetti, who treated the above-noted Niccolò Orsini after he was shot, is among the practitioners whose silence on the matter concurs with von Pfolspeundt's text. Instead, Benedetti outlines a very diagnostic approach to such injuries, asking questions and performing logical tests, such as examining Orsini's urine. When he found it contained no blood, he concluded that the bullet had done no damage to his bladder and kidneys.[98]

It would not be long, however, before surgeons began to believe that poison was associated with gunshot wounds. This thinking led to some quite drastic treatments being employed by doctors in an effort to counteract it. In his 1497 text, Hieronymus Brunschwig insisted that surgeons should remove the gunpowder from a wound by whatever means they could employ.[99] Theriac, or treacle in English, a highly revered, multi-ingredient remedy containing vipers' flesh, was to be administered to the victim.[100] It was believed that the venom or poison in the vipers' flesh would neutralise the poison presumed to be in the wound.[101] The Genoese surgeon Giovanni de Vigo was another of those who believed that gunshot victims suffered from poisoning because of these wounds. He was a man of considerable influence, and his surgical text of 1514 proved to be very popular among surgeons for many years. In it he describes a method of treatment that must have been far worse than the injury itself.[102] It involved pouring boiling elder oil, combined with theriac, directly into the bullet wound to cauterize it and remove the supposed poison.[103]

In 1537, during Ambroise Paré's time with the French army in Turin, he observed that the senior surgeons continued to employ de Vigo's method.[104] He noted that this approach resulted in French soldiers suffering from fever and excruciating pain, with wounds that were swollen and scorched.[105] Being just a young surgeon himself, Paré had no choice but to follow the example of the more experienced practitioners. Eventually, during one surgical session, Paré found that he had more patients than boiling oil. When he ran out, he decided to try a new approach. He dressed the gunshot wounds using only a mixture of egg yolk, rose oil and turpentine.[106] Paré was far from convinced that he had done the right thing, and that night he struggled to sleep, fearing that in the morning he would find his patients dead or clinging to life. He arose early the next morning and quickly made his way back to the ward, where he was surprised to find the soldiers resting comfortably, having slept well. Additionally, he discovered that the men were not in pain, nor were their wounds swollen.[107] Encouraged that gunshot wounds were not poisoned after all, Paré confirmed his initial findings by continuing to test his new technique on other soldiers who suffered similar injuries. After this period of testing, he stated quite strongly, 'When I had many times tryed this in divers others, I thought thus much, that neither I nor any other should ever cauterize any wounded with gunshot'.[108]

Undoubtedly, there was an element of luck, and perhaps even a touch of recklessness, in Paré's initial discovery of an improved technique of treating gunshot wounds. Nonetheless, despite his young age, it was he who chose to seize on the opportunity to try something different and then test it further until he was certain that his method was better than what was being used at the time.[109] In the decades that followed, numerous soldiers with both simple and complex gunshot wounds benefited from Paré's new treatment method, as did surgery as a whole. One account comes from the Battle of Dreux, at the start of the French Wars of Religion (1562–98), when Paré, '. . . dressed fourteen in one chamber onely all hurt with Pistol-shot, and other instruments of diabolical fire and not one of the fourteen died'.[110] In a more difficult case, he treated the Marshal of Brissac at the Siege of Perpignan in 1542, when the officer was hit in the right shoulder by a bullet.[111] Other surgeons had already investigated Brissac's injury, believing that the ball had disappeared into his body. Paré examined him and requested that the Marshal replicate his posture at the moment of the bullet strike.[112] By pressing gently with his fingers, he was able to locate the ball under Brissac's shoulder blade.[113] Paré then directed the dauphin's surgeon, Nicole Lavernault, to remove it by making a small incision in that area.[114]

As weapons of fire and arrows gave way to gunpowder and cannons, it ushered in a far more lethal era of warfare, one that still exists today.[115] Compellingly, one of the engagements described by Paré, the Siege of Thérouanne in 1553, includes a French attack on enemy trenches as well as a mistimed grenade that set fire to an arsenal, causing many soldiers to be badly burnt.[116] Words such as 'trenches' and 'grenade' would become synonymous with the horrors that were seen again in places like Thérouanne some 400 years later during the First World War.[117] With that in mind, an excerpt from the poem titled *The Next War* by First World War soldier and writer Osbert Sitwell offers a fitting tribute to those who suffered some of the most devastating injuries of war, not only in the last century but also during the period under review:

> We think perhaps we ought
> To put up tombs
> Or erect altars
> To those brave lads
> Who were so willingly burnt,
> Or blinded,
> Or maimed,
> Who lost all likeness to a living thing,
> Or were blown to bleeding patches of flesh.[118]

Chapter 5

BONES, TEETH AND SKULLS

> . . . with mighty maces they break the bones.
>
> *The Canterbury Tales – The Knight's Tale*[1]

The Iberian chivalric romance *Amadís of Gaul* features a tournament scene in which the title character, disguised as a Greek knight, jousts with Salustanquidio, the towering Prince of Calabria.[2] The hero Amadís arrives at the lists clad in gleaming snow-white armour, with a multicoloured surcoat, helmet and shield. In contrast, the prince is dressed in black armour adorned with serpent emblems.[3] The two men eventually take to their horses, one at each end of the lists, and gallop toward each other at full speed. With lances levelled and shields at the ready, they clash in the centre, each landing a blow, but only Salustanquidio is unseated from his mount:

> . . . he was a large man and bulky, and had fallen from a high horse, and his armour was heavy and the ground was hard, and moreover the left arm upon which he had fallen, was broken near the wrist, and the greater part of his ribs put out.[4]

Although the story of *Amadís of Gaul* is a work of fiction, passages like this one, depicting warriors with broken and battered bones, offer a glimpse into the harsh realities faced by soldiers during the late medieval period and the decades that followed. Indeed, in his fourteenth-century poem *Livre*, which describes the life of a knight, Geoffroi de Charny acknowledges that broken bones were an expected risk in tournaments, combat and training.[5] Another poem, *Of Knyghthode and Bataile*, a Middle English adaptation of the seminal Roman military treatise *De Re Militari* by Flavius Vegetius Renatus, includes the phrase 'often breaks bones and bruises flesh', here again highlighting the sorts of injuries that were commonly sustained in battle.[6] The risk of bone fractures and dislocations only increased as the presence of gunpowder weapons became more common on the battlefield.[7] Ambroise Paré, who treated many of these injuries during his career as a battlefield surgeon, noted, '. . . Souldiers have had arms and leggs broken, and shot off by Cannon-bullets . . .'.[8]

Fractures and dislocations were a regular part of a military surgeon's work during this period. According to Paré, treatment of such injuries aimed to achieve three main objectives: to realign the bones, maintain their proper positioning, and prevent complications such as pain, gangrene, and inflammation.[9] Among soldiers, fractures of the arms and legs remained particularly common. Methods such as traction, bandaging and splinting continued to be used to treat them, showing little advancement from the techniques practiced by doctors in earlier centuries.[10] Since these procedures were discussed in detail in the previous volume, this provides an opportunity to explore the therapies used to treat other common types of fractures and bone injuries sustained by warriors of the period, including those affecting the ribs and back.[11] These treatments can be found in the texts of most of the men of medicine under examination here, with the exception of Henri de Mondeville, who died before he was able to complete his work on bone fractures and dislocations.[12] His surgery does, however, include procedures for treating the skull, including trepanation, which is examined in the final section of this chapter.

Ribs

> . . . he has broken my hip and my ribs . . .
>
> *Amadís of Gaul*[13]

Numerous tales and poems composed by warriors who turned their hands to the pen as well as the sword feature scenes in which their characters find themselves with broken or damaged ribs. It seems likely that they were simply reflecting on their own experiences and observations. In *Le Morte d'Arthur*, for instance, the eponymous king has his ribs crushed by a club being wielded by a giant early in the story.[14] During a tournament in the Spanish tale *Tirant lo Blanc*, Tirant unhorses a Greek lord called the Grand Noble, who breaks two of his ribs in the fall.[15]

Away from tales like these, surgeons found such injuries to be considerably more difficult to treat than the long bones of the arms and legs, which could be managed fairly routinely. The shape and position of the ribs meant that when they were broken, practitioners had to find more ingenious methods of treatment. Jehan Yperman, in his succinct advice, offers an imaginative approach employed by some medical practitioners. He begins by discussing fractures with inward-bent ribs, recommending that surgeons first apply a covering of resin or thick honey to their hands. They were instructed to repeatedly apply small, heated cups over the fractures, which were to be pulled away swiftly. This cupping technique, along with the surgeon's sticky hands, was intended to realign the damaged rib bones. Following this, the popular antiseptic ointment known as apostolicon was to be applied to a piece of leather and bandaged over the broken ribs until they healed.[16] Also known as Apostles' Ointment, its name derives from the fact that it traditionally contained the same number of ingredients as there were apostles of Christ, although the specific components often varied between practitioners.[17]

Guy de Chauliac included much more detail in his surgical text, describing treatments for rib fractures that deformed in both directions. However, before any procedure could take place, patients were to be bled, given laxatives to evacuate their bowels and fed a light chickpea broth.[18] If the ribs were broken outwardly, he would carefully manipulate the bones back into their natural position using his fingers. He would then apply a plaster of egg whites and wheat on a soft cloth before placing a thick strip of shoe leather over the area and bandaging it into place.[19]

Ribs that were broken inwardly were looked after in a manner not unlike that suggested by Yperman. Chauliac's patients were first placed in a warm bath or beside a hearth while he covered his hands with glue. He then placed his sticky appendages on the areas where the depressed ribs were located, lifting them gently as the patient coughed or held their breath.[20] In more serious cases, de Chauliac proposed making a small incision in the chest so that a hook could be inserted to lift the broken bones back into place. As anyone who has ever experienced cracked or broken ribs can attest, the accompanying pain can be severe, somehow seeming to get worse before getting better. Chauliac used rose honey to help reduce the patient's discomfort.[21] Plasters made with egg whites were also applied to the ribs and bandaged only lightly. New plasters made from honey and bean paste were to be applied later in the healing process. Patients' dressings were to be changed every five days, with the expectation that the ribs would be healed in about 20 days.[22]

Ambroise Paré argued against the cupping and sticky hands methods suggested by Yperman and de Chauliac. In addition to causing the patient more pain, he felt that these procedures attracted bad humours to the area of the fractures.[23] In cases where the rib fractures were simple, Paré dispensed with bloodletting, evacuating the bowels, or any special diet. However, when patients did have more complicated breaks, he would employ these measures, just as de Chauliac had done.[24] Paré's treatment technique involved first placing the patient on their side. Next, a mixture of turpentine, mastic, black pitch and other sticky substances was spread onto a piece of sturdy cloth and placed over the patient's fractured ribs. Once the cloth had time to set, and with the patient holding their breath, it was suddenly ripped away, '. . . with great violence'.[25] Frighteningly, this was not just a one-time procedure; it was to be repeated as many times as it took for the ribs to return to their natural position and for the patient to be able to breathe more comfortably.

Since the ribs protect many of the body's important organs, when they are broken, bone fragments can lead to damage and infection in these structures.[26] With the increasing prevalence and power of gunpowder weapons, such injuries became more widespread and problematic. In fact, they would pose challenges for battlefield surgeons for many centuries to come.[27] If the surgeon could feel that the rib bones had splintered, Paré suggested they make an incision in the patient's chest, which would provide the opportunity to try and remove the offending pieces. Still, as one of Paré's accounts suggests, this could be a difficult and often unsuccessful process. In 1553, a soldier called Monsieur de Martigues was shot in the chest while trying to locate the enemy. The bullet broke two of his ribs, carrying splinters from the bones into his lungs. Despite the surgeon's best efforts to save de Martigues, the serious nature of his injuries meant that he did not survive.[28]

Back

> With frequent falls and bruises and other misfortunes, such a weakness came upon him . . .
>
> Miracles of St Thomas of Hereford[29]

In addition to *Of Knyghthode and Bataile*, Vegetius' influential *De Re Militari* was the basis for many of the books and manuals of war that were written during the late Middle Ages, including Christine de Pizan's *The Book of Deeds of Arms and of Chivalry*.[30] In his original text, Vegetius strongly recommended that daily military exercises be carried out by soldiers to help keep them fit, healthy and battle ready.[31] It is a notion that is reiterated by de Pizan in her fifteenth-century text:

> The continual exercise of arms provides all the necessary skills, as is the case with anyone who has on many occasions experienced a variety of military adventures in various countries and nations.[32]

Alongside tournaments and battles, this demanding routine of training and exercise often took its toll on the necks and backs of soldiers. Take, for instance, the condottieri, mounted captains of mercenary troops from many of the medieval republics that now make up Italy. These men are known to have regularly suffered back problems because of their rigorous regime of training, riding and fighting.[33]

The archaeological record provides several examples of injuries that likely led to chronic back problems for those who were dedicated to a military lifestyle. An excavation in 1997 at Stirling Castle in Scotland exposed the skeleton of one such well-built English warrior. Investigation revealed that the bones were quite likely those of a knight called John de Stricheley, who died on 10 October 1341.[34] It was clear that a lifetime of riding, military exercise and battle had not been kind to his body.[35] A number of issues with his teeth and bones were uncovered when they were examined, including impact trauma to some of his vertebrae.[36] Another case involves Sir Hugh de Hastyngs, a tall and muscular English knight who died in 1347. He served in Edward III's forces in France for most of the 1340s and participated in several major battles, including Sluys, Crécy and Calais.[37] When his skeleton was studied in the mid-1980s, numerous problems were identified, including osteoarthritis in his spine, right hip, shoulder and elbow. The damage clearly pointed to an individual whose days had been spent on horseback, exercising and fighting with heavy weapons.[38]

It was not just heavily armoured knights who suffered persistent back problems. There is also evidence that indicates that regular soldiers, mainly archers, experienced similar sorts of back issues. In England, where mandatory archery training began as young as age seven, the strain that a lifetime of practicing this arduous skill could put on an individual's spine and dominant shoulder was considerable.[39] Confirmation of such issues can be found among the skeletons recovered from Henry VIII's flagship, the *Mary Rose*, which sank in 1545. Several have been identified as those of skilled archers and display degeneration in the shoulder and lower spine, which is attributed to the physical demands of archery over many years.[40]

Depending on the severity, chronic back issues can at best be uncomfortable and, at their worst, completely debilitating.[41] Despite this, very few remedies to treat long-term issues, such as a bad back, can be found in the texts of medieval surgeons.[42] This is not to say that therapies did not exist, as there were a number of oils and plants that could be used to provide short-term relief from pain. Rose oil, to which other pain-relieving ingredients could be added, was a particularly popular topical analgesic.[43] Medicinal baths were also commonly used to obtain temporary respite from such problems.[44] Just as in modern times, it was believed that the waters aided in the treatment of a sore back and other similar ailments. It is known that fifteenth-century Venetian condottieri regularly spent time at the baths at Abano, not far from Padua. One officer, Erasmo Gattamelata da Narni, was even granted permission to travel as far away as the baths of Petriolo, near Siena, to try and find relief for his back problems.[45]

When it came to more serious injuries to the neck and back, some could be life-changing or even fatal.[46] A late thirteenth-century knight called Miles, 'a famous warrior, renowned far and near for his exploits in tilting' is recorded among the miracles of St Thomas of Hereford.[47] The numerous falls and injuries he sustained while competing in tournaments eventually left him paralyzed. Physicians tried everything in their power to treat the knight, but despite their efforts, he remained in that condition for six years. What occurred next is difficult to determine, but according to the text, on Easter Eve, during the translation of the bones of St Thomas of Hereford to a more prominent place, Miles was carried to the saint's tomb. It was there that he prayed to St Thomas for a cure for his paralysis. The next morning, he found himself healed, so much so that he was able to wait on the bishop's table that evening, serving the senior cleric and his guests.[48]

Yperman did not include anything on the subject of such serious neck and back trauma. This is perhaps unsurprising, as his teacher,

Lanfranchi of Milan, wrote very little about the subject, other than to caution against trying to treat such injuries, '. . . if the grave signs are recognized'.[49] These so-called grave signs are described in the work of Henri de Mondeville's mentor, Theodoric, who said of serious injuries to the neck:

> . . . examine his hands to see if they are flaccid and numbed and deadened, and if the patient cannot move them nor flex them, and if there is no feeling in them when they are pressed, then you should know that something awful has happened. But if he moves them and feels the pressure of your fingers, then you may know that the spinal cord is safe.[50]

Equally, when the vertebrae of the back were damaged, Theodoric advised that the feet should be checked in the same way as the hands when the neck was injured. He noted that if the patient experienced problems with urinating or rectal incontinence, the injury was likely to be fatal.[51] When these signs were not present it meant a more positive diagnosis was possible. Theodoric suggested that the surgeon could remove any bone splinters or fragments that resulted from the damaged vertebrae.[52] Beyond that, he does not provide much detail, stating only that the back was to be, '. . . set with all the physician's ingenuity'.[53]

Guy de Chauliac's text bears resemblance to that of Theodoric, primarily in the notion that there is hope for patients with relatively serious back injuries, provided they do not experience paralysis or incontinence.[54] He was able to offer more in terms of patient care, including a healing ointment containing pain relief. A salve composed of rose honey and cooked egg yolks, supplemented with analgesics, was applied to the patient's back using bandages. Rest and restricted movement, maintained through careful bandaging, were crucial to the patient getting better. As their condition improved, healing plasters could be applied to support further recovery.[55]

Not much had changed by the sixteenth century in terms of the understanding or treatment of such severe trauma to the vertebrae and spine. The limits of a surgeon from this time can be seen in an entry from Paré's casebook involving a fatal spinal injury suffered by an officer at the Battle of Saint Denis in November 1567. At the request of the French king, Charles IX, Paré was sent to treat a general named Monsieur le Connestable who had been hit in the middle of his back by a shot from a pistol.[56] When he reached the officer's home, Paré discovered that the ball had broken some of le Connestable's vertebrae and crushed his spine, leaving him without the use of his legs or the ability to control his bodily functions. At that point, Paré understood there was little he could do to assist him. Connestable soon experienced significant cognitive decline and died within just a few days.[57]

Shoulder Dislocations

> . . . gave him so violent a blow on the shoulder that ever after the said Lyonnel was lame on that side.
>
> *Chronicles of Enguerrand de Monstrelet*[58]

The *Miracles of Charles of Blois* provide an account of a 25-year-old knight called Geoffrey Budes. He was part of French forces attempting to reclaim the small walled town of Ussel, in central France, from the English and their allies in February 1371.[59] As they attacked the town, Geoffrey attempted to scale the walls but was knocked into the ditch below by the large rocks being pelted at him from above. He lay there with several injuries, including a broken right arm and dislocated shoulder, until his comrades, who used a cloak to drag him from the ditch, removed him to a place of safety.[60] After pledging his devotion to Charles of Blois, Geoffrey was taken away on horseback through snow-laden mountains and valleys to Clermont, where his bones were set, perhaps by the same soldiers who had escorted him that far.[61] The text notes that when Geoffrey later reached Paris, he still required further medical attention, but the surgeons there praised the work that had already been done to treat him.[62]

This record of Geoffrey Budes highlights one of the most commonplace injuries suffered by warriors of the time: a dislocated shoulder, which occurs when the humerus is displaced from the shoulder joint.[63] There are many such examples among the annals and texts of the day, including the *Chronicles of Froissart* and the later *Diaria de bello Carolino*.[64] It is a phenomenon that persists in modern military forces. According to a 2018 study conducted by the US Military, soldiers experience shoulder dislocations at a rate twenty times higher than civilians.[65] An earlier report also found that, in addition to those in the military, participants in contact and overhead sports were at a greater risk of suffering such an injury.[66] Modern findings such as these provide context for why this injury was so common during the late medieval period and early sixteenth century. Although their sporting activities and fighting styles differ, the characteristics of athletes and warriors effectively illustrate the lives of soldiers during the medieval era, particularly those belonging to the knightly classes.[67]

Several treatment methods for a dislocated shoulder identified during the period under investigation here are notably absent from key twelfth and thirteenth-century surgical texts and were therefore not addressed in the previous volume.[68] Most of these techniques were not necessarily new; rather, they were rediscoveries that drew on the teachings of ancient physicians such as Hippocrates.[69]

Guy de Chauliac's surgery includes several methods for reducing a common shoulder dislocation.[70] The first procedure began with the surgeon raising the patient's arm while simultaneously using their shoulder or other hand to guide the head of the humerus back into the socket. As the arm was gradually lowered, the surgeon needed to ensure that the humerus remained securely positioned within the shoulder joint.[71] The next of de Chauliac's techniques required the help of two assistants who each held one end of a bar or rod. A ball was placed under the patient's armpit before their arm was draped over the bar. While the assistants lifted the bar, the surgeon pulled the patient's arm in a downward direction, returning the humerus back into the shoulder joint.[72] Another of his methods was a riskier variation of the previous procedure, with this one using a ladder and a footstool to get the job done. The patient would stand on the footstool, with a ball tucked under their armpit and their arm dangling over a rung of the ladder. The surgeon would then hold the patient's arm down while an assistant removed the stool from beneath them. The patient's weight would cause their humerus to go back to its proper position.[73] Whatever method was used, de Chauliac advised that once the humerus bone was back in place, the shoulder was to be tightly bandaged. These bandages were to be changed every nine days. The arm was to be placed in a sling that was to remain on for the first nine days or until the swelling had reduced.[74]

Much of von Pfolspeundt's text on dislocations focuses on the shoulder, which he uses as something of a template for the other joints of the body. His advice is to have the shoulder reduction done as quickly as possible. As far as von Pfolspeundt was concerned, any dislocation that had gone untreated for more than a year was deemed to be incurable. He believed that even a dislocation that had been left untreated for a few weeks could pose serious challenges for a surgeon. Von Pfolspeundt's concerns about looking after such injuries at this stage are underscored by the fact that the surgeon was to hear mass before completing the procedure.[75] In these instances, the patient required several warm baths and softening compresses before the surgeon could attempt to return the humerus to its proper position in the shoulder joint.[76] Unfortunately, von Pfolspeundt's account provides only a vague description of the actual reduction procedure. However, once it had been completed, a wooden ball wrapped in lint material was placed under the patient's armpit to keep the head of the humerus fixed in place while it healed.[77]

One of the most comprehensive works on shoulder dislocations is found in the text of Ambroise Paré. He included a multitude of treatments for reducing such injuries, including those techniques found in the surgery of Guy de Chauliac. He also added detailed illustrations for each of the many procedures.[78] One of his methods required an assistant who was roughly the same height as the patient. They were to stand with their shoulder under the patient's armpit while the surgeon, who was on the opposite side, wrapped his arms around the patient, his hands meeting at the injured shoulder. As the surgeon shook the patient, the shoulder reduction was completed by the assistant with a sudden downward motion of the patient's arm.[79]

Paré recommended preparing a salve to reduce the discomfort and swelling brought on by such an injury. It was made from flour, an egg, Armenian bole, pitch and myrtle. After it had been applied, the armpit was filled with wool or cotton cloth that had been soaked with oil of rose or myrtle. To prevent the cloth from adhering to the hairs of the body, other components, such as vinegar and rose perfume, were added.[80] A bandage, about 2.7m long and five fingers wide, was needed to stabilize the shoulder:[81]

> The midst thereof shall be put immediately under the arm pit, and then crossed over the lame shoulder, and so crossing it as much as shall be fit, it shall be wrapped under the opposite arm.[82]

This initial dressing was to be left alone for the first four or five days before it was changed, provided there were no other problems with the injured shoulder. A sling was also to be provided to keep the patient's arm in an elevated position.[83]

Teeth

> . . . the blood spirted out from under the steel — he lost some teeth . . .
>
> *The Story of Grey-Steel*[84]

In the epic *Tirant lo Blanc*, published just before the sixteenth century, the hero loses some of his teeth during combat, the text noting, '. . . since Tirant had no visor, the Saracen smote his jaw and dislodged four teeth'.[85] Like Tirant, soldiers of this period frequently concluded battle with fewer teeth than they possessed at the outset of the fighting. The modern analysis of the skeleton of Sir Hugh de Hastyngs, the battle-hardened fourteenth-century English knight noted earlier in this chapter, revealed that osteoarthritis was not the only problem he faced in later life. He suffered a significant impact, or possibly several impacts, to his mouth, which resulted in the loss of seven or eight of his front teeth.[86] As well as changing his appearance quite considerably, such damage would have severely hampered Sir Hugh's capacity to speak and eat properly.[87]

A surviving review of a company of soldiers in the Provençal army from the autumn of 1374 has left a small but valuable window into the state of regular fighting men during this period.[88] The information contained within the roll provides an idea of the appearance of many of the soldiers, including the state of their dental health. Only three categories were needed in the medieval survey, 'missing one tooth, missing some teeth and teeth uncommon'.[89] In addition to those that were lost to age or disease, the various trauma-related scars and deformities observed on these individuals provide evidence that many of their teeth were knocked out due to violence. Additional corroboration of such trauma to the mouths of typical soldiers can be found in the mass burial at the location of the fifteenth-century Battle of Towton. Approximately 50 per cent of the crania that were excavated and analysed showed at least some traumatic tooth loss or destruction.[90]

Tournaments were another place where warriors often lost their teeth. In 1390, during the reign of Richard II of England (1367–1400), a good-looking English knight called Piers Courtenay was affronted when a Scottish knight, William Dalzell, turned up at the royal court dressed intentionally in a fashion nearly identical to that of Courtenay.[91] The offence created by Dalzell caused a serious disagreement between the knights. To settle their differences, the two ended up jousting, and as their horses came together for a third time, Courtenay had two of his front teeth taken out by Dalzell's lance.[92]

When it came to replacing smashed or broken teeth, both de Chauliac and Paré had similar ideas on the subject. Chauliac suggested using human teeth or carved replacements made from cow bones, which could be fastened into place in the patient's mouth.[93] Recommending that the false teeth be fashioned from bone or ivory, Paré offered a comparable plan to that of de Chauliac, but with more detail about the actual process of fitting them into the mouth:

> . . . teeth artificially made of bone or Ivorie may bee put in the place of those that are wanting, and they must bee joined one fast unto another, and also so fastned unto the natural teeth adjoining, that are whole; and this must chiefly bee don with a thred of gold or silver, or for want of either, with a common thred of silk or flax . . .[94]

Such teeth would not have been without their problems. Ivory substitutes had the tendency to decompose in the mouth over time, leading to ulcers and infections. While they would continue to be used for a few hundred years, by the end of the eighteenth century, false teeth made from ivory began to go out of fashion.[95]

Soldiers' teeth were not always broken or knocked out by violent strikes from fists and weapons; sometimes, they were just loosened by such an impact. These types of blows could cause their own problems in the form of abscesses. This was the situation with John de Stricheley, the fourteenth-century English knight already mentioned in this chapter. Among the many issues he had accumulated during his life as a soldier was a painful abscess that had formed around his gums, the result of an impact to his mouth that loosened several of his teeth.[96]

The surgical texts of Yperman and von Pfolspeundt contain almost nothing regarding trauma-based damage to the mouth. Instead, their attention is given to things such as tooth decay and bad breath.[97] Contrarily, de Chauliac included substantial detail about dental surgery in his work, incorporating treatments for abscesses and loose teeth caused by damage to the mouth. To begin, the surgeon recommended using vinegar or rose water to cleanse the area of infection.[98] Then, the patient would require bloodletting, an evacuation of their bowels and a reduction of saliva in their mouth before the loose teeth could be treated.[99] A mixture of cinnamon, cypress tree nuts, frankincense and alum could be spread on the patient's gums. If this treatment failed to secure the teeth properly, gold wire could be used to bind them to the nearest healthy teeth.[100]

Paré also devoted a considerable amount of space in his text to the teeth and mouth. He cited the example of a tailor called Antoine de la Rue, who had been hit in the mouth with the pommel of a dagger. The blow had broken his jaw and loosened three of his teeth. In addition to looking after de la Rue's jaw, Paré attached his loose teeth to healthy ones using waxed thread. He also prepared an astringent using cypress tree nuts, myrtle berries and a small amount of Armenian bole, mixed with water and vinegar, which was held in the patient's mouth for an extended period. Paré notes that de la Rue was eventually able to use the teeth just as he had before he was struck by the dagger's pommel.[101]

Skulls

> . . . one of whom received so terrible a blow as clove his head asunder . . .
>
> *The Memoirs of Philip de Commines*[102]

During the period under investigation in this volume, the head remained one of the most vulnerable parts of a soldier's body. This was partly because it continued to be a primary target in both battle and tournament.[103] Additionally, the social hierarchy among warriors meant that only a select few were equipped with adequate protection for the head and face, while many went into battle with little or nothing to shield them.[104] The three mass graves from the Battle of Visby (also Wisby) in 1361, which were discovered on the Swedish island of Gotland, are indicative of the disparity in head wounds between those who went into battle wearing helmets and those who lacked such equipment. In the first grave, which contained the bones of soldiers who benefitted from head protection, only 6 per cent of the crania showed any damage. The other two graves contained the bones of those who were unprotected, with nearly 50 per cent of the skulls showing battle damage of some sort.[105] Similarly, skulls excavated from mass graves at other known battle sites dating to the 250-year period investigated here, such as Sandbjerget in Denmark, Towton in England, and Uppsala in Sweden, appear to show a pattern like that observed at Visby.[106]

While the very nature of head wounds meant that they were frequently fatal, there are examples from across Europe that show that occasionally combatants did manage to survive even the most horrific damage. An excavated grave from St Mary Spital, London, contained the skull of a male between 26 and 35 years of age, from the period between c.1250 and c.1400. The left side showed clear signs of a forceful strike with a heavy, bladed weapon. The blow left a very obvious wound, penetrating both the left frontal bone and the rim of the orbit. This individual would have been left blind in that eye and otherwise disabled, as damage to that part of the brain tends to impact memory and communication skills and can result in behavioural problems. It seems probable that he would have required care and assistance for the remainder of his life, something he may well have received from the monks in the infirmary of St Mary Spital.[107]

The mid-fifteenth-century chronicle *La Cronaca di Cristoforo da Soldo* describes how an officer called Giannantonio di Gattamelata (c. 1415–56) was struck in the head by a lead bullet from a handheld gun at the Battle of Ghedi in Lombardy in 1453. The ball passed through both his helmet and skull.[108] Gattamelata managed to get to the town of Lonato, where he was examined and treated by several unnamed doctors.[109] The severity of the wound left him unable to speak and paralysed on one side of his body. Remarkably, he survived for another three years, despite disbelief that anyone could endure such a serious injury.[110]

The Battle of Good Friday is a lesser-known conflict that took place on 6 April 1520, near Uppsala, Sweden. The fighting occurred between a Swedish peasant army and a Danish force, largely made up of mercenaries who were stationed at Uppsala.[111] In 2001, the skeletal remains of individuals who fought in the battle were unearthed, including two crania, documented as A4:12 and A4:26. In addition to the damage that killed them that day in the spring of 1520, the skulls also showed evidence of healed, depressed fractures caused by bladed weapons.[112] While these injuries may not have been quite as severe as the two previous examples, the individuals still would have required significant medical attention.[113]

The surgical texts of Yperman and Paré give us an understanding of how men like these may have survived such terrible trauma. Beginning with Yperman, his surgical text includes detailed treatment plans for a couple of head injury cases, including that of a soldier who had suffered a severe blow from a blunt weapon. The warrior was still unconscious when Yperman began to attend to him. The Flemish surgeon exposed his skull by cutting a cross through his scalp using a razor. Once he peeled back the flaps of skin, Yperman discovered that the soldier had a depressed skull fracture. He applied cloth dressings to the area, soaking them first in three parts olive oil and one part rose honey, changing them regularly during the man's time in his care.[114] Although it was a struggle during these early stages, Yperman kept his unconscious patient nourished with barley broth, egg yolks, a whipped mixture of milk and flour and applesauce.[115] The soldier eventually regained consciousness, and the damage to his skull began to heal, with new bone forming. After a period of six weeks, he began to speak once more, rather humorously referring to Yperman as 'Uncle' when he spoke to him.[116] As the man's speech continued to improve, so too did his injury. The damage to his skull mended well, leaving no real depression or bony projection.[117] When it was time to close the wound, Yperman had to carefully realign the sections of skin. Using an individual thread of silk or linen, each line of the incised cross was sutured separately, ensuring that the edges of skin were brought together properly to avoid the formation of ugly scars.[118]

Like other types of wounds, head injuries, some of which were especially difficult to detect, became increasingly prevalent with the introduction of gunpowder weapons.[119] The text of Paré contains the case of a cavalryman who was defending a breach in a castle wall when he was struck on the top of his head by a bullet. The helmet he was wearing seemed to protect him, ending up dented but not penetrated by the bullet. While there was no apparent damage to the cavalryman's head, he died six days later from a stroke. A postmortem investigation by Paré disclosed that the ball had struck him where the suture lines met at the top of his skull.[120] He discovered that the force of the bullet's impact had caused tiny fractures to the inner table of the soldier's skull, creating the sharp bone splinters that damaged his brain and resulted in a stroke. This case made Paré determined to understand how such an injury could be revealed in the future.[121] He decided that when a soldier was struck in the head by a bullet, the first step would be to shave their scalp. A plaster made with wax, pitch, tar, turpentine and powdered iris would then be applied to the affected area. If tenderness or swelling persisted, it would be taken as a sign of possible internal damage. To save the patient's life, a hole would be drilled into that area of his skull so that a search for any bone fragments could be conducted. This last step would only be done after other physicians and the patient's friends had been consulted.[122]

The process of drilling or scraping through the skull is known as trepanation. Having been practised for millennia, the technique continued to be employed during the period under review here. It could be used for several reasons, including the removal of bone fragments and weapons, the treatment of disease and issues of mental health, or to relieve pressure on the brain.[123] Instructions for the procedure are found in the works of Yperman, de Mondeville, de Chauliac and Paré.[124] Theodoric's mid-thirteenth-century preparatory measures to aid the patient during this operation by blocking up their ears were bolstered by men like Yperman, who included something for the patient to bite on:[125]

> . . . cover the wounded's man's ears with wads of cotton or the like, and give him a glove to bite on. This is how you control the disturbing noise that is part of the operation and how you prevent the chattering of the victim's teeth.[126]

Indicative of the increase in head injuries caused by gunpowder weapons are the many examples of trepanation found within Paré's text. At the Siege of Metz in 1552, he operated on Monsieur de Pienne, who was struck in the temple by a stone bullet.[127] At the Battle of St Quentin in 1557 Paré notes that he had to trepan many injured French soldiers.[128] During the Siege of Rouen, in 1562, he stated, '. . . I trepanned eight or nine, who were hurt at the breach with the strokes of stones'.[129] These experiences gave Paré a profound understanding of what was necessary to perform the procedure successfully and ensure the patient's survival. He went on to design numerous surgical instruments to better perform the operation, including some with enhanced safety features, such as a drill with an adjustable guide to prevent penetration beyond the thickness of the skull.[130]

Chapter 6

MUTILATED AND MAIMED

> . . . many I have maimed all utterly that they might never after help themselves . . .
>
> *Le Morte d'Arthur*[1]

There are several chroniclers and writers who did not hold back in their descriptions of the horrors of conflict, recording a vivid picture of the sort of miserable and debilitating injuries many warriors suffered in battle.[2] The *Chronicle of Geoffrey le Baker* is certainly no exception, with its report on the condition of English sailors as they returned from the Battle of Winchelsea at the end of August 1350. Also referred to as the Battle of les Espagnols-sur-Mer, this vicious naval fight during the Hundred Years War ended in victory for Edward III of England's forces over a Castilian fleet allied with the French. What is clear from le Baker's account is that several among the English were left with wounds that gave them very little to celebrate:[3]

> They brought back their wounded, with heads covered in linen bandages to hold their injuries together, arms and legs had been punctured by crossbow bolts and darts, and teeth were torn out, noses also had been cut off, lips cleft, and eyes ripped out . . .[4]

Certainly, there would have been some whose wounds were not nearly as serious. Their treatments would likely have left them with little more than scars that resulted in a new nickname or symbol of bravery.[5] Since the first volume examined such cicatrices in detail, this chapter focuses on more severe facial injuries, such as those described by le Baker.[6] Additionally, amputations are revisited, with an emphasis on the innovations and rediscoveries that enhanced the effectiveness of surgeons and made patients more comfortable. The late Middle Ages through the early sixteenth century also saw significant progress in prosthetic devices, many of which restored dignity and mobility to soldiers who had been mutilated or maimed in battle.[7] Several of these advancements, especially those developed by Paré, are explored throughout these pages.[8] In the final section of this chapter, the lives of soldiers who suffered such debilitating injuries are investigated.

The Ears and Hearing Loss

> . . . on pain of having his ears cut off . . .
>
> Trial of William Pykemyle, London 1379[9]

There are numerous accounts of soldiers who sustained injuries to their outer ears, with many having them severed entirely. John Barbour's poem *The Bruce* explains how Robert the Bruce, while being assailed by three men, used his sword to slice away the ear and cheek of one of them.[10] Even those whose heads were protected by steel were at risk of injury, as the story of *Amadís of Gaul* describes, 'Galaor made at him, and with his sword struck him upon the helmet; it cut away all it touched, and lopt off his ear . . .'.[11]

It seems that opposing warriors were not the only ones who could cause a soldier to lose an ear. It was also possible for such injuries to be initiated by those fighting on the same side. According to the chronicle *Gesta Henrici Quinti*, or *The Deeds of Henry the Fifth*, on the day prior to the Battle of Agincourt, King Henry V of England demanded complete silence amongst his ranks. He ordered severe penalties for anyone who disobeyed this order:

> . . . rex indixit silentium per totum exercitum, sub pœna amissionis equi et harnasii in generoso si delinqueret, et auris dextræ in valettum et inferiorem quemlibet, sine spe veniæ exequendâ qui edictum regium præsumeret violare.[12]

> . . . the king imposed a silence throughout the entire army, under the penalty of losing a horse and harness if the offender

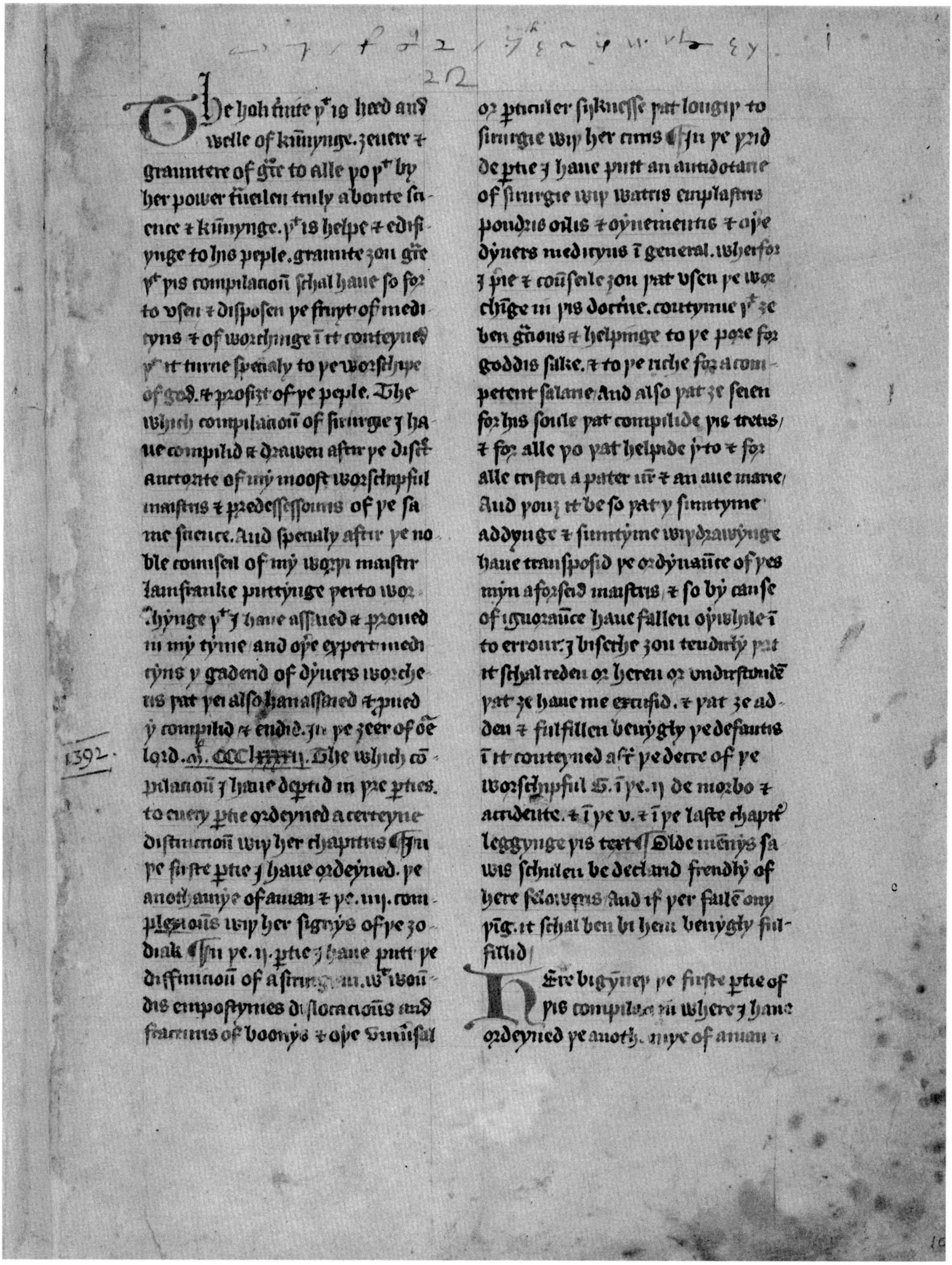

1. Opening folio from an anatomy based on Henri de Mondeville and Lanfranchi of Milan, which precedes a surgery. From an incomplete and abridged English translation, originally written in 1392, by an unknown surgeon who seems to have practised in London. It begins: 'The holi trinite that is heed and welle of knowynge . . .'. (Created c. 1475, Henri de Mondeville, *Chirurgia*, plus miscellaneous receipts, MS.564, f. 10r. Courtesy of the Wellcome Collection)

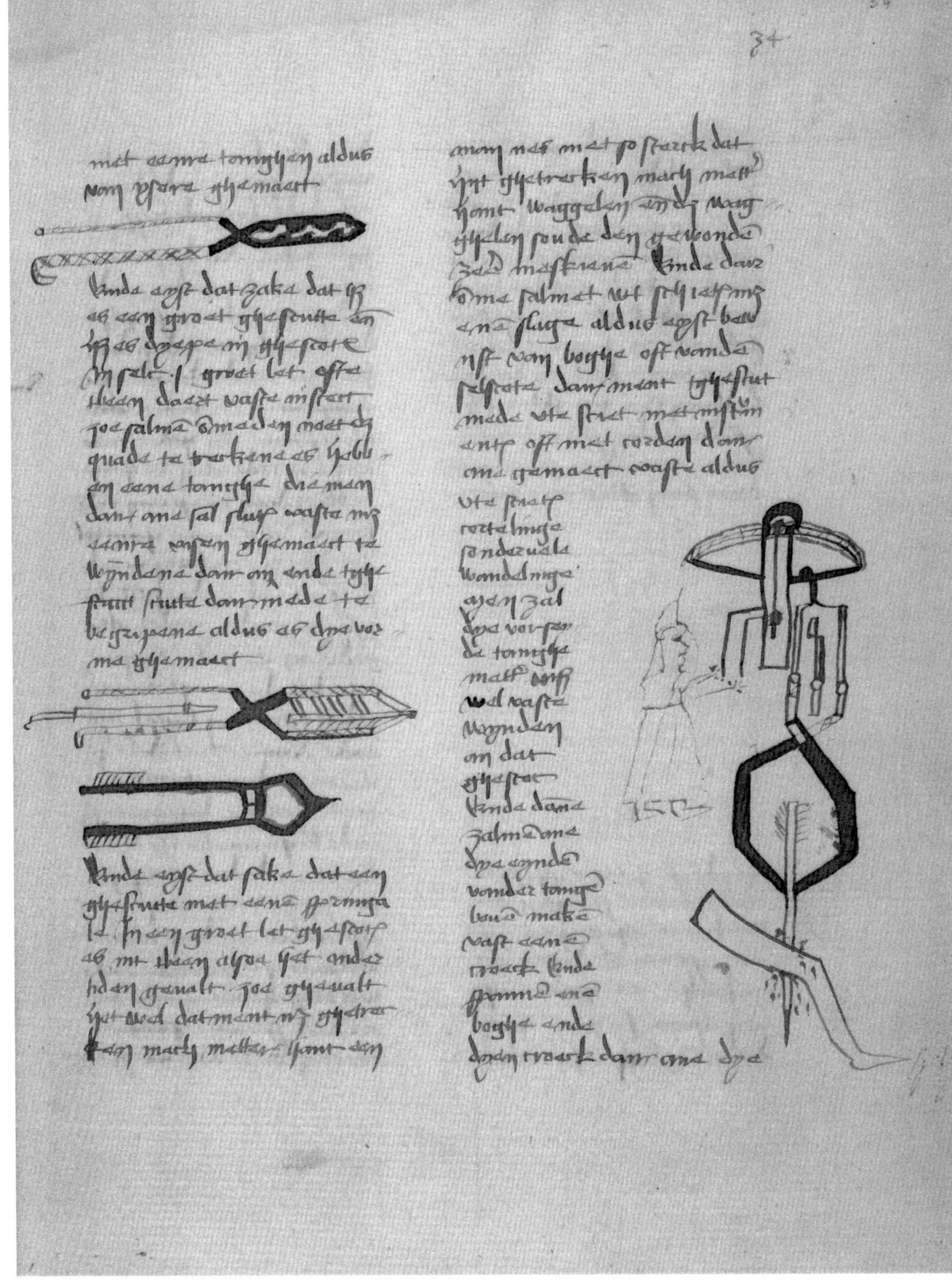

2. From a fifteenth-century copy of the Surgery of Jehan Yperman. The illustration on the right shows how a crossbow could be used to remove a stubborn arrow from a patient's limb. At the bottom is an injured leg and at the top the crossbow, with a clamp in the centre connecting the two. When the empty crossbow was fired the action forcefully withdrew the arrow. (Cyrurgie van meester Jan Yperman, Courtesy of Universiteitsbibliotheek Gent, HS. Gent, UB1273, f. 34r)

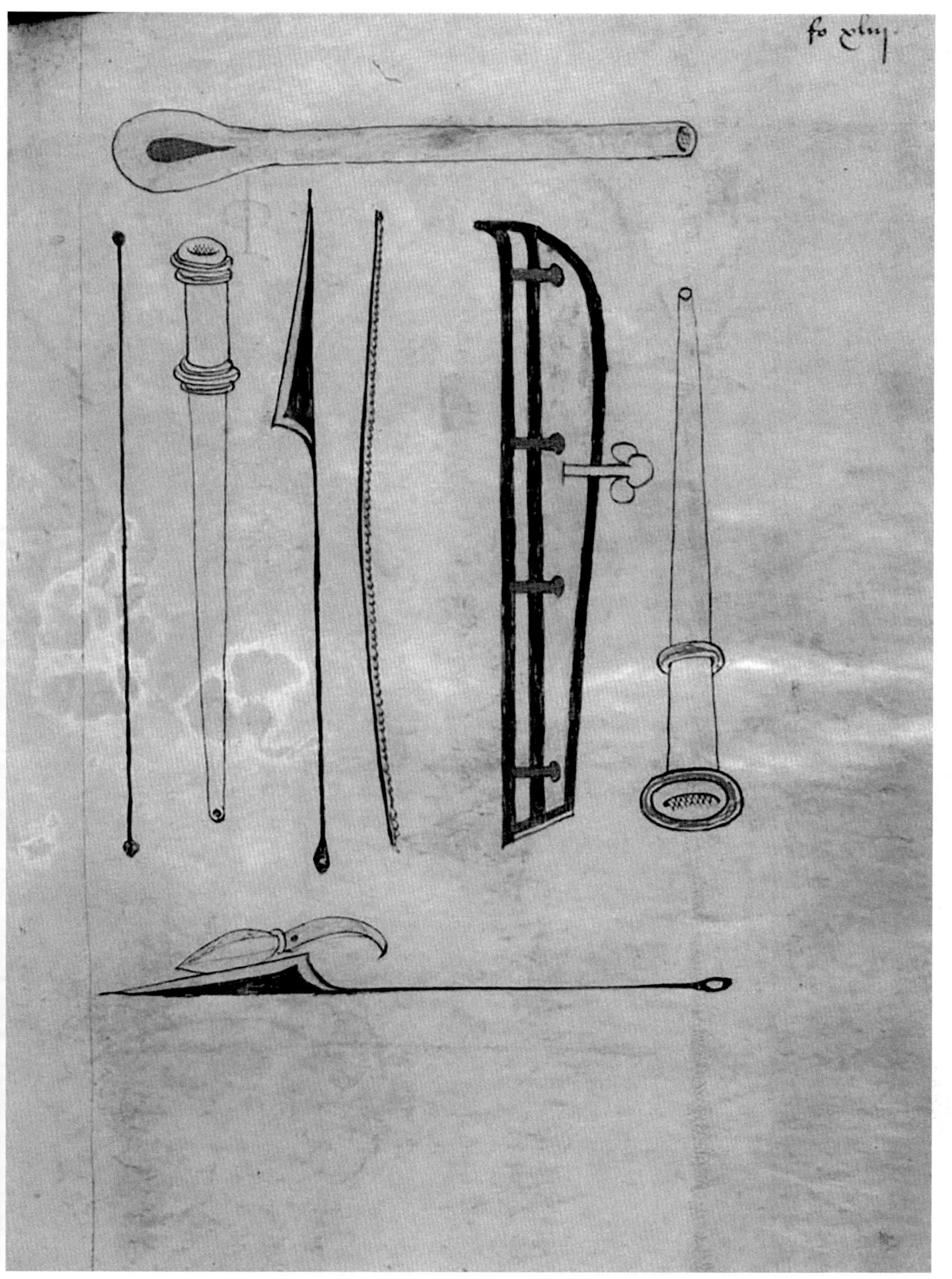

3. From a late fifteenth-century copy of John Arderne's work. Surgical instruments used to treat anal fistulas. (Courtesy of University of Glasgow Archives & Special Collection, MS Hunter 251 (U.4.9), folio 43 recto)

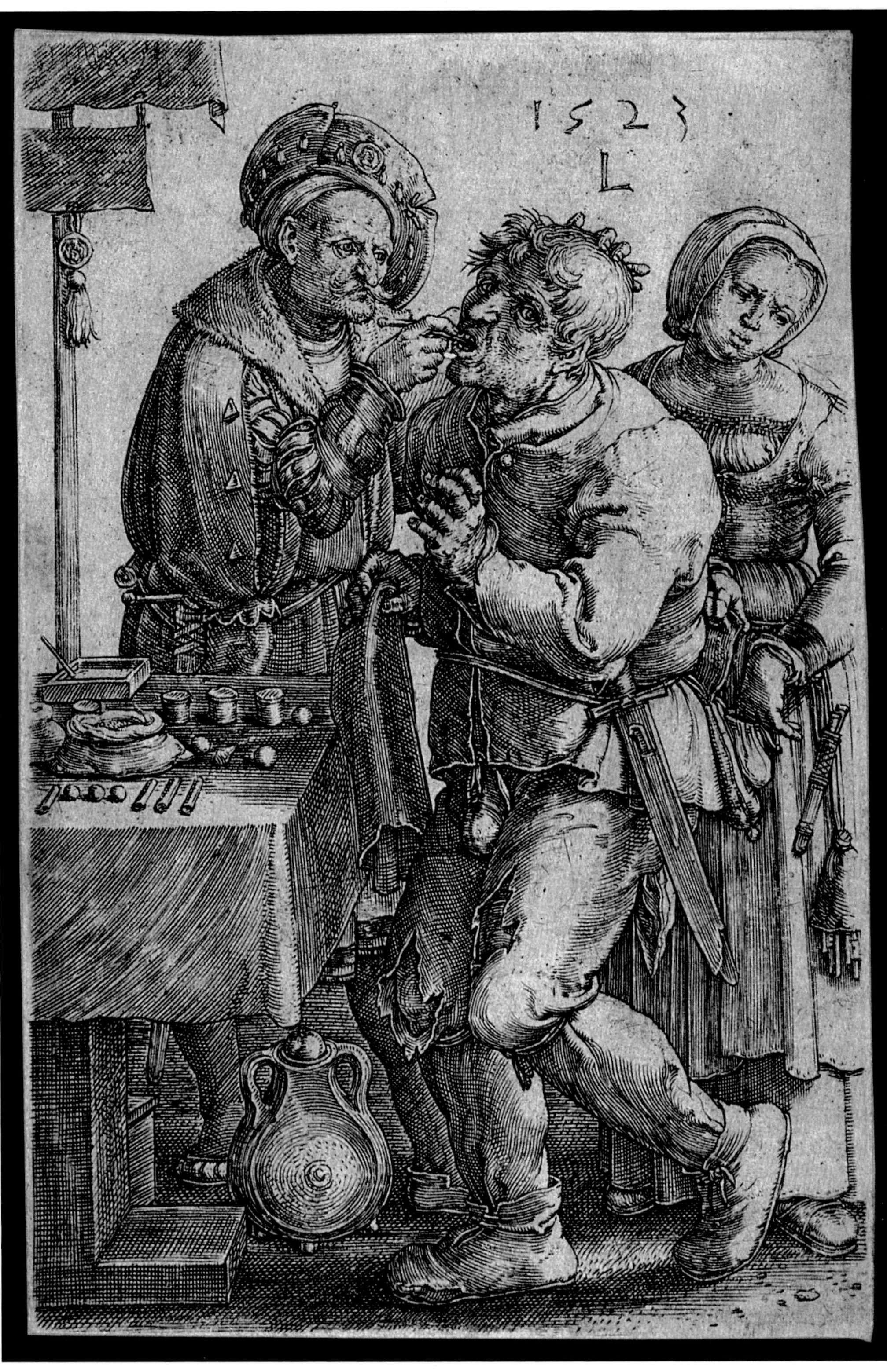

4. A tooth-drawer extracting a tooth from a standing patient, who is being pick-pocketed by a woman. (Line engraving after L. van Leyden, 1523. Courtesy of the Wellcome Collection, Reference: 16423i)

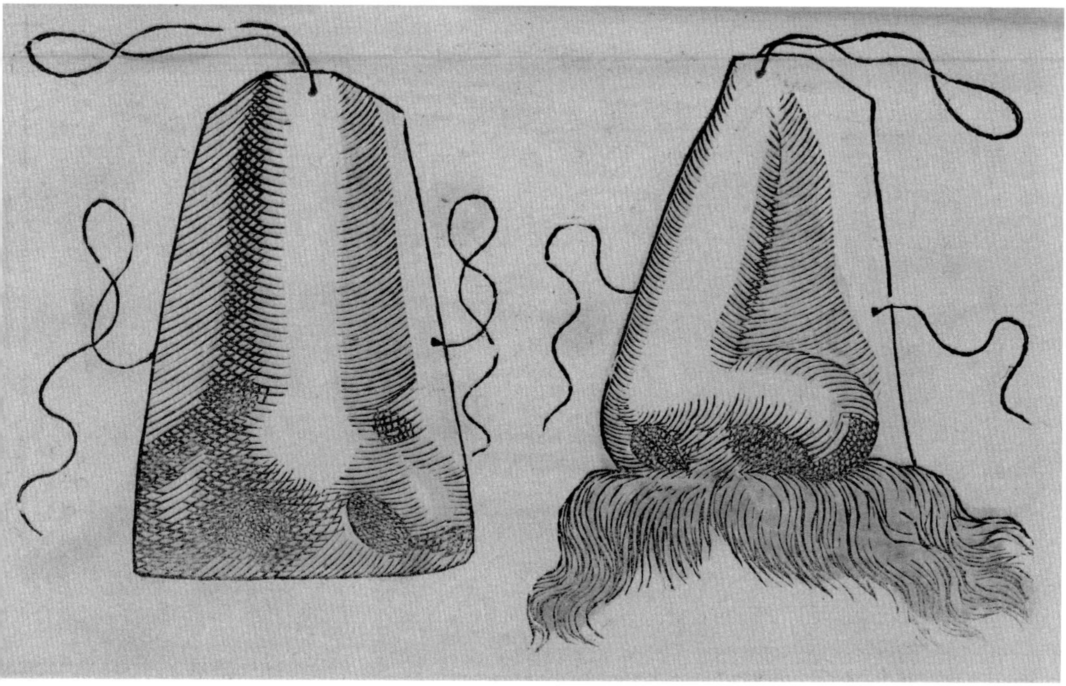

Above: **5.** Two types of artificial noses produced by Ambroise Paré, including one with an attached moustache to hide any evidence of injury to the patient's upper lip. (1564 – *Instrumenta chyrurgiae et icones anathomicae* / [Ambroise Paré], p. 199. Courtesy of the Wellcome Collection)

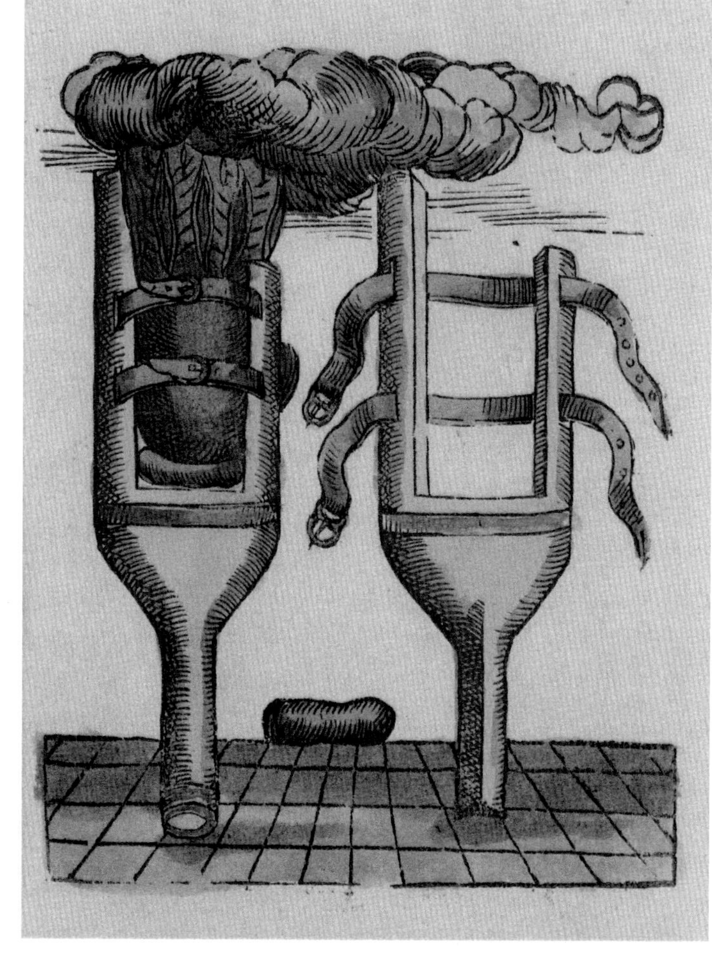

Right: **6.** Paré's design for his so-called 'woodden Leg made for poor men'. (1564 – *Instrumenta chyrurgiae et icones anathomicae* / [Ambroise Paré], p. 79. Courtesy of the Wellcome Collection)

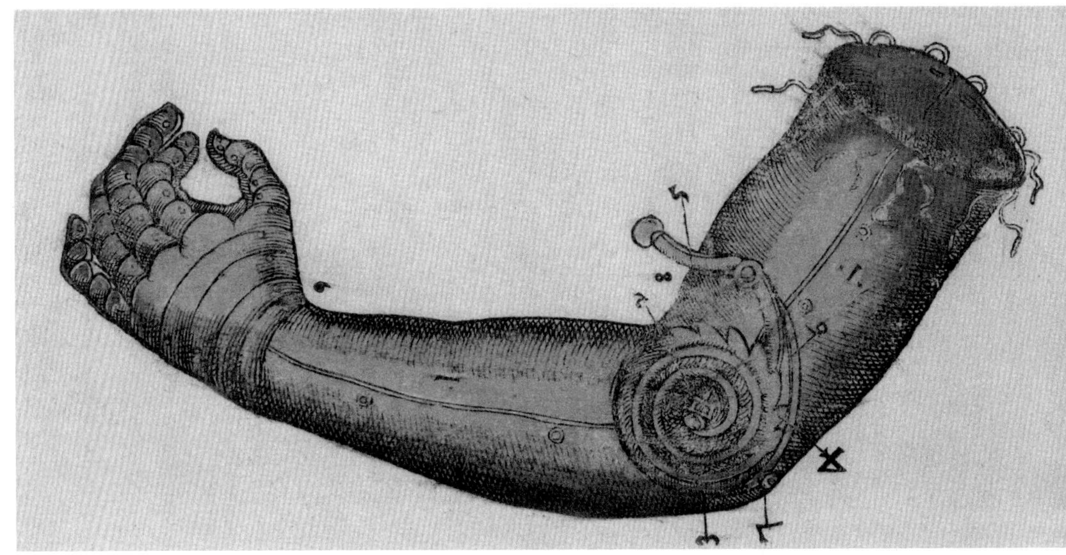

Above: **7.** Articulated prosthetic arm made of iron, designed by Paré. (1564 – *Instrumenta chyrurgiae et icones anathomicae* / [Ambroise Paré], p. 105. Courtesy of the Wellcome Collection)

Below: **8.** An apothecary publicly preparing the drug theriac, under the supervision of a physician. It was used to treat both wounds and diseases, including the bubonic plague. (From Hieronymus Brunschwig, Woodcut – 1500–99, Reference: 16050i. Courtesy of the Wellcome Collection)

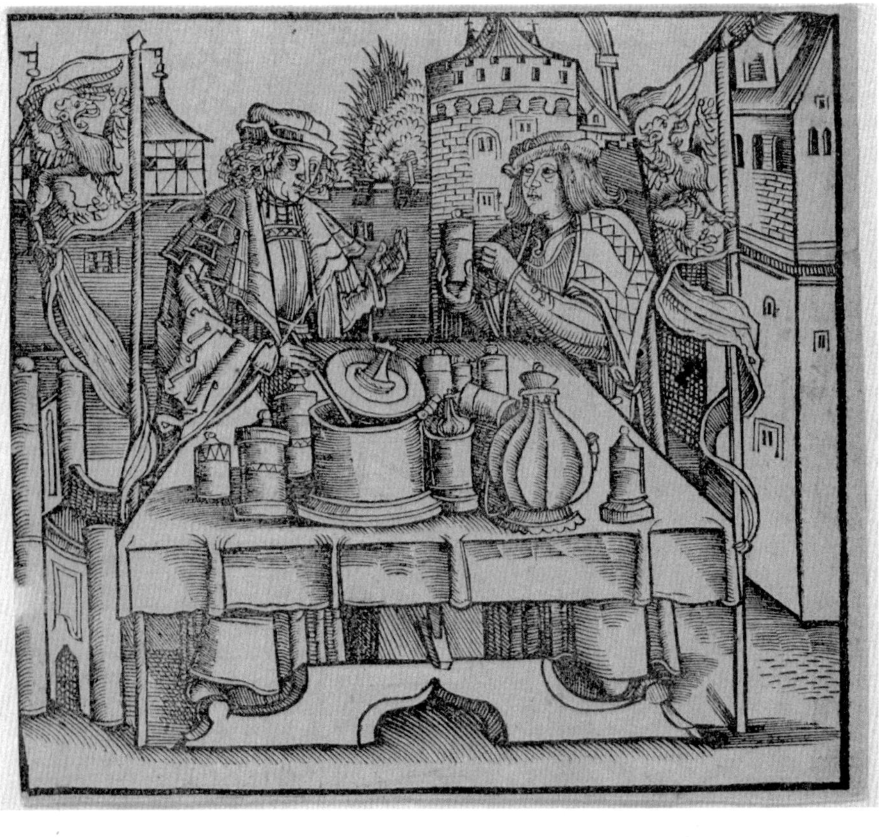

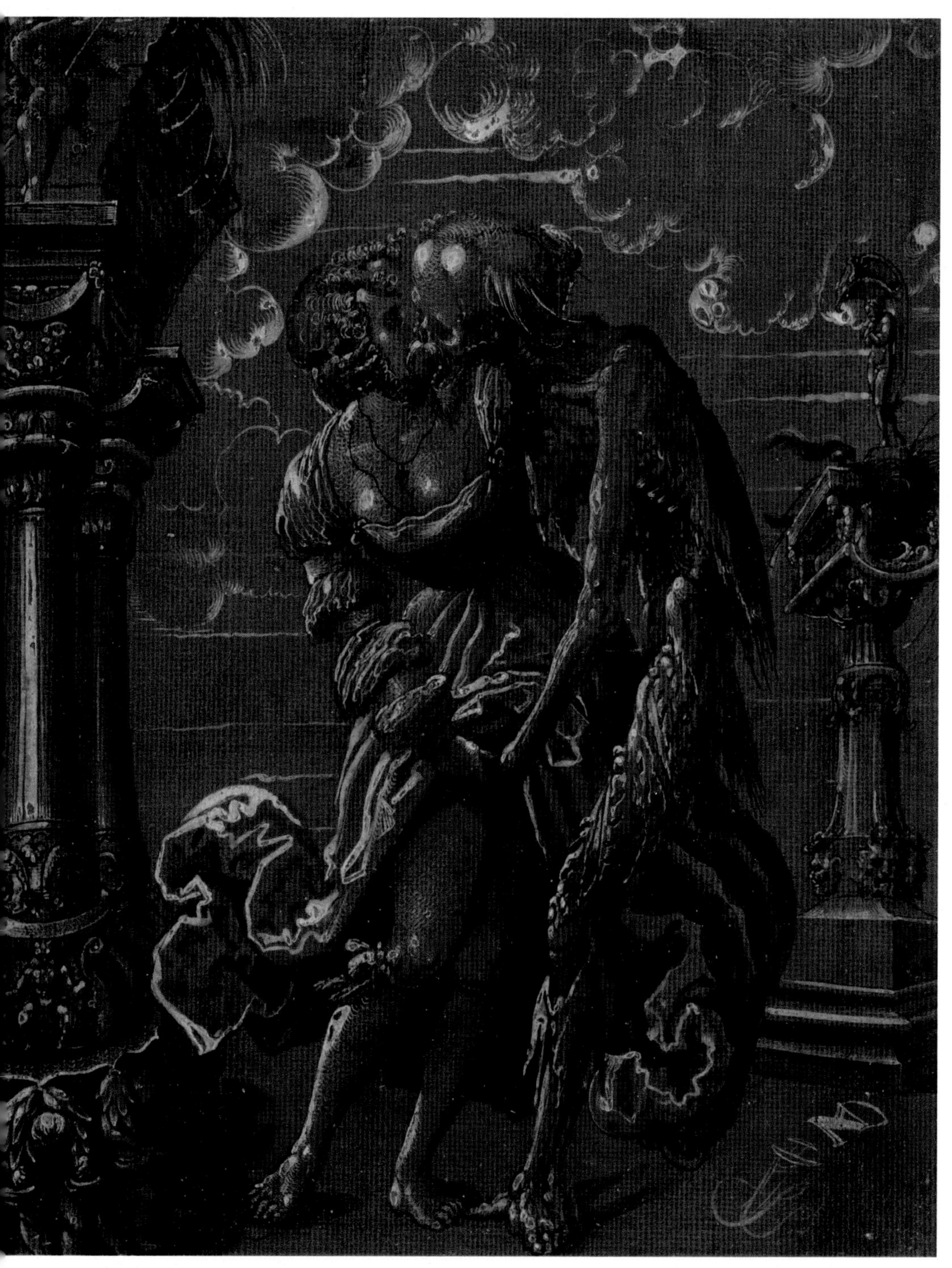

9. An image called *Der Tod als Kriegsknecht umarmt ein Mädchen*, or *Death as a soldier embraces a girl*, depicting Death as a syphilitic soldier groping the genitals of a woman (Artist: Niklaus Manuel Deutsch, mixed media on fir, 1517, Courtesy of Kunstmuseum Basel, Amerbach-Kabinett (Martin P. Bühler))

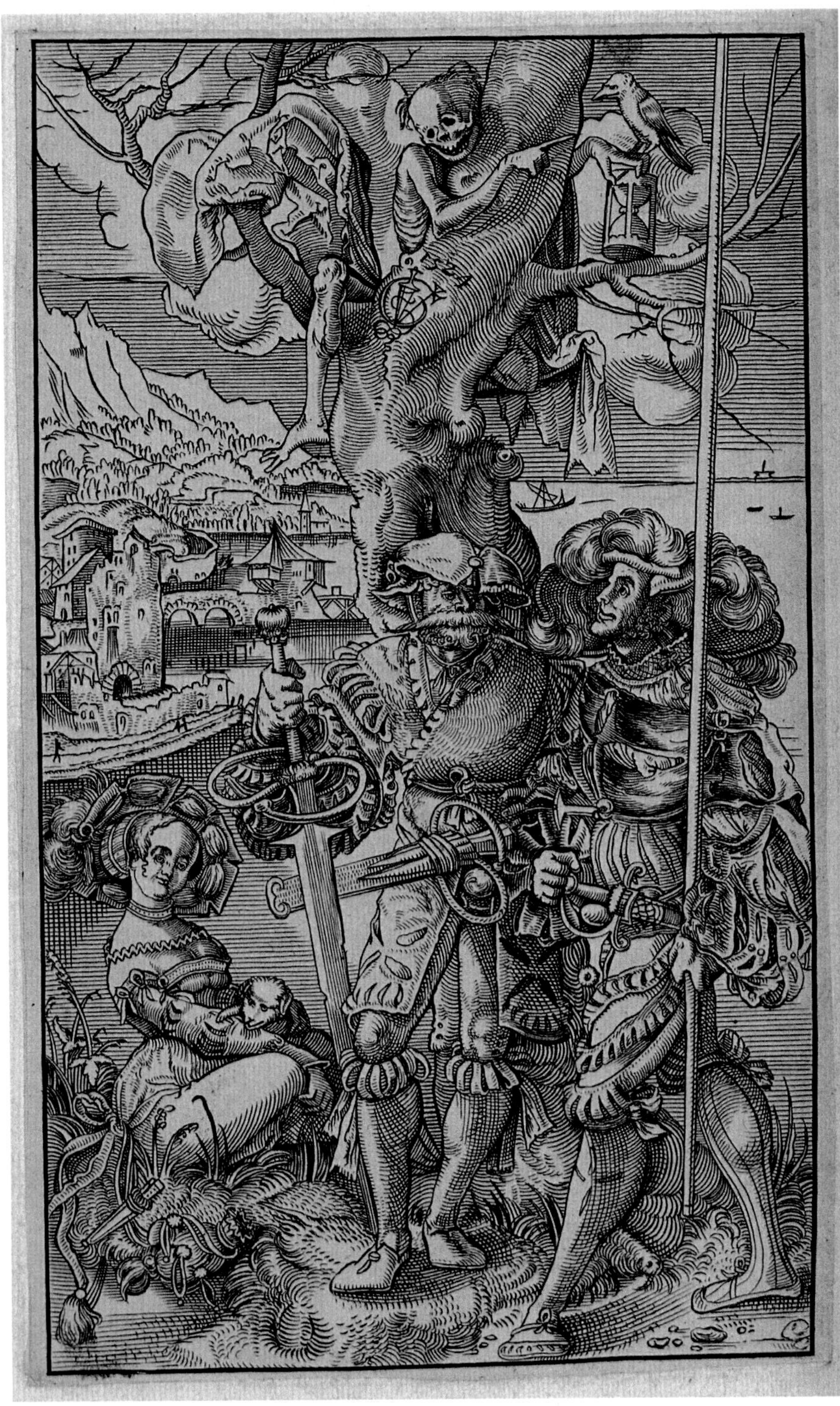

10. Two mercenary soldiers approach a seated sex worker while Death sits in a tree pointing to an hourglass indicating that syphilis will soon take its toll. (Etching after Urs Graf, 1524, Reference: 33730i. Courtesy of the Wellcome Collection)

> be a nobleman; and the right ear would be taken from those of lower rank, if any were to presume to violate the royal edict, without any hope of a pardon.

Rejoining a detached outer ear or even a piece of it was simply not possible at this time. As Yperman noted, it was the sort of thing that could only be done in fables.[13] What was possible, however, was to surgically repair part of the outer ear that had recently been cut but was still partially attached, provided it had a viable blood supply. Yperman's treatment for such a wound began with an examination of the damage. If the cut was large, he would first insert a wick into the patient's ear canal. It provided a guide for repositioning the damaged portion of the outer ear when it was sutured back into place while helping to keep scar tissue from impairing the patient's hearing afterwards.[14] A single length of waxed silk, red or white in colour, was used to close the wound with a running suture.[15] Next, Yperman noted that red powder should be applied to the area of the wound before it is dressed using a pad of oakum, a fibrous material made from the hemp plant. This dressing was to be changed every nine days, with warm wine being applied to keep the area moist during healing. The application of the final bandage was done using just an oakum pad that had been soaked in warm wine.[16]

Two and a half centuries later, Paré was treating wounds to the outer ear in much the same manner as Yperman. He was careful to explain that when suturing the partially disconnected portion of the ear, the needle should never touch the cartilage, only the skin and the small area of flesh that covered the tough tissue. He believed that if the surgeon damaged the cartilage, it could lead to gangrene setting in.[17] Like Yperman, Ambroise Paré was also concerned about the possibility of 'superfluous flesh' growing around the ear canal during healing and causing impairment to the patient's hearing. Instead of a wick, he recommended that a piece of sponge be placed there to keep this from occurring.[18]

Many soldiers who did lose their outer ears during wartime found themselves facing further challenges once they returned home. This was because, in many parts of Europe at this time, the mutilation of the ear was a common punishment for many types of crimes, including theft.[19] Consider the example of a French thief called Thassin-aus-oz from Bazeville who had his ear cut off on 12 August 1355, at St. Martin, as a penalty for stealing two sheets.[20] Disfigurements such as this were meant to bring humiliation to thieves like Thassin-aus-oz, marking them out as criminals for the rest of their lives. Since the public could not immediately differentiate between a soldier who had suffered the loss of an ear and a criminal who had been duly punished for their crimes, it created obvious difficulties for the wounded warrior. One answer to the problem was to obtain an official letter, which could be immediately produced as proof that a soldier's physical appearance was related to war and not an act of lawlessness.[21]

In his medical text, Paré proposed a variety of solutions for those who experienced this kind of disfigurement. One involved wearing a cap over the damaged or missing ear and stuffing it with cotton to mimic its structure.[22] If just a portion of the ear was missing, the answer could be to create holes in whatever natural flesh was left using a bodkin needle. Once these openings had healed, some 'convenient thing' could be shaped into the missing piece of the ear and tied to the natural portion using the holes.[23] When the entire outer ear was missing, an ear-shaped prosthesis could be fashioned '. . . made of paper artificially glewed together, or els of leather . . .'.[24] Once the paper or leather had been formed to match the missing ear, it could be painted to make it look as natural as possible. It was held in position either by means of laces or by a piece of wire that wrapped around the back of the head.[25] The loss of the outer ear can impact certain aspects of hearing, especially sound localization. Remarkably, it has been discovered that a well-shaped and correctly positioned paper or leather replacement, such as those described by Paré, may have partially restored this function in some individuals.[26]

Soldiers faced not only the risk of losing their outer ears but also the very real danger of hearing loss, as the deafening noise of sieges and battles could cause lasting damage. In *The Book of Deeds of Arms and of Chivalry*, Christine de Pizan describes the thunderous sounds of an early fifteenth-century siege, including, '. . . bombards, cannon shots, the terrible din of stones being thrown by engines against the walls, the shouts of attackers, the sound of trumpets . . .'.[27] Much of what she describes can be seen in the German-language *Spiezer Chronik*, which includes an illustration of the siege of the fortress at Baden in 1415. Among the besieging army is a cannoneer wearing green who can be seen igniting a large cannon with his right hand while futilely attempting to block the noise from his left ear with the other hand.[28] Men like this cannoneer were especially susceptible to hearing loss. Surgeons like Paré were certainly aware of the harm that gunpowder weapons were causing to soldiers' hearing, but there was little they could do about it.[29]

In much the same way, medieval surgeons had no way to properly treat hearing loss. Sadly, there is still no known cure, and aids such as cochlear implants are only very recent innovations.[30] Even before the proliferation of gunpowder weapons, Yperman recognized that nothing could be done if an individual's hearing loss was due to internal damage.[31] However, this was a departure from what other doctors, including his mentor, Lanfranchi of Milan, believed. He suggested putting the fat from green frogs into the ears of deaf patients to help improve their hearing.[32] John Arderne claimed he could treat hearing loss using the following remedy:

> Eggs of ants and earthworms beaten up with white wine and distilled in an alembic and, after cleansing the body, injected into the ear makes the deaf hear and stops tinnitus.[33]

At best, these so-called cures and remedies may have had some effect in clearing blockages, such as a buildup of wax, but they would have been useless for soldiers whose hearing had been permanently damaged by the noise of battle.[34]

The Nose

> When the nose suffers an oblique cut leaving an attached piece, sew it back in place with sutures precisely edge to edge.
>
> Jehan Yperman[35]

As noted at the end of Chapter 3 and in le Baker's account of those returning from the Battle of Winchelsea, a soldier's nose was particularly vulnerable to the weapons of the period.[36] Here again, a helmet was not always impenetrable, as portrayed in the tale of *Amadís of Gaul*, 'Agrayes made a blow at him that only struck his vizor, but it went through and sheared his nose clean away . . .'.[37] As with the ears, medieval practitioners had no means of reattaching any part of the nose once it had been severed. Nevertheless, folklore claiming such restorations were possible persisted throughout the period, prompting many surgeons and physicians to dismiss these beliefs outright. Guy de Chauliac called such claims 'old wives' tales', while Mirfield said that those who told such stories were 'just plain lying', and Paré simply noted that such an injury 'cannot bee restored or joined again'.[38]

As with the ear, the successful repair of a lacerated nose also required some attachment to the face and a viable blood supply.[39] Guy de Chauliac's text describes the meticulous care that was required to repair such a wound. The surgeon started by heating and bending some straight suture needles to match the contours of the laceration that was to be stitched. Tubes made from cloth or the hollow portion of a goose's feather were sprinkled with wound powder and placed inside the patient's nostrils to enable them to breathe properly as the stitches were going in, as well as during the healing process.[40] Once the nose was sutured, pads for the exterior of the wound were to be soaked in egg white, sprinkled with wound-healing powder and placed over the stitches. Another pad, also soaked in egg white, was applied to the entire area of the nose.[41] During subsequent bandage changes, white wine and healing ointments were to be spread around the area of the stitches. The method of bandaging the nose differed among surgeons, but de Chauliac took a pragmatic approach, stating that each case should be judged on its merits. The one thing he insisted on was that every patient wear a skullcap so that bandages could be attached to it to keep everything in its proper place. If the damaged flesh did not survive the procedure, it was to be removed. What was left of the nose could then be bandaged.[42]

The form of rhinoplasty suggested by von Pfolspeundt and Paré in Chapter 3 provided a surgical solution for an individual whose nose had been cut off, but it did not represent the only available alternative. Speaking about the young man from St Thoan who had received this surgery, Paré mentions a silver prosthesis that he had worn after he first lost his nose.[43] The French surgeon described a similar device that he devised in two different types: one without facial hair and another that included a moustache to hide any damage that had been done to the victim's upper lip.[44] According to Paré's instructions, a practitioner could make such a replacement using a small sheet gold or silver or by glueing together pieces of paper or linen cloth. In order to accurately resemble the lost nose, the selected material would be sculpted and painted. Strings or laces were used to secure these prostheses in place. They were threaded through tiny holes made in the artificial nose and fastened at the back of the wearer's head or hat.[45]

Like the nose, the hard palate in the roof of the mouth is linked directly to breathing. In Paré's time, it was frequently damaged by syphilis or bullet wounds, often leaving individuals struggling to breathe or speak clearly.[46] To replace the damaged palate, Paré designed a device made from a thin piece of silver or gold, about the thickness of a coin and slightly larger in circumference than the cavity itself. The metal was hammered into the shape of a small dish, carefully moulded to fit the contours of the roof of the mouth, with the convex side facing upward. A piece of sponge was attached to that side of the device before it was positioned into the roof of the mouth, and as Paré described:

> . . . when it is moistened with the moisture distilling from the brain, will becom more swoln, and puffed up; so that it will fill the concavitie of the Palat, that the artificial Palat cannot fall down, but stand fast and firm, as if it stood of it self.[47]

The Eyes

> He plunged his dagger into the champion's eye . . .
>
> *Tirant lo Blanc*[48]

The eyes were perhaps the most vulnerable part of a medieval soldier's face, being susceptible to everything from fists and sword butts to the many edged weapons of war. Even things such as powdered quicklime and coal dust were adapted to damage the eyes of combatants.[49] In *The Book of Deeds of Arms and of Chivalry*, Christine de Pizan describes the sort of harm that quicklime could cause:

> . . . suitable vessels full of quicklime should also be provided so that these can be thrown down if the enemy comes close to the walls. When these break, the quicklime will enter the eyes and the mouth and thus do some of the attackers in.[50]

There were other, less expected hazards, that could also cause injuries to the eye.[51] An account from the *Miracles of Charles of Blois* offers an example of this type of minor eye wound. It involves a 26-year-old soldier named John Hervey from Nantes, who was part of a group of warriors under the leadership of a knight called Yvon de la Jailla in the year 1369. Hoping to evade confrontation with enemy forces located near Derval in western France, Sir de la Jailla opted to lead his men on a nighttime detour, navigating through a wooded area to circumvent them. As they rode in the darkness, Hervey's face struck the branch of a tree, leaving a thorn lodged in his left eye. Since it was dark and the group wanted to keep their movements secret, they could not stop and help him. When they finally arrived at a place of safety, there was significant concern for Hervey, as it seemed certain that he would lose his eye. A man called Perrotte was called to examine him, and he confirmed that the eye was badly damaged. He offered to try and remove the thorn, but fearing an even greater injury, Hervey was reluctant to have it treated. Instead, he put his faith in God and Charles of Blois to help him. A day or so later, when Sir de la Jailla next saw Hervey, all seemed to be well with his eye. The knight asked the soldier what had happened, and he explained that he had made a vow to visit the grave of Charles of Blois before rubbing his eyes. By doing this, he caused the thorn to become dislodged, leaving his eye undamaged.[52] It seemed to Sir de la Jailla that there was only one answer for the cure, stating, '. . . since the thorn was in such a dangerous place, it could not have been cured except miraculously'.[53] The knight would later be one of the many witnesses who confirmed the details of this incident to those investigating the miracles attributed to Charles of Blois.[54]

In the absence of something miraculous, there were many ointments and remedies that could be used to treat less serious types of eye injuries. Several of them came from an influential thirteenth-century oculist named Benvenutus Grapheus (also Grassus), who wrote a seminal treatise on the eyes called *Ars probatissima oculorum*, or *The Best Art of the Eyes*.[55] His work quickly gained popularity with surgeons such as Yperman and continued to be accepted by many in the medical community.[56] The treatments suggested by Grapheus, especially those relating to scratches, blows and foreign matter, would be repeated in several medical texts. One such remedy was referred to as the 'supreme treatment' by Yperman and 'God's given gift' by de Chauliac.[57] It was made using twelve eggs laid by white ducks, which were beaten with a lead pestle and mortar until they produced a thick, creamy substance. This could be placed under the patient's eyelid three times a day. As the eye began to improve, cotton pads soaked with the whites of hens' eggs could then be applied.[58] According to Yperman's surgery, Benvenutus Grapheus claimed this technique helped to reduce inflammation, extract pus and remove bad humours from the eye.[59] Although he does not acknowledge Grapheus by name, Ambroise Paré advocated a similar method using a dozen egg whites beaten in a lead mortar, but with the addition of rose water to the mixture he produced.[60]

The remedies of other oculists and even skilled tradesmen can also be found in the surgical texts from the period. Guy de Chauliac included the work of an Islamic oculist named Ali ibn Isa al-Kahhal (fl.1010) in his major surgery.[61] He recommended that eye injuries be washed with the milk of a lactating woman or with soft water. If these liquids failed to remove the irritants, then the upper lid of the eye should be folded back and the particles removed with a soft cloth or tweezers before being rinsed again with breast milk.[62] Tiny fragments of metal posed another significant danger should they make their way into a soldier's eye on the battlefield. The surgeon Hieronymus Brunschwig proposed the use of magnetic iron ore to extract such minute metal particles. It was a technique he had picked up from stonemasons, for whom this sort of injury was something of an occupational hazard.[63]

The damage caused by chemical irritants, like quicklime, was not always treatable and could result in permanent blindness.[64] There is also considerable evidence to show that the prevalence of arrows and other projectiles regularly took soldiers' eyes out.[65] The *Lanercost Chronicle* offers the example of English archers harrying Scottish forces near Dupplin Moor in 1332 and '. . . so blinded and wounded the faces of the first division of the Scots by an incessant discharge of arrows . . .'.[66] The same annal reports a similar situation at Berwick the following year.[67] Of course, there were many other weapons, including lances, swords and daggers that were equally capable of blinding a soldier. Surgeons like Guy de Chauliac understood that there was nothing that could be done when irritants or wounds caused the eye to stop functioning.[68] Ambroise Paré was also clear that when the eye had been put out or was badly damaged, there was '. . . no hope to restore the sight or functon of the eie . . .'.[69]

There are many recorded cases of soldiers who lost the use of one of their eyes yet not only survived but continued their military careers. The *Scalacronica* of Sir Thomas Gray points to the Siege of Berwick in 1318, stating, 'The constable, Roger de Horsley, lost there an eye by an arrow', yet he carried on in his capacity for more than two decades.[70] The *Chronicles of Froissart* mention Thomas Holland, an English knight who had lost one eye.[71] Others, like William Montagu and Jean de Chalon IV, endured similar injuries but were nonetheless able to continue their military service.[72]

While most medical practitioners suggested little or nothing in terms of a cosmetic fix for the loss of an eye, Ambroise Paré offered a couple of solutions.[73] He recommended an artificial replacement be made from polished gold or silver, overlaid with enamel to mimic the shape and colour of the eye. It could be placed into the empty socket where the eye had once been. Paré understood that some may not be able to tolerate such a prosthesis, so he suggested encasing the artificial eye with a piece of iron wire wrapped in silk, which was then worn like one half of a pair of modern glasses secured around the ear.[74]

Limb Loss and Prostheses

> Don Guilan lopt off his right arm.
>
> *Amadís of Gaul*[75]

Just as it had been throughout the earlier centuries of the Middle Ages, the risk of losing fingers, a hand, or a leg in battle continued to be considerable, something that is regularly reflected in the literature of the time. The late medieval poem *The Story of Grey-Steel* offers the illustration of Sir Eger, who lost a digit to the knight Grey-Steel, 'I glanced at my right hand and perceived that the little finger was gone'.[76] The author of *Le Morte d'Arthur* added several battle scenes in which warriors lost limbs, including this passage from early in the story:

> . . . then Brastias smote one of them on the helm that it went to the teeth, and he rode to another and smote him that the arm flew into the field. Then he went to the third, and smote him on the shoulder that shoulder and arm flew in the field.[77]

Equally, severely damaged or badly infected limbs and appendages could lead to complications that, in some cases, made amputation necessary for a soldier's survival. Miguel de Cervantes, who wrote *The Adventures of Don Quixote de la Mancha*, was maimed at the Battle of Lepanto in 1571 while fighting on the side of the allied Christian forces against the Ottoman Empire. He suffered a serious injury to his left hand, likely inflicted by either a sword or a gunshot wound.[78] The injury was severe enough that de Cervantes required surgery to amputate the appendage, a procedure that was undertaken at a hospital in Messina. Unfortunately, the operation was done so poorly that he ended up losing the complete use of his left arm. Despite his severe injury, de Cervantes continued serving as a soldier for a few more years.[79]

As has so often been shown, the arrival of gunpowder weapons increased the harm that could be done to soldiers and their limbs.[80] In the preamble to his writings on *Wounds made by Gunshot and Other Fiery Engines*, Paré expressed his grave concerns about gunpowder weapons, saying '. . . that these engines were made for no other purpose, nor with other intent, but only to be imployed for the speedy and cruell slaughter of men . . .'.[81] He includes several examples within his texts that show just how common the loss of a limb or appendage could be during the wars of the mid-sixteenth century.[82] In one instance, he described being sent from Paris to Dourlan by the king of France to assist with the treatment of wounded soldiers, many of whom '. . . escaped quite with the loss of a leg, or an arm, or the loss of an eie, and they said they escaped good cheap . . .'.[83]

There were many potential dangers when a soldier lost a limb, be it on the battlefield or during surgical amputation. They could go into shock or very quickly lose a large percentage of their blood volume and expire before any treatment could be administered or completed. The sixteenth-century Portuguese epic *Palmerin of England* details what happened when the character Florian of the Desert cut off the arm of an assailant:

> Florian alighted, and taking off the helmet from him whose arm he had cut off, found that between loss of blood and terror, he had yielded up the ghost . . .[84]

Of the twelfth- and thirteenth-century surgeons examined in the previous volume, only Theodoric provided instructions on the amputation of limbs. He recommended cauterizing the stump to stop the flow of blood after the surgery had been performed.[85] Unfortunately, it is not a terribly effective method, and tends to inflict more pain and discomfort on the hapless patient.[86] Ligation, a technique employed by ancient surgeons, is a much better and less painful method.[87] It involves the use of a needle with thread or wire to close the blood vessels at the stump rather than applying heat. Although ligation is considered a more effective method, its use in amputations became largely obsolete among European surgeons during the Middle Ages. It is worth noting that a limited number of doctors, including Henri de Mondeville, did employ ligation for amputations, but like Theodoric, the majority seem to have opted for cauterization.[88] Guy de Chauliac recommended the use of a red-hot cautery instrument or boiling oil to halt blood flow during these operations, and Paré initially utilized red-hot irons for the same purpose.[89]

Although Paré used cauterization, his writings clearly express a deep dissatisfaction with the practice. He had witnessed the tragic mishaps and the terrible pain it could cause to patients, along with other side effects, including convulsions and fever. In his search for a better option, he decided to apply Galen's wound ligation method on his patients who had lost limbs. While it is clear that Paré was not the first to employ the technique in this way, he was the one who reintroduced it and promoted it widely.[90] By doing so, especially at a time when the number of battlefield casualties was on the increase, he managed to save the lives of many.[91]

Paré's vast experience enabled him to gain a valuable understanding of the needs of soldiers who had undergone amputations. For instance, he observed that those individuals who were left with long stumps below the knee often faced challenges with their mobility. The unnecessary length and weight of the lower limb were awkward and caused them to tire more quickly. He cites the example of an officer named Captain Francis Clerk, who had lost his foot to an iron bullet, but when he was first treated, his lower leg was left intact above the ankle.[92] Paré ended up performing an operation to remove most of it, leaving just '. . . five fingers breadth below his knee . . .'.[93] The successful procedure enabled Captain Clerk to move around in a much more comfortable manner.

The French surgeon also established the existence of phantom limb pain, which occurs when an amputee still experiences sensation in a missing limb.[94] While he did not completely understand the phenomenon, he wrote the following nearly 500 years ago:

> A most clear and manifest argument of this false and deceitfull sense appears after the amputation of the member; for a long while after they will complain of the part which is cut away. Verily it is a thing wondrous strange and prodigious, and which will scarse be credited, unlesse by such as have seen with their eyes, and heard with their ears the Patients who have many months after the cutting away of the Leg, grievously complained that they yet felt exceeding great pain of that leg so cut off.[95]

In terms of prostheses for the common soldier who had lost a limb, primarily a leg, the evidence points to the continued use of wooden supports and crutches.[96] In Paré's text, there is an example of one such device being given to a soldier after he had his lower leg amputated:

> The Camp beeing broken up I returned to Paris with my Gentleman whose leg I had cut off, I drest him and God cured him; I sent him to his hous merrie with his wooden leg, and was content, . . .[97]

Individuals who were of higher social standing often benefited from more sophisticated metal devices. The innovative designs for articulated hands, arms and legs, many of which were created and developed by Paré, resulted in a variety of advanced replacements.[98] A couple of protheses that predate Paré's work are worth examining, if only briefly. The first belonged to a young knight called Götz von Berlichingen, who lost his right hand to a small cannonball at the Siege of Landshut in 1504. He had a heavy metal replacement made that could be attached to his armour with leather straps. It had fingers that could be manually flexed into several positions, enabling him to hold his weapons and the reins of his horse during battle. The device allowed him to continue his military career for a further four decades.[99] Another prosthesis belonged to a Turkish pirate named Horuk Barbarossa, who lost his right hand in battle around 1517. He too had a metal replacement fitted, which allowed him to continue fighting.[100]

Damaged Lives

. . . hath been maimed and bruised in the wars . . .
A Caveat or Warning for Common Cursitors[101]

In 1958, a large group of disarticulated bones was discovered in a communal grave at Aljubarrota, in Central Portugal, where the battle of the same name was fought in August 1385, between the Kingdom of Portugal, supported by the English, and the Crown of Castile, allied with French forces. When the soldiers' bones were reanalysed in the late 1990s, they revealed signs of previous healed injuries, some of which would have been life-changing. One individual who was at the battle was missing most of his right arm, while another had only a portion of his left leg remaining.[102] While bones such as these provide more evidence that individuals in this period could survive serious physical trauma, they are also proof that at least a few of them answered the call in times of war, despite the nature of their injuries.[103] Of course, not everyone who formed part of an army or navy was necessarily a warrior. There were important support roles, such as food preparation and transportation, that could accommodate a disabled former soldier without them having to be directly involved in battle.[104]

This is not to say that everyone was accepted into the armies and navies of these centuries. In Honoré Bonet's seminal late fourteenth-century treatise on war and its rules, *L'arbre des batailles*, or *The Tree of Battles*, there is a section entitled *What Persons Cannot and Must Not Be Compelled to Go to War* that lists those who should not be forced to fight in times of conflict. It includes the deaf, blind and sick, along with women, the young and the elderly. Interestingly, Bonet does note that if a man is unable to speak but is strong and valiant, he could still become a soldier, provided he had his lord's approval.[105] Christine de Pizan's *The Book of Deeds of Arms and of Chivalry* offers quite a scathing critique of any blind man who aspires to take up arms.[106] In England, during the years 1415 and 1416, as King Henry V prepared his forces for war against France, he took the opportunity to have his potential soldiers vetted, which led to several being '. . . rejected on account of age or weak health . . .'.[107]

Generally, life could be extremely challenging for soldiers who returned home from war with crippling injuries. Many found it difficult to reclaim their previous roles in society and only a fraction of them were entitled to receive any form of pension.[108] In England, such allowances tended to be reserved for individuals who had previously been in the employ of the crown in some capacity.[109] Richard Leveson of Wolverhampton serves as an example of a soldier who benefitted in this way. Formerly an esquire to King Henry IV of England, he was wounded and left disabled at the Battle of Shrewsbury. He received compensation from the crown in the amount of ten pounds annually.[110] John Kent, a yeoman of the royal kitchen, is another who had served Henry IV. He too was maimed at the same battle and received a pension for the balance of his life.[111]

Equally, the English crown might choose to support a disabled servant-turned-soldier by placing them in the care of a religious establishment, such as St John's Hospital, Brakle (also Brackele or Brakkeley). On 23 April 1316, Edward II of England petitioned the brothers of St John's to look after Nicholas Russel, who had served the king for many years before being badly injured while fighting in Scotland.[112] St John's continued to be used in this capacity under the reign of Edward III as well. In October 1327, the king requested they care for Laurence le Charetter '. . . in consideration of his good services to the king and because he was maimed in the king's service . . .'.[113]

On the continent, in places like Venice, a more formalized system of compensation for soldiers who sustained debilitating injuries began to gain popularity. This was especially true of mercenaries, whose contracts commonly stipulated such benefits.[114] Ferrando da Spagna, a Venetian corporal who lost his right arm to a type of cannon called a bombard in 1446, was offered a lifetime pension of six *lire* every month.[115] A century later, a Spanish mercenary named Gonsalo de Villa Panda fought on the side of Henry VIII against the Scottish when his legs were badly wounded. He was left crippled by his injuries, and in 1546, he was awarded the sum of four pounds.[116]

Institutions that catered specifically for disabled warriors were few in number, and those that did exist often had limited capacity or could only care for individuals over short periods of time.[117] One such establishment was St George's in Windsor. After funds were made available in 1348, it had the capacity to provide care for twenty-four poor or infirm knights.[118] Sick and elderly Teutonic knights were looked after by other members of the order. Those who had been in the Holy Land were typically sent back to Europe to spend their remaining days in homes that had been specially set up to care for them.[119] By the mid-sixteenth century, the institution built at Winchester and dedicated to St John in 1275 was still caring for sick and disabled soldiers.[120]

With no pension or other means of support, numerous disabled ex-soldiers were forced to beg or turn to some other means of fending for themselves, often with dire consequences.[121] A criminal court case from France in August 1390 provides a noteworthy example. It involves a defendant called Jehannin Machin, who bore the nickname 'Court-Bras' or 'Short-Arm'.[122] He had been a baker in Paris before joining a French campaign against Duke William of Gelderland in 1388. It was there that Machin sustained the wound to his arm that earned him the alias. His injury was severe enough that when he returned home, he could no longer make bread and pastries, so he took a job as a porter at the gates of Paris.[123] When he found that this did not pay enough, Machin began supplementing his income. At first, he tried begging, but eventually he turned to crime, which is how he became known to the authorities and ended up facing a judge at the end of the fourteenth century.[124]

A letter from 1422, sent by a rank-and-file soldier called Thomas Hostell to the council of Henry VI of England, paints a dismal picture of life for a former soldier who had been left incapacitated by war and who had no place to turn for help. He was a veteran of the armies of Henry VI's son and grandson and had been present at sieges and battles like Harfleur and Agincourt.[125] Hostell's injuries included a broken cheekbone and the loss of an eye, both caused by a crossbow bolt.[126] By the time he wrote his letter, Thomas was a destitute old man with no way of supporting himself other than through 'men's gracious almasse', as he phrased it in his missive.[127] In the absence of a welfare state, Thomas saw no other option but to throw himself on the mercy of the crown and ask for assistance.[128]

The author Robert Copland was a man who knew early sixteenth-century London well, having walked its streets as a watchman.[129] His poem, called *The Hye Way to the Spyttell Hous*, or *The Highway to the Spital-House*, which was written between 1535 and 1536, indicates that things had changed very little for the disabled soldier by this time. The text is set up as a conversation between the author and the porter of a London hospital or almshouse.[130] In one verse, the porter describes the kinds of people likely to arrive seeking help, including mutilated soldiers living on the margins of society:

> And honest folk fallen in great poverty
> By mischance or other infirmity,
> Wayfaring men and maimed soldiers
> Have their relief in this poor house of ours.[131]

Later in the poem, Copland explains the grim existence for those disabled ex-soldiers who were not lucky enough to be looked after by others who cared. They were left to move about from one place to another, trying pick up what scraps they could:

> Ragged and lousy, with bag, dish and staff,
> And ever haunteth among such riff-raff,
> One time to this spital, another to that.
> Prowling and poaching to get somewhat
> At every door, lumps of bread or meat . . .
> And in such misery they live day by day
> That of very need they must come this way.[132]

The life of an infirm and destitute former soldier living 500 or 600 years ago was undoubtedly far worse than can be imagined. Yet, as highlighted in the previous volume, it remains strangely difficult to feel much emotion for those who endured such pitiful lives so long ago because of what they experienced during times of war. The passage of time seems to remove the sympathy we might otherwise feel for a modern soldier or a relative who fought in the wars of the last century. The chapter surrounding the subject of disability in the first book ended with an excerpt from the poem *Disabled* by one of the First World War's best-known poets, Wilfred Owen. Its themes helped to connect the lives of those who had been wounded in battle nine or ten centuries ago with soldiers who ended up in the same position because of the First World War. Another verse, this one by Ivor Gurney, a soldier and poet from the Gloucester Regiment who was gassed at Passchendaele in 1917, may serve a similar purpose by highlighting the parallels between the lives of more modern soldiers left disabled by war and those of the warriors discussed in this chapter. Entitled *Strange Hells*, the poem mirrors several of the ideas explored by Copland in his *Highway to the Spital-House*:

> Where are they now on State-doles, or showing shop-patterns
> Or walking town to town sore in borrowed tatterns
> Or begged. Some civic routine one never learns.
> The heart burns – but has to keep out of face how heart burns.[133]

Chapter 7

TWO PLAGUES

O Iesu! Iesu! our helthe, our medycyne,
Our hevenly leche, our socour in syknesse,

The Fifteen Oes of Christ[1]

The first few decades of the fourteenth century were not kind to Europeans. Appalling weather, famine, disease and financial instability put tremendous pressure on rulers and their people.[2] The many wars being fought across the continent only served to increase the demands on already stretched human and financial resources. Indeed, by the middle of the fourteenth century, conflicts seemed to be everywhere.[3] Among them, the Hundred Years War had just begun what would become more than a century of violence and destruction across much of Western Europe. In the north of the continent, the Swedish-Novgorodian Wars continued to be fought and same was true of the Teutonic Order's crusade against Lithuania. Elsewhere, the central European ruler Louis I, King of Hungary and Croatia (1326–82), attacked Naples.[4]

This catalogue of misery and war made Europeans all the more unprepared for what was to come next – one of the worst catastrophes in human history, the Black Death.[5] This disease, the bubonic plague, is caused by the bacterium *Yersinia pestis*, or more simply *Y. pestis*, the same one that resulted in further outbreaks of the illness in the decades and centuries that followed the mid-fourteenth century.[6] The plague was transmitted to human hosts by infected fleas, ticks and lice that thrived on rats and other animal carriers of the disease, a fact not understood at the time nor for centuries to come.[7] During the late thirteenth and early fourteenth centuries, the plague spread from Asia to Africa and Europe, reaching the latter by way of the Mediterranean in 1347. It appears to have arrived in Cyprus during the late summer of that year and then Sicily in early October.[8] The friar and chronicler Michele da Piazza describes the twelve pestilence-laden Genoese trading vessels that limped into the Sicilian port of Messina:

> They brought with them a plague that they carried down to the very marrow of their bones, so that if anyone so much as spoke to them, he was infected with a mortal sickness which brought on an immediate death that he could in no way avoid.[9]

Their deadly cargo spread quickly, killing a large proportion of the city's population. The frightened citizens who were left soon drove the sailors back to their ships and away from the island, which only caused the disease to be spread further afield.[10] Throughout the rest of 1347 and the beginning of 1348, ships continued to arrive from the Black Sea and elsewhere, carrying the disease to unsuspecting ports all along the coasts of Italy and southern France.[11] By then there was no turning back; the Black Death had taken hold among Europe's population, spreading rapidly in every direction.[12]

The *Chronicle of Jean de Venette* describes the nature of the plague, including the swellings or *buboes* that give the disease its name:

> He who was well one day was dead the next and being carried to his grave. Swellings appeared suddenly in the armpit or in the groin—in many cases both—and they were infallible signs of death.[13]

Plague sufferers experienced other symptoms as well, including vomiting, fever, confusion and impaired mobility.[14] As cases proliferated, new types of the disease emerged, giving it even greater impetus. These variants are still classified as *Y. pestis*, but they differ in infection patterns, symptom onset, and rapidity of death.[15] One of these, known as pneumonic plague, is generally transferred by inhaling aerosolized fluids emitted from the lungs of an infected carrier by way of a cough or sneeze. It was first recognized by Guy de Chauliac, who was able to describe its symptoms and differentiate it from the bubonic variety of the plague.[16]

By 1351, the disease had found its way into nearly every corner of the continent before finally abating, at least for a time.[17] The devastation it caused was staggering. It is difficult to gain a firm grasp on the death toll attributed to the plague in Europe between 1347 and 1351, but it appears to have been much larger than once thought. When Ziegler wrote his seminal text on the Black Death in the late 1960s, it was believed that between 30 and 35 per cent of Europe's population had lost their lives to the pestilence.[18] Since then, advances in science and research suggest that the plague must have been far more deadly than that, perhaps having been responsible for killing between 40 and 60 per cent of Europe's inhabitants.[19]

Death on Every Side

> Because the battles and wars
> Were so great in all the lands
>
> *The Judgement of the King of Navarre*[20]

Plague sufferers frequently died alone without the comfort of a physician, priest or family members.[21] At times, the massive loss of life meant that there were barely enough of the living to bury the dead.[22] Defensive fortifications surrounding towns and cities were left to crumble, crops went unplanted and there was barely enough manpower to gather fish from the sea.[23] Despite apocalyptic scenes like these being played out across Europe during the years of the Black Death, wars continued to be fought between countries and states, costing many more lives and assets. In his poem called *Le Jugement dou Roy de Navarre*, or *The Judgement of the King of Navarre*, the French poet and composer Guillaume de Machaut (c.1300–77) wrote of this time:

> The earth and sky have been
> Showing the signs of war,
> Of pain and pestilence.[24]

Sometimes, the plague only slowed the pace of conflict, as it managed to do for a short time in the war that was fought between Lithuania and the Teutonic Order.[25] During the Swedish-Novgorodian Wars, when the pestilence reached Sweden in 1349, it delayed King Magnus Eriksson (1316–74) from exacting retribution against the Novgorodians, who had wrested back control of the important island fortress of Orekhov, now Shlisselburg, in north-western Russia. However, by the summer of 1350, the king was able to gather enough men together to form another army and renew hostilities.[26] In 1347, during the Hundred Years War, the Truce of Calais was signed between the sides and was renewed more than once during the period of the Black Death.[27] Nevertheless, there were times when the fighting carried on, both on land and at sea, even with the truce in place and the plague raging.[28]

Elsewhere, the disease would have a more devastating impact on armies involved in battles and sieges. In England, the pestilence wreaked havoc from the time it arrived in 1348 until it began to dissipate 18 months later.[29] An entry in the *Chronicle of Henry Knighton* describes the moment when news of the plague's devastation in England reached Scotland in 1349. The Scottish, believing firmly that God was on their side, saw the destruction in England as an opportunity to overpower their weakened enemy and so gathered an army in the forest around Selkirk in the Scottish borders in anticipation.[30] However, before they could press home their perceived advantage, the plague struck the Scottish camp, killing many of the soldiers.[31] The survivors, some of whom were very unwell, were soon overrun and killed by the English as they tried to retreat.[32]

In August 1349, at the height of the Black Death, Alfonso XI, King of Castile (1311–50), began besieging Gibraltar in an attempt to reclaim it from Muslim control. The area was well fortified, and Alfonso's army struggled to make much headway. As the year came to an end, plague began to decimate the Castilian camp. The *Corónica del Muy Alto et Muy Católico Rey Don Alfonso el Onceno*, or *Chronicle of the Very High and Catholic King Don Alfonso the Eleventh*, explains that King Alfonso was advised by his lords and knights 'to leave the siege, as many companies of his soldiers were dying from the pestilence and that he was also in grave danger from the disease'.[33] The king refused to listen, citing the men and money that had already been lost in the venture. Alfonso's men continued the siege until 26 March 1350, when the king himself was killed by the plague, leaving the Castilians with no choice but to halt their attempt to capture Gibraltar.[34]

The outbreak of bubonic plague that occurred between 1347 and 1351 was not the last time the disease wreaked havoc in Europe, not even close. Over the next few centuries, it would return repeatedly, with its first resurgence occurring just a decade later in 1361.[35] These subsequent outbreaks are typically referred to as the plague or the pestilence, rather than the Black Death, and while none of these reoccurrences reached the death toll of the catastrophic eruption of the disease in the mid-1300s, they still managed to cause large losses of life each time.[36] To make matters worse, reappearances regularly intersected many of Europe's sieges and battles. The Portuguese chronicler Fernão Lopes explains in his *Cronica de El-Rei D. João I*, or *The Chronicle of King John I*, the situation among Castilian soldiers when the plague broke out in their camp as they besieged Lisbon in September 1384:

> . . . começou de se atear a peste tão bravamente em elles, assim por mar, como por terra, que dia havia que morriam cento e cincoenta e duzentas, assim mais e menos, como se acertava, de guisa que o mais do dia eram os do arraial occupados em enterrar seus mortos.[37]

> . . . the plague began to spread so fiercely among them, both by sea and by land, that between 150 and 200 died each day so that soldiers spent most of their time in camp burying the dead.

Verona, then part of the Venetian Republic, suffered an outbreak of plague between 1438 and 1439, while war with the Duchy of Milan raged all around. City officials were eventually forced to admit pitifully, '. . . we are battered and dispersed by a combination of war, plague and famine'.[38] At the Siege of Perpignan in 1542, Ambroise Paré was a surgeon with the French army when the pestilence struck many of their soldiers. The ferocity of the disease was partly to blame for the withdrawal of French troops from the action against the Spanish, who held the reinforced town.[39]

An Unbearable Burden

> . . . so impoverished by the said pestilence and other adversities in these times of war . . .
>
> *Calendar of the Close Rolls, England 1350*[40]

As seen above, the combined horrors of war and plague regularly brought with them a third disaster, famine. These times must have seemed positively biblical to those experiencing them, both soldiers and civilians alike.[41] It was as if the world was nearing its end. Writers, especially those on the continent, expressed the hopelessness of the situation.[42] In 1464, the anonymous Castilian poet who wrote the poem *Las coplas de Mingo Revulgo*, or *The Barbs of Mingo Revulgo*, likened the devastation of war, plague and famine to 'mad wolves' who prowled the land in pursuit of their victims:

> I dreamt this very night
> And tremble at the thought
> That this time neither beards
> Nor beardless would be spared.
> So go to bed and sleep!
> For, as far as I can see,
> About the way things are,
> I guess the three mad wolves
> Will hunt throughout the land.[43]

The unimaginable loss of life and the economic destruction brought on by this lethal combination often placed an unbearable burden on those who were left to try and pick up the pieces.[44] Entire communities suffered greatly, and many settlements were ultimately left abandoned due to the widespread devastation.[45] The resultant population decline made it increasingly difficult for those in power to raise sufficient manpower and taxes for the needs of the nation, state or republic.[46]

Throughout England, cities, towns and counties found themselves overwhelmed by the three mad wolves.[47] Great Yarmouth, a port town on England's east coast, offers an example. It had been one of the country's best sources of tax revenue prior to the Hundred Years War. However, the conflict with France and the arrival of the plague in 1349 nearly caused its downfall. Deaths from the pestilence, plus the constant requirement to supply the English war fleet with ships and sailors, put a considerable strain on its thriving fishing industry and population as a whole. Suddenly, there were fewer and fewer men left to catch herring, the valuable commodity that made the town the success it was.[48] Any that were caught became increasingly difficult to sell due to rampant inflation and a smaller market for the fish. The situation worsened as significant increases in taxes, along with the cost of defending the town against marauders, added to the misery endured by the remaining inhabitants. The lack of available funds and the town's general decline at that time are evidenced by the stoppage of major building works on the local Minster Church of St Nicholas.[49] Subsequent outbreaks of the plague, along with other factors, meant that it would take nearly a century and a half for Great Yarmouth to begin its recovery from the devastation inflicted during those years.[50]

The situation in France was among the worst anywhere in Europe.[51] In addition to the Black Death, most of the early battles of the Hundred Years War had been fought on its shores and ended in defeat for the French.[52] Extensive damage and destruction were inflicted on vast areas of the country by marauding soldiers and the disaffected, resulting in the deaths or displacement of countless French civilians.[53] The circumstances in the property market in Caen are indicative of the profound losses experienced by the nation, the effects of which were felt for many years. A reduced population and more available buildings and land led to a decrease in demand. Between 1352 and 1360, about a third of lessors still struggled to rent their properties for even half the value they did before these events had occurred.[54] Numerous others were simply left vacant or in ruins, as described in many rental contracts of the time:

> As because of the English our enemies and because of the mortality that God recently sent on his people, the households of the city of Caen and the other heritages are depleted of revenue and several remain wasted and empty places, and several have become worthless . . .[55]

During the fifteenth and sixteenth centuries, these cycles of warfare and plague continued to significantly impact civilian populations. One such conflict, the War of the Pazzi (1478–80), saw Pope Sixtus IV and Naples fighting against the Medici family and Florence. The city of Arezzo, not far from Florence, was engulfed in the violence when a severe outbreak of the plague struck the area.[56] A letter dated 17 January 1479, from Abbott Jerome Aliotti in Arezzo to a law student called Antonio de Geriis, away at university in Bologna, indicates the gravity of the situation:

> As regards our city's calamity, it is incredible to state how many citizens, especially heads of families, have died of this

> pestilence . . . Besides, we are anxiously expecting a siege of the town, so that, implicated in so many and so harsh evils, I deem blest you and our other countrymen who are absent at this calamitous time.[57]

Cannons, Goats and Prayers

> By the grace of God there schall be no perell of no dethe.
>
> From the plague cure of Edward IV of England[58]

Amongst all this carnage, war was hard enough to escape, but the plague was even more difficult to avoid. Most Christian Europeans believed that the disease was 'voluntat Dios', or 'God's will', as the *Corónica del Muy Alto et Muy Católico Rey Don Alfonso el Onceno* puts it, sent as a punishment for the sins of the people.[59] There were some who tried to appease God with their acts of penance and therefore escape his retribution. Among them were the Flagellants, groups of men and women who travelled from town to town, whipping themselves into a violent self-righteous frenzy in an attempt to avert God's wrath.[60] In Sweden, as the Black Death approached, King Magnus Eriksson's penitential measures were far less severe than those of the Flagellants yet still reflected a sense of self-righteousness. His desire to save his country from the plague was driven in large part by his ambition to continue his military campaign against Novgorod. The king addressed his people:

> God for the sins of man has struck the world with this great punishment of sudden death. By it most of the people in the land to the west of our country are dead. It is now ravaging in Norway . . . and is approaching our kingdom of Sweden.[61]

Trying to prevent such a death sentence, Magnus asked the people of Sweden to pray earnestly to the Virgin Mary that the plague might not strike their nation.[62] As penance for their sins, he also ordered them to eat just bread and water on Fridays, or 'at most to take only bread and ale'.[63] They were also to walk barefoot to their churches and parade around the cemeteries holding holy relics.[64] When the Black Death inevitably arrived in Sweden, the death toll was large and included the king's brothers Knut and Hacon. Magnus took the arrival of the plague to mean that God was outraged at him for pausing the campaign against the Novgorodians.[65]

Having no real idea what caused the disease, let alone how to cure it effectively, the medical community was only marginally more successful in preventing and treating the plague than those who thought to placate God with whips and bare feet.[66] Looking after the infected only increased practitioners' exposure to the plague and killed large numbers of them. At the time, the astrologer Simon de Covino said about Montpellier, the great seat of medical learning in the Middle Ages, '. . . there are a greater number of physicians than in any other place, barely one of them survived the plague'.[67] Naturally frightened by these terrible events, many doctors fled the sick or hid themselves away in their own homes.[68] Remarkably, however, most of the surgeons and physicians under review in this volume do not appear to have shied away from the illness. Both de Chauliac and Paré ended up contracting the disease, yet both managed to survive. Despite there being no proper treatments for the plague, it did not stop men like these, along with other physicians, surgeons, quacks and even kings, from trying to find one.[69]

The English surgeon John Arderne returned from France around 1348 and settled in Newark, where he seems to have escaped the Black Death unscathed.[70] Among his treatises is a salve for the buboes that were associated with the plague. It required three ounces of old hog's lard, which was mingled with a caustic substance called vitriol.[71] The ingredients were placed over a fire, and when they had been removed from the heat, more lard was added. Once the resulting ointment had cooled, it could be smeared onto a patient's buboes.[72]

Guy de Chauliac describes the outbreak of the Black Death in some detail, noting of his own experience:

> I did not want to be accused of shirking my responsibilities, so, I never left. I lived in fear of the disease and did what I could to preserve myself . . . Even so, toward the end of the plague, I became one of its victims. I suffered with fever and had an abscess on my groin. I was ill for six weeks and my colleagues feared for my life. I treated my pus filled buboe . . . and I survived, as God willed it.[73]

He believed the plague could be prevented by what has come to be known in modern times as social distancing. Those who were able to escape the disease stood the greatest chance of evading its grasp. For most individuals, however, this would have been easier said than done. In this case, he recommended various other preventative measures including regular bloodletting, the use of theriac and the continual maintenance of a fire to purify the air.[74] When the pestilence did strike, bloodletting, laxatives and medicines sweetened with honey were advised. Buboes could be treated with an ointment made from boiled onions, ground figs, butter and yeast. If they became infected, as de Chauliac's did, they were to be cupped or cauterized.[75]

A century on from de Chauliac, von Pfolspeundt also included several suggestions in his surgery, for both the prevention and treatment of the pestilence.[76] Quite a useful piece of advice in von Pfolspeundt's text was to avoid the damp breath of a person sick with the plague.[77] A supposed prophylactic could be made by mixing thyme, juniper, rue, laurel, white nut, betony, angelica and gentian. No measures are given for the ingredients in the barber-surgeon's text, but they were to be combined with honey and consumed in the morning and evening.[78] Included among his treatments for plague sufferers is a rather unusual cure. Garlic was to be boiled and then mixed with white clay before being formed into little cakes. The plague victim was then to stand as close to the hot oven as possible while the cakes were baked at a high temperature.[79]

Having suffered symptoms such as a buboe on his stomach and an infected abscess under his right armpit, Ambroise Paré also survived the plague.[80] He would go on to compose a detailed, 42-chapter book on the subject in 1568.[81] First and foremost, just as de Chauliac had done, Paré endorsed distancing oneself from the plague whenever there were outbreaks. If this could not be done, he had a long list of suggestions to help strengthen the body against the disease. It included taking clean air and moderate exercise prior to meals. In order to maintain a balance of the humours, he recommended regular bloodletting and the use of laxatives to ensure proper bowel evacuation. Paré cautioned against gluttony, excessive drinking and the consumption of sweets, as he believed these habits could undermine one's health. One of the most intriguing ideas in his treatise was to keep a live goat in the house. Its pungent odour was believed to stop any plague-filled air from entering the home.[82]

Paré's catalogue of cures and remedies for patients who contracted the disease is even more comprehensive than his preventative measures. Fresh, clean air was important in ridding the plague from the body. Windows were to be left open to blow away any air polluted with the pestilence. The patient's bedchamber was to have a fire, predominantly at night, to help purify the air.[83] Wine and spicy foods were to be avoided, but bread, easily digested meats and water with honey or lemon syrup were advised to be eaten and drunk.[84] He deemed the best antidotes to be theriac and mithridate, both of which worked on the principle that the poison contained within them would counteract the disease. The patient was to consume them, as well as apply them externally.[85]

The Dutch physician Levinus Lemnius suggested what is arguably the most warlike idea to eradicate plague from a town or city. Recorded in Paré's text, soldiers pointed cannons loaded only with gunpowder towards the plague-infested place. It was believed that by firing them in both the morning and evening, the contaminated air would be forced out of the area. Additionally, it was claimed that the burnt gunpowder from each firing helped to purify and revitalise the air.[86]

Syphilis

> Then, this terrible disease known since then among us by the name of Syphilis does not take long to spread in our entire nation . . .
>
> *Hieronymus Fracastorius*[87]

Sexually transmitted infections (STIs) such as gonorrhoea persisted in much of Europe during this period.[88] In England, it was known by names like the *running sore* and the *brennynge* (burning), while in France, *chaudpisse* (hot piss) and *clap* were just two of the names used to identify this venereal disease.[89] Examples of the STI in a military context are not terribly common, but not completely unknown. In the fourteenth century, the army surgeon John Arderne recorded a treatment for the disease, one that was intended to be injected into the sufferer's urethra.[90] An entry in the *Brut Chronicle* offers a stronger martial link to gonorrhoea in the fifteenth century. It details how during his invasion of France in 1475, many of Edward IV of England's soldiers contracted the disease:

> And in þat Iorney our Kyng lost many a man þat fylle to þe lust of women, & wer brent by them; & þere membrys rottyd away & þey dyed.[91]

> And in that journey, our King lost many men that fell to the lust of women, and were burnt by them; and their members rotted away and they died.

This practice of blaming women for the spread of STIs, as indicated in the example above, is sadly not unusual. Indeed, it is a tendency that has changed little over the centuries.[92]

If specific military examples of gonorrhoea from this time are difficult to come by, then syphilis presents something altogether different. In the mid-1490s, it surged to epidemic levels across Europe and beyond, remaining widespread for several decades, with soldiers playing a crucial role in the spread of the disease.[93]

The name *syphilis* likely comes from a poem called *Syphilis sive morbus Gallicus*, or *Syphilis or the French Disease*, by a Venetian named Hieronymus Fracastor (c.1478–1553). Written no later than 1530, this fictional work tells the story of a shepherd called Syphilis who upsets the god Apollo. The deity soon takes his revenge by afflicting people with a terrible disease, which ends up being named after the offending shepherd.[94] Decades before it was called syphilis, it had been known by many other aliases like *gor* (also *gore*), *grandgore*, and the *great pox*, a name that was meant to differentiate it from smallpox.[95] It had even more monikers that relied on one country's dislike for another, enabling blame for the illness to be placed on enemies and neighbours. In France, the infection was called the *Neapolitan disease* or the *Pox of Naples*, while those from Naples named it the *French disease*. In Portugal and Denmark, it was labelled the *Spanish disease*, but the Russians considered it the *Polish disease*.[96]

The origin of syphilis in Europe has been the subject of a long-running debate, with a few competing theories having been suggested. There is the belief that it was brought back to Europe from the Americas with Christopher Colombus and his men in the last decade of the fifteenth century, although this argument has lost a lot of the strength that once made it the leading hypothesis.[97] Others are of the opinion that it may have come to Europe by way of another continent or was perhaps already present, having been misidentified or confused with another disease like leprosy.[98] Whatever the case may be, a conclusive answer remains elusive.[99]

Syphilis is caused by a type of spiral-shaped spirochaete bacterium called *Treponema pallidum* that is transferred through the mucous membranes of the genitals, anus or mouth during sexual contact. Alternatively, it can also be spread to the foetus by an infected mother during pregnancy.[100] Having taken on a virulent form that the continent of Europe and places beyond were wholly unprepared for, this cruelly deceptive disease was far worse during the late fifteenth and early sixteenth centuries than it is today.[101] A lack of immunity among the population and no proper cure meant that the illness spread rapidly, with very aggressive symptoms.[102] The primary stage of the disease usually began two or three weeks after sexual contact. At this point, the victim developed ulcers around the mouth or groin, which disappeared after a month or two. The secondary stage then followed not long afterwards, making the individual feel very unwell.[103] Sufferers experienced headaches, pain, fever and a rather unpleasant rash, usually around the hands, feet and face. Perhaps worst of all, were the pustules containing a putrid-smelling discharge that developed on the skin of some individuals. One of the earliest descriptions of some of these symptoms is found in a poem by the Spanish court physician Francisco Lopez de Villalobos entitled *Tratado sobre las pestiferas bubas*, or *On the Contagious and Accursed Buboes*, published in 1498:

> On all the whole skin and the face we observe.
> And here a vast foulness of eruption is displayed.
> And with it pain of joint that is felt very bad
> And measureless siccidity in vein and nerve.[104]

The symptoms of the second stage of the disease would also begin to disappear on their own, potentially making the individual believe they had been cured. Usually, though not always, after lying dormant for weeks, months, or even years, the final (tertiary) stage of the illness would begin. It could cause terrible disfigurements, with the nose and palate being especially vulnerable to damage and loss.[105] Writing in the early part of the sixteenth century on the nasal ulcerations caused by syphilis, Giovanni de Vigo noted how they '. . . left behind very distressing deformations for the sick'.[106] The disease also left large tumour-like growths, called *gummas*, on the bodies of the infected. Many succumbed to the disease at this stage, while others went blind, suffered permanent damage to their bones and internal organs, or were institutionalized because of their deteriorating mental health.[107] *The Highway to the Spital-House*, Robert Copland's poem from the early sixteenth century, indicates that many '. . . sore men eaten with pox' ended up living on the streets of London with the poor, the abused and the former soldiers.[108]

There are signs that syphilis had begun its reign of terror in Europe before the mid-1490s. Von Pfolspeundt's surgery, written three and a half decades earlier, contains intriguing references to the disease among some of the soldiers he was treating.[109] In places such as Denmark, England and Ireland, there are also indications that disease existed prior to 1494–5. However, these later dates, along with the city of Naples, are frequently cited as the epicentre for the epidemic.[110] While coinciding with the unsuccessful attack on the city by the army of Charles VIII of France, it is widely acknowledged that a significant outbreak of this highly contagious strain of syphilis occurred here during this time, affecting soldiers, camp followers, sex workers and local citizens.[111] In early July 1495, as the French began pulling their defeated army back towards the Alps, they found themselves embroiled in a clash with Venetian forces and their allies near Parma. The Battle of Fornovo, as it is known, represents one of the earliest reports of syphilis. Indicative of the rapid spread of the disease, Marcello Cumano, a physician with the Venetian army, wrote that some of their soldiers had sores on their genitals and others had pustules on their faces and bodies. After several days, many of them were struggling with terrible pain in their limbs and even larger pustules on their bodies.[112] They were not the only ones; the truth was that large numbers of Charles VIII's retreating army were also infected. These were men who had come from all over Europe, France, Spain, England, and elsewhere.[113] Crucially, once they began disbanding and making their way back home in their thousands, they unwittingly took the 'contagious poison' with them.[114]

Spread Far and Wide

> 1495: This disease was brought to Germanic lands by mercenaries, who were later called Landesknect . . .
>
> *Nürnberger Chronik von 1580*[115]

Of course, soldiers were not the only ones responsible for the proliferation of the disease; sailors, merchants, camp followers, those in the sex trade and others also shared some of the blame.[116] With that said, the role that fighting men played in spreading and sustaining syphilis across Europe cannot be understated.[117] Unfortunately, as history has shown time and again, when there is conflict, a significant increase in STIs can usually be expected among warriors.[118] During the First World War, syphilis would never be far from soldiers' lives, as highlighted by the poets in their ranks. In his poem *'They'*, Siegfried Sassoon's soldier named Bert had 'gone syphilitic', while E. E. Cummings describes how 'the son of man goes forth to war with trumpets clap and syphilis'.[119]

In November 1495, Lyon would be among the first places in France to be impacted by the disease since the city lay in the path of Charles VIII and many of his infected soldiers as they returned from Naples.[120] Soon, Paris and other parts of France would also begin to feel the wrath of the illness.[121] An early example of the disease involving a specific French warrior was recorded by Cardinal Peter of Avignon in a miracle story from 1499.[122] The account describes a French knight, Reynprecht de la Flors, who had been bedridden with syphilis for approximately five years, suggesting that he may well have contracted the disease in Naples in or around 1494–5.[123] By this time, he was in severe pain, and his body was badly marked by the sores and gummas associated with the disease.[124] The account states that de la Flors had lived a life of sin, but in his suffering, he was visited by an old priest called Macharyus (formerly Stephen), who provided the knight with spiritual encouragement and guidance.[125] The knight took the priest's advice and turned to God before humbly confessing his sins. One evening, after finishing a particularly fervent prayer session, he saw a vision of Christ being whipped.[126] Mary, the mother of Jesus, was nearby, wringing her hands and weeping at the sight. Flors turned to her and asked if she could intercede with Christ on his behalf so that his sins might be forgiven. He then fell at the feet of Jesus as she pleaded for him.[127] Once the vision was over, he awoke to find himself kneeling beside his bed, crying for joy.[128] In disbelief, his servants discovered him, having been healed of most of the damage and pain caused by the disease that had afflicted his body. The account suggests that he was left with some spots and other remnants of syphilis, at least for a time.[129] Reynprecht de la Flors was apparently so moved by what had happened to him that he went on to become a monk.

There are signs that syphilis had spread even further than France in 1495, arriving with Germanic mercenaries known as Landsknechts (also Lansquenets) in places like Augsburg, Nuremberg and Nördlingen.[130] Over the next few years, infected soldiers and sailors would continue to spread syphilis as they travelled the terrestrial roads and nautical routes across Europe.[131] Reports show that the disease was soon spreading with ferocity across England and areas that now make up the Netherlands and Switzerland.[132] By the spring of 1497, the illness had emerged as a significant problem as far north as Scotland. This may have been due to some of the 500 returning Scottish mercenaries who had formed part of Charles VIII's army.[133] The disease reached towns and cities across the land, particularly those with large seaports like Aberdeen and Edinburgh.[134] On the continent, syphilis continued to push further north and east, reaching the North Sea by 1498 and Prague and Hungary in 1499.[135] As it continued its relentless march to just about every corner of Europe and many places far beyond, soldiers were feared as some of the most common carriers of the disease.[136]

Syphilis, Soldiers and Art

> Unless you're . . . decorated with the French pox besides, hardly anyone will believe you're a knight.
>
> Erasmus[137]

The notion that soldiers were among the primary culprits responsible for the spread of syphilis is reflected in the works of various European artists of the time.[138] Visual artists were some of the first to make this connection, with one of the earliest and most widely known images being a woodcut by the famous Nuremberg artist, Albrecht Dürer (1471–1528). Dating from 1496, it shows a syphilitic mercenary covered in the large gummas associated with the disease.[139] In addition to this, there are many other lesser-known works of art, including a painting from 1517 by the Swiss artist Niklaus Manuel Deutsch, called *Der Tod als Kriegsknecht umarmt ein Mädchen* or *Death as a soldier embraces a girl*. It depicts Death wearing a shabby soldier's uniform while groping the genitals of a young woman.[140] The tattered trouser leg on his left thigh seems to cover the venereal sores that afflict him in the last stage of the disease.[141] A woodcut from 1524 by another Swiss artist, Urs Graf, shows two Landsknechts passing a sex worker sitting by a tree with a figure of Death perched in the branches. Death looks slyly at the soldiers as he points to an hourglass he holds in his left hand.[142] It is just a matter of time before the disease spreads between the two familiar groups and takes its toll.

There are several European poems and works of literature from the late fifteenth and early sixteenth centuries that relate specifically to fighting men, the spread of syphilis, and the harm the disease caused. Returning to Hieronymus Fracastor's, *Syphilis sive morbus Gallicus*, it opens with the accusatory lines:

> I sing of that terrible disease, unknown to past centuries, which attacked all Europe in one day, and spread itself over a part of Africa and of Asia. I will tell what concourse of influences, what occult germs have caused it, how it arose in Latium at the time that the French armies rendered desolate that unhappy country, what reason caused it to be called the French disease.[143]

Among the works from France is an anonymous poem, almost certainly written before 1530, called *The Seven Merchants of Naples*.[144] The story recounts the misfortunes of seven men, all labelled 'merchants', who contract syphilis. In truth, they are not merchants; the term is used ironically, as each had pursued encounters with sex workers in Naples:[145]

> On me vendit ung dangereux caterer
> Lequel on dit la maladye de Naples[146]
>
> I was sold a dangerous sickness
> Which is called Naples disease

The men, who include a blind man, a monk, a student, and others, take turns explaining to the reader how they contracted syphilis. The first to tell his story is identified as an adventurer, but he is actually a soldier who had fought with the French army in Naples. While he was there, he says he bought a terrible disease that left him little more than a sad beggar and a horrible, deformed monster.[147]

The Rotterdam-born scholar Erasmus (c. 1469–1536) wrote several colloquies or conversations that contain references to syphilis and the warriors of Europe. Taking the colloquy entitled *The Soldier and Carthusian* as an example, it is structured as a dialogue between a warrior and a Carthusian monk who lead very different lives. Near the end of their discourse, the monk recognizes the ravages of syphilis on the soldier's face and body and begins to question him about the disease:

> **Monk**. And I see I can't tell what Sort of Rubies on your Chin.
>
> **Soldier**. Oh, they are nothing.
>
> **M.** I suspect that you have had the Pox.
>
> **S.** You guess very right, Brother. It was the third Time I had that Distemper, and it had like to have cost me my Life.
>
> **M.** But how came it, that you walk so stooping, as if you were ninety Years of Age; or like a Mower, or as if your Back was broke?
>
> **S.** The Disease has contracted my Nerves to that Degree.[148]

Reflecting European society in the late fifteenth and early sixteenth centuries, the arts recorded a disease that had caught the population completely off guard. Suddenly, sex had become much less safe; even lethal and fighting men were seen among the main carriers of the disease. While the images and words from this period served to entertain the public, they also educated, warning soldiers and civilians to refrain from a life of promiscuity.[149]

From Venus to Mercury

> . . . the important thing is for us to try to treat and cure this disease.
>
> Giovanni de Vigo[150]

Syphilitics were despised by those who were not afflicted with the disease. The public clearly feared contracting the STI, but also believed that sufferers got what they deserved, having displeased God with their wickedness.[151] Institutions began to close their doors to those with syphilis or segregate them from the rest of society. As early as 1496, hospitals, like the Hôtel

Dieu in Paris, refused to treat patients suffering from the illness. Other Paris hospitals banished syphilitics to former leper houses, stables, or anywhere else that was away from those not stricken with the disease.[152] In Aberdeen, the Town Council introduced some of the earliest measures that recognized sexual contact as the main method by which the 'infirmitey cumm out of Franche' was being spread so quickly.[153] On 21 April 1497, brothels were ordered to be closed. Sex workers were forced to cease practising their trade and look for other work or face serious punishment.[154] Under orders from King James IV of Scotland, the Edinburgh Town Council took a different approach in September 1497. All those infected with syphilis and anyone who claimed to be able to cure the disease were banished to the Island of Inchkeith in the Firth of Forth, not far from the city.[155] Across Europe, from London to Geneva, similar measures were taken, but despite well-meaning efforts, the spread of syphilis continued unabated.[156] It seemed that once the disease reached a populated area, it was nearly impossible to eradicate, making a cure of some sort a desperate necessity.[157]

It would not be long before mercury-based ointments became the remedy of choice being prescribed by those who practised medicine.[158] These thick salves were made by mixing mercury with lard and other ingredients, such as sulphur and various herbs. They were applied liberally over the entire bodies of patients, who were then made to sweat profusely by wearing extra clothing or sitting in front of a fire.[159] Also known as quicksilver, mercury had been used in the treatment of skin problems for many centuries. Avicenna recommended its use to cure lesions, acne and boils.[160] In his twelfth-century surgical text, Roger Frugard suggested using mercury to treat scabies, and Roland of Parma unsurprisingly followed suit in the next century.[161] Surgeons from the late medieval period were no different. Jehan Yperman recommended quicksilver in the treatment of ringworm, lice and scabies, as did Guy de Chauliac and others.[162]

Not all the medical community, however, was immediately on board with the use of mercury to treat syphilis. In his 1514 treatise on the subject, Giovanni de Vigo questioned why some practitioners were so hasty to apply quicksilver to issues like scabies yet refused to use it on patients with a disease as dangerous as syphilis.[163] Quacks, often called *pox-greasers*, who were looking to make as much money as quickly as possible, created almost the opposite problem when it came to the use of mercurial ointments.[164] By using mercury in considerably higher doses than those being applied by more responsible surgeons and barber-surgeons, these charlatans were able to obtain what seemed to be much quicker and more efficacious results for their patients, all the while poisoning them to death.[165] This forced some rational practitioners to reconsider the strength of their salves in order to compete with the pox-greasers.[166] Whether any of these ointments ever struck a balance between a safe level of mercury and a positive impact on the disease is up for debate.[167] What is hard to ignore, however, is that even low levels of mercury exposure can cause serious health problems, including organ damage, neurological impairment and harm to developing foetuses.[168]

The poetry of time paints a grim picture of the syphilis sufferer who underwent these mercurial treatments. In his poem *Syphilis sive morbus Gallicus*, Fracastor refers to these sessions as 'disgusting', while still believing them to be a better alternative to the disease.[169] Other, less well-known works describe the mental and physical harm to which the syphilis patient was subjected at the hands of both quacks and more established practitioners. An anonymous poem written before 1533, called *Ballade de la verolle*, or *Ballad of Syphilis*, repeats the notion that the syphilis sufferer wished they were dead instead of having to incur the wrath of the disease and its supposed cure:

> . . . these scourges of anointing and ointment have rubbed and greased me at each joint, and have made my mouth so hot—I am greased so much that I wish I was dead a hundred times a day . . . to be in some grave is what I desire; a hundred times a day I wish I were dead.[170]

Contrasting the barbarous nature of mercury treatments, the end of the second decade of the sixteenth century brought with it a different sort of remedy from the New World: a hard, heavy wood called *guaiacum*. Originating in the Caribbean and northern parts of the South American continent, guaiacum quickly became the in-vogue treatment.[171] The basic method of preparation involved grinding the wood into a fine powder and soaking it in water. The liquid was then drained, boiled, and the residue skimmed off. This scum was dried and made into a powder that could be applied to the sores associated with the disease. After being boiled once more, the water used in the initial process could be given to syphilis patients to drink.[172] Ambroise Paré wrote a chapter on guaiacum and its use against syphilis in his book on venereal disease.[173] He did not believe that it was effective enough on its own to cure the STI. He was of the opinion that stronger treatments, such as mercury, were required alongside it.[174] Other concoctions made from imported flora, such as sarsaparilla, cinchona, and *Smilax china* (commonly known as china root), were also believed to possess healing properties.[175] The knight Ulrich von Hutten (1488–1523), himself a syphilis sufferer, outlined a treatment made using quicklime, which he says he, '. . . learned of a Soldier in Italy'.[176] Although fairly harmless, guaiacum and these other natural remedies were eventually found to be of little value against the disease and consequently faded into obscurity.[177]

Throughout the early modern period and right up until the twentieth century, despite the obvious dangers, mercury remained the prevailing treatment for soldiers and civilians suffering from syphilis.[178] Over the many centuries, it was administered not just as an ointment, but in several other forms as well, including orally and by inhalation.[179] It was not until the Second World War that a breakthrough in treatment finally came in the form of penicillin, which was found to be much safer and more effective against both syphilis and gonorrhoea.[180]

The true death toll attributed to syphilis during the outbreak that began in the mid-1490s is difficult to determine, but it is likely to have been considerable, perhaps in the low millions.[181] While a significant number, it is dwarfed by the devastating loss of life caused by the bubonic plague during the period examined here, which probably numbered in the tens of millions.[182] Even so, the impact of these two diseases extends far beyond the initial figures, as they can be increased dramatically by the huge number of victims that succumbed to them in the ensuing decades and centuries.

Survivors of these diseases, particularly from so long ago, are sometimes the overlooked victims in all this. It seems only right to leave the final words of this chapter to the syphilitic former soldier at the end of the poem *Les sept marchans de Naples*, who is left with shameful and agonizing reminders of the terrible disease and no other choice but to beg for charity:

> With tears and more tears, I must leave my weapons and battles. So take heed yourselves, fellow soldiers, to avoid such illnesses . . . Instead of a pike I now carry a noose, and hold down the field out in front of a monastery, begging for alms from charitable people.[183]

Chapter 8

DAMAGED PSYCHES

> And all because melancholy
> Extinguishes every happy thought
> *The Judgement of the King of Navarre*[1]

While they are less common than texts containing physical injuries, there are those from the late Middle Ages and the first part of the sixteenth century that provide poignant reminders of the psychological scars left on both soldiers and civilians in the wake of conflict. Certainly, mental health was not acknowledged in the same manner it is today, yet individuals nonetheless endured suffering in ways that remain strikingly familiar. Terms such as *battle-grief* and *melancholy* were used to describe combatants and noncombatants in these centuries-old works, indicating mental health challenges that align with present-day terms like post-traumatic stress disorder (PTSD).[2]

PTSD has undoubtedly become a familiar acronym, but perhaps precisely for that reason, its true meaning has been somewhat diluted. It is a psychological condition that is typically triggered by witnessing or experiencing a traumatic or life-threatening event, such as combat or a serious accident. An excerpt from the *Chronicle of Geoffrey le Baker* vividly depicts the distressing conditions of the Battle of Poitiers in 1356, highlighting the very real potential for individuals to be affected by such threats and horrors:

> Then the standard-bearers fell, their banners falling with them; some of the French stepped on their own guts which had fallen out of their bellies, others spewed out their teeth, there were many who were fixed to the ground, while there were others who could be seen standing with their arms missing.[3]

During such an occurrence, the body's self-defence system goes on high alert, and large quantities of stress hormones are released, causing the so-called 'fight, flight or freeze' response. In some trauma sufferers, this state of hypervigilance takes considerably longer to shut down and return to normal. The body may repeatedly go into overdrive and release more stress hormones during this period in response to much less traumatic stimuli. This prolonged state of hypersensitivity can begin to significantly alter the way the brain works and can lead to intense, long-term or permanent mental health challenges, including insomnia, nightmares, fatigue, feelings of detachment, flashbacks, depression and the risk of suicide.[4] Consider the letter written by the London-based Hanseatic merchant Gerhard von Wesel to Cologne soon after the Battle of Barnet on Easter Day 1471. In his correspondence, he observed that some of the returning soldiers now 'preferred to stay indoors'.[5] While they represent just a few simple words, they are noteworthy because they signal the familiar sense of withdrawal from the world around them that so many warriors experience as a symptom of PTSD.[6]

Compellingly, there are echoes of the modern definition of PTSD in Geoffrey II de Charny's late fourteenth-century *Book of Chivalry*, as he portrays the psychological challenges faced by men-at-arms '. . . enduring fearful physical perils and the loss of friends whose deaths they have witnessed in many great battles in which they have taken part; these experiences have often filled their hearts with great distress and strong emotion'.[7] Although less detailed than those of Geoffroi II de Charny, even the writings of his father, Geoffroi de Charny, and the much earlier Roman author Vegetius acknowledge the 'fight or flight' response experienced by warriors in combat.[8]

In recent centuries, before PTSD entered the lexicon, various terms such as battle fatigue, shell shock and soldier's heart were used to denote the psychological struggles encountered by individuals who endured the trauma of war.[9] In the seventeenth century, this condition was referred to as nostalgia or the 'Swiss disease', as it was identified among Swiss mercenaries.[10] Soldiers described experiencing feelings of profound sorrow, physical weakness and exhaustion, along with challenges in maintaining focus and fulfilling their military responsibilities, all of which are common symptoms of PTSD.[11] The *Miracles of King Henry VI* features a soldier who displayed signs of similar psychological injury long before the term 'Swiss disease' was coined. He was an Englishman from Salisbury named Robert Warton who was attached to Henry VII's army in Brittany in 1489.

While he was there, he became very unwell, 'And so it was very obvious that his mind was disturbed, and he was deeply grieved at the fact that he had seen himself further isolated from his country'.[12] Over a short period of time, he found his strength waning and he became unable to perform any of the tasks of a soldier.[13] Surgeons were stumped by his situation and were unable to offer anything that might help him.[14]

The *Chronicles of Froissart* contain an earlier case of a mind wounded by trauma. It comes from the mid-1380s and involves a French knight called Sir Peter de Béarn. Although he had become a seasoned warrior by the time the details were recounted, the original trauma seems to have been a life-threatening event that occurred while he was a young knight.[15] It took place while he was in a forest hunting an enormous bear. When his dogs cornered the animal, it killed four of them and injured several more. To defend his hounds, de Béarn drew his sword and attacked the creature. The two of them fought one another, and when the bear nearly overpowered him, the knight found himself in genuine fear for his life. However, de Béarn eventually managed to overcome the bear and kill it.[16] The following night, he began having recurrent nightmares, an early sign that psychological trauma had occurred.[17] It appears that his subsequent wartime experiences only served to exacerbate his already damaged psyche.[18] By the time he was an older man, he feared sleeping alone, and his terrifying nighttime episodes had intensified significantly:

> This sir Peter of Bearn hath an usage, that in the night time while he sleepeth, he will rise and arm himself and draw out his sword and fight all about the house and cannot tell with whom . . . he dare not sleep alone in his chamber . . .[19]

To protect de Béarn from himself during these episodes, and to ensure he was not left alone at night, his servants slept in the same room as the knight. They were tasked with waking and disarming him whenever he experienced one of these frequent bouts with his sword.

Nightmares and episodes like those experienced by de Béarn are extremely common among individuals who have experienced trauma. They can quickly become a part of the traumatized individual's life and can carry on unadulterated for decades.[20] Unsurprisingly, terrible dreams feature regularly among the poetry and prose of soldiers from the First World War.

Charles Hamilton Sorley, who was killed in action at Loos in October 1915, wrote a haunting poem titled *When You See Millions of the Mouthless Men*, inspired by the images that plagued his nightmares.[21] Siegfried Sassoon penned something similar in a verse called *Sick Leave* that begins:

> When I am asleep, dreaming and lulled and warm, –
> They come, the homeless ones, noiseless dead.
> While the dim charging breakers of the storm
> Bellow and drone and rumble overhead,
> Out of the gloom they gather about my bed.[22]

Depression is among the most usual symptoms associated with psychological trauma.[23] Far more than mere sadness, persistent depression can profoundly affect many aspects of a person's life, including sleep, appetite and relationships. Charles, Duke of Orléans, appears to have endured it for decades, having witnessed and survived the slaughter of numerous comrades among the French nobility at the Battle of Agincourt. Unsettlingly, the *Chronique de Jean Fèvre, seigneur de Saint-Remy*, notes that he was found alive beneath a pile of dead French men-at-arms before being taken prisoner by the English.[24] As gruesome as it may sound, such seemingly miraculous extrications were not unknown. In fact, the Count of Richemont was also found in a similar predicament that day, not far from the duke.[25] The poem *The Battle of Crécy* likewise recounts some of those who were recovered alive after the fierce fighting of that conflict had ended:

> Guillaume, however, was discovered
> Among the dead, wounded in the face and body,
> The night after the battle,
> And then indeed Huet Cholet, without doubt,
> Was found on the third day after the battle,
> Which was certainly directly confirmed.[26]

Having not yet seen his 21st birthday, the horrors of Agincourt were far from the beginning of the trauma that shadowed Charles' life. In 1407, when he was just 13 years of age, his father, Louis I, Duke of Orléans, was assassinated.[27] Barely a year later, Charles suffered another devastating blow when his mother, the Duchess of Orléans, passed away while at her chateau in Blois.[28] In September 1409, his young wife Isabelle of Valois died while in childbirth.[29] Bearing such a considerable burden at a young age was undeniably challenging, particularly in the wake of what he experienced at Agincourt. When his captivity in England is added to this litany of trauma, it is hardly surprising that he suffered with depression and anxiety for much of his life. Charles was a prolific poet, and these themes recur frequently throughout his work.[30] The first verse from his poem *Dedens mon livre de pensée*, or *In the Book of My Thought* provides an example of the melancholy that troubled him so deeply:

> In the book of my thought
> I found my heart writing
> Sorrow's true story
> Illumined with tears.[31]

Potential treatments and remedies for the mental health challenges experienced by men such as Robert Warton, Sir Peter de Béarn and Charles, Duke of Orléans, are explored later in this chapter. As for how others perceived soldiers who suffered from such conditions, it is difficult to determine with certainty. However, some evidence suggests that these individuals may have been met with some degree of sympathy. Honoré Bonet, the author of *The Tree of Battles*, developed a deep understanding of the nature of warfare. His insights were shaped in part by the many conversations and debates about war he was exposed to during his youth, particularly among knights. He had also witnessed first-hand the impact conflict had on France during the second half of the fourteenth century.[32] The author's work includes a chapter exploring the various facets of soldiers' struggles with mental health issues. Entitled 'Whether a Soldier Who Goes Out of His Mind Should Be Imprisoned', he delves into some of the complexities surrounding the treatment and perception of warriors such as these:

> Suppose a duke or a count sets out from England with a great company of Englishmen, and comes into the Duchy of Guienne to make war on the lands of the King of France. But, having arrived in this duchy, he becomes raging mad, leaves his soldiers, and then goes off like a madman alone, by woods and hedges, and is found by a soldier of the French King . . .[33]

Scenarios like this one, which was later reiterated by Christine de Pizan in *The Book of Deeds of Arms and of Chivalry*, have played out on the battlefields of Europe throughout history.[34] Bonet and de Pizan both agreed that compassion was necessary in such cases. They concluded that a soldier in a disturbed mental state should not be labelled as an enemy, nor should they be imprisoned or ransomed. Since such individuals could not fully understand or control their behaviour, they were not to be held responsible for the consequences of their actions either, even if they caused harm to others.[35]

Similar leniency and understanding can be found in an English case from the early months of 1306. It involves a soldier named Nigel Coppedene (also Coppendene), who was in prison in Chichester for killing a man named Henry Rosselyn of Bradewatre. An entry in the *Calendar of the Patent Rolls* for 20 February of that year notes that when the murder occurred, Coppedene '. . . was at the time and for some time after in a state of madness'.[36] The cause of his poor mental health was ascribed to his experiences as a prisoner of war, where he endured severe trauma and abuse at the hands of his captors.[37] Due to these extenuating circumstances, the Crown ultimately pardoned Coppedene for the murder.[38]

Civilian Suffering

> In the hope of finding some sort of remedy and medicine for the grievous illness, bitterness of heart, and sadness of mind that manifests itself in floods of tears . . . and still do not cease (which is a great pity) on the part of queens, princesses, baronesses, ladies, and maidens of the noble royal blood of France, and among all the women who are suffering from such great misfortune in the kingdom of France, because of so many deaths or the captivity of those near to them – husbands, children, brothers, uncles, cousins, other relatives and friends, some of them killed in battle . . .
>
> *Epistle of the Prison of Human Life*[39]

The loss of loved ones to conflict, the ongoing threat or experience of physical and sexual violence, and the destruction of property, together with exposure to traumatic and distressing events, resulted in severe psychological issues for many civilians during wartime in this period.[40] Despite their usual exclusion from the sources, the number of those affected must have been staggering. Nowhere was this truer than in France. The deep sorrow experienced by the French population in the wake of their calamitous defeat to the English at the Battle of Agincourt is vividly captured in the opening lines of Christine de Pizan's *Epistre de la prison de vie humaine*, or *Epistle of the Prison of Human Life*, referenced above.[41] This letter, completed on 20 January 1418, was written to Marie of Berry, Duchess of Bourbon, who had lost several family members at Agincourt.[42] It is hardly surprising that the epistle notes the lingering emotional pain of so many French civilians across all walks of life, even two and a half years after the battle, given the decades of traumatic and life-threatening events that had affected their mental well-being.[43] Before Agincourt, the French had suffered losses at Crécy and Poitiers, which were major setbacks in early part of the Hundred Years War. The bubonic plague had returned more than once, while civil war between the Burgundian and Armagnac factions divided the population in the early part of the fifteenth century.[44] Making matters worse were the unemployed soldiers, mercenaries and criminals who banded together in gangs known as *companies* and *écorcheurs* in the fourteenth and fifteenth centuries. They terrorised France through robbery, murder, and sexual violence, often causing more suffering and devastation than the wars of the time.[45]

The psychological impact of Agincourt on French civilians is explored in another poem of the time, *Le Livre des Quatre Dames*, or *The Book of the Four Ladies*, written by the French poet Alain Chartier not long after the battle. In a style common to the period, it takes the form of a debate. Four women who have, in various ways, lost their partners in the Battle of Agincourt present their arguments to the narrator, each claiming that their mental suffering is the most severe. The first woman's beloved was a knight who died on the battlefield, while the second's, quite possibly Charles, Duke of Orléans, was taken prisoner. The fate of the third woman's partner is not known, as he is still missing, and the fourth's seemingly deserted the army.[46]

Such suffering was not unique to the citizens of France. In England, there is the example of Katharine de la Pole, who lost both her husband and son in quick succession in the autumn of 1415 as they took part in

King Henry V of England's expedition to France. Her husband, Michael de la Pole, the Earl of Suffolk, died of dysentery on 17 September, during the Siege of Harfleur.[47] Their son, who was also named Michael, survived Harfleur but was slain at Agincourt, just 38 days after the death of his father.[48] The grief Katherine suffered must have been immeasurable, not to mention that of the three daughters of the younger Michael de la Pole who lost both their father and grandfather.[49] The medieval church of St Peter and St Paul in Fressingfield, Suffolk, contains a grand south porch, a gift from Katherine de la Pole, Countess of Suffolk, in memory of the husband and son she lost.

The first verse of the poem *Duelo de la madre de Lorenzo Davalos*, or *Mourning of the Mother of Lorenzo Davalos*, by the fifteenth-century Spanish poet Juan de Mena, reflects the lifetime of mental anguish felt by so many women like Marie of Berry and Katherine de la Pole who lost sons, husbands, fathers and brothers to war:

> With jagged nails she tore her face
> And rent her breasts with little measure.
> She kissed her son's dead lips grown cold
> And cursed the hands that wrought his murder.
> She cursed the war and its beginning
> And wrathfully spewed cruel complaints
> Denied herself her due reprisal
> And close to living death, she stopped.[50]

The self-harm depicted in the poem's opening lines reflects a recurring motif in medieval literature and imagery and functions as a powerful symbol of a wounded mind.[51]

Sexual Violence

> . . . he hath slain her in fulfilling his foul lust of lechery.
>
> *Le Morte D'Arthur*[52]

Civilians endured and witnessed horrific acts committed by marauding soldiers, companies and écorcheurs.[53] Many lived in a constant state of hypervigilance, fearing for their lives and the safety of their families. Sleep, when it could be found, was often taken in fortified churches, while entire families sought refuge in caves for months on end, desperately searching for security.[54] Of the crimes perpetrated against civilians, one of the most common and deeply feared was sexual assault. For millennia, invading armies and rogue factions have used sexual violence as a weapon of war to terrorise populations, destabilize communities and assert dominance.[55] Primarily targeting women and children, these brutal acts inflict deep psychological and physical harm on survivors, with long-lasting consequences.[56]

In 1414, the town of Soissons, in Northern France, was in Burgundian hands, with English support, when it was besieged and taken by Armagnac forces. The attackers showed little mercy to the town's citizens or those soldiers who were garrisoned there. Many were hanged, churches and houses were looted, and crimes of serious sexual violence were committed against the women of the town.[57] The fifteenth-century French chronicler Enguerrand de Monstrelet provides a harrowing account of the incident:

> There is not a Christian but would have shuddered at the atrocious excesses committed by this soldiery in Soissons: married women violated before their husbands, young damsels in the presence of their parents and relatives, holy nuns, gentlewomen of all ranks, of whom there were many in the town: all, or the greater part, were violated against their wills, and known carnally by divers nobles and others, who, after having satiated their own brutal passions, delivered them over without mercy to their servants . . .[58]

As de Monstrelet suggests, the Church condemned such despicable acts, as did the ideals and laws that supposedly governed the warriors of the period examined here.[59] In the latter part of the fourteenth century, Geoffroi II de Charny wrote that it was the responsibility of men-at-arms to protect the honour of all women.[60] There are surviving English statutes from around the same time that state that no soldier or sailor shall rape or violate any woman, under penalty of death.[61] In the early fifteenth century, under Henry V of England, soldiers were strictly forbidden from harming women and children. Those who committed such crimes could be put to death.[62]

The regulations of 1544 that governed the English army under Henry VIII continued to make rape by a soldier a capital crime.[63]

Stringent rules and principles that prohibited sexual violence were one thing, but the reality of war and the resulting breakdown of the rule of law often meant something very different.[64] Given the reluctance of many Christian writers to note or even acknowledge such matters, it is likely most wartime atrocities went unrecorded.[65] Yet, like de Monstrelet's chronicle mentioned above, some of these incidents were documented in annals and court records; and, as with his account, they make for very disturbing reading:

- A deeply troubling case from 1333 concerns a 10-year-old girl, Jeanette Bille-heuse, who was invited into the house of a woman called Jacqueline la Cyrière under the false pretext of performing domestic work for her. Cyrière's real intention was to supply the little girl to a soldier from the Lombardy region of what is now northern Italy so that he could have sex with her. Once the crime was uncovered, it proceeded to trial, where Jeanette was examined by two court-appointed matrons. When they discovered the extent of the soldier's crimes against the girl, including torture, rape and serious abuse, Jacqueline la Cyrière was sentenced to be burnt to death for her role in the offences. Just what became of the soldier is not known, as no punishment for him is recorded.[66]
- An account from June 1389 in Paris recounts the rape of a young French woman who had been violated in the presence of her husband by an English soldier stationed at the fortress of Château de Châlucet, near Limoges.[67] Outraged by the assault on his wife, the husband retaliated by killing the soldier. Together, the couple hid the body and set his horse free to avoid suspicion. They fled the area immediately and went to live in a village called Montevrain, where they stayed for about five years until the woman's death. It was only later, while her husband was in prison for an unrelated crime, that he confessed to killing the English soldier.[68]
- A French manuscript records the case of a married woman who was taken and sexually violated by a group of men belonging to one of the companies that roamed the country at the time. She stated the experience left her feeling deeply humiliated and terrified that her

husband would despise her if he found out what had occurred.[69] The entry also notes that, in the aftermath, she later became 'mad and demonic'.[70]

- Between 1469 and 1474, Sir Peter von Hagenbach (c. 1420–74) was put in charge of the region of Alsace on behalf of Charles the Bold, Duke of Burgundy. During that time, he and his soldiers committed crimes of sexual violence on a mass scale.[71] On one infamous occasion, Hagenbach is known to have invited several couples to a party. During the evening, the husbands were sent out of the room, while their wives were stripped naked and had a hood placed over their heads.[72] When the men returned, they were ordered to identify their wives by their bodies. Those who failed to recognize them were tossed down a long flight of stairs, while the husbands who succeeded were poisoned with alcohol, all for the perverse pleasure of von Hagenbach and his men. In 1474, he was brought to trial for a series of crimes, including sexual assault, committed by both himself and his soldiers. The proceedings took place in Breisach before more than two dozen judges from the Holy Roman Empire, in what is considered by some to be the forerunner to modern-day war crimes trials. Hagenbach was ultimately found guilty and executed.[73]

Hearing the voice of a sexual assault survivor, such as the woman who endured the brutal gang rape by the men from the company, is rare for the time. Her poignant remarks offer a powerful glimpse into the psychological torment experienced by countless survivors of sexual violence, both in her time and throughout history.[74] The feelings of embarrassment and humiliation she describes are natural responses to the trauma of sexual assault and are commonly reported by survivors of such violence.[75] Although terms like 'mad' and 'demonic' are no longer employed to describe mental health conditions, their use in reference to her psychological state provides an indication of the emotional devastation she experienced.[76] It is only in relatively recent years that a clearer understanding has emerged regarding the strong correlation between sexual assault and its impact on survivors' mental health. Extensive research has established that such violence is closely associated with a high prevalence of serious mental health conditions, including PTSD, severe depression and an increased risk of suicide.[77]

The number of women and children who experienced emotional trauma as a result of sexual assault during the conflicts of this period is impossible to determine, though the available evidence suggests it was alarmingly high.[78] In a time with little understanding of psychological trauma, many survivors were likely left to endure severe mental health consequences, burdens that neither they, their families, nor contemporary medical practitioners were properly equipped to manage.

Suicide

> . . . it is full great pity, alas! to read how thy daughters died, that slew themselves . . .
>
> *The Canterbury Tales - The Franklin's Tale*[79]

Wilfred Owen's First World War poem *S. I. W.*, an abbreviation for Self-Inflicted Wound, tells the harrowing story of a young English soldier, stationed on the Western Front, who takes his own life with his rifle. Owen reveals that the soldier acted out of a 'crisis of his soul', a poignant expression of the significant psychological harm inflicted by the war, which had severely damaged his mind.[80] Regrettably, such crises of the soul have led to the suicides of far too many soldiers throughout history.[81] Recent studies reveal that in many modern armed forces, suicide has now become the leading cause of death, surpassing the risk of being killed in combat by a significant margin.[82]

Although less frequently documented, particularly in historical sources, many noncombatants have also taken their own lives after suffering the psychological effects of war.[83] The chronicles and literature of this period are full of accounts of villages, towns and cities being attacked, set ablaze and looted, often resulting in the death, injury, violation or capture of civilians.[84] The *Chronicle of Jean de Venette* recounts many such incidents from fourteenth-century France during the Hundred Years War, including a notable example from 1358:

> Both the English who had escaped from Paris and the Navarrese overran the fields and vineyards, slaying or taking captive anyone they found in the fields and burning several

> villages, among others La Chapelle-Saint-Lazare, the town of Saint-Laurent near Paris, the granary of Lendit, Saint-Cloud, and some others nearby . . . Losses and injuries were inflicted by friend and foe alike upon the rural population and upon monasteries standing in the open country. Everyone robbed them of their goods and there was no one to defend them.[85]

Even if unspoken, the psychological toll caused by such harrowing scenes, repeatedly witnessed and experienced across France, must have weighed heavily on noncombatants who had been exposed to years of violence, disease and moral collapse. This is certainly reflected in many of the recorded cases of civilian suicide from the time:

- Jean Lunneton was a tenant farmer on the estate of the monastery of Chaalis, north of Paris, where he lived with his wife Perotte and their three children. The Hundred Years War had taken its toll on the family, particularly Jean. His mental health had suffered badly and would only become worse. Soldiers had plundered their property in the past, and just before Christmas 1386, word came that more were on their way. The family's possessions were loaded onto a cart, and Jean asked his wife to take them, along with their children, to Senlis, a safer location a few miles away. By this point, Jean's mind was in such a poor state that he was bedridden, barely able to move, let alone take the journey with his wife, who begged him repeatedly to leave with the family. Left with no choice but to take their children and property to Senlis, she did so with the intention of returning to retrieve Jean. Once the children and the family's property were safe, she came back to get her husband but could find no trace of him.[86] After more than a week, her worst fears were realized when Jean was discovered, having hanged himself from a tree in the woods not far from their farm.[87]
- In 1418, a man named Perrin la Vachier, a butcher from Sarcelles near Paris, died by suicide. He had lived with his wife and family before being adversely affected by the prolonged hardships caused by the Hundred Years War, which by then had been ongoing for over 80 years. According to court records, la Vachier had, '. . . lost the major part of his goods by the fact and occasion of the wars . . .'.[88] Already burdened by personal and family tragedies, the devastation

caused by the conflict appears to have been the breaking point: 'For which things or otherwise, he, because of the turmoil caused by the enemy, he went away, to hang on a tree, where he died . . .'.[89]

- In 1424, a woman named Henriette, who was the wife of Jehan Charnel, took her own life at Montagny-Sainte-Félicité, a town near Senlis. Those close to her explained that while her husband was away working, a group of soldiers came and stole one of their horses and two robes. When Henriette tried to stop them, they beat her terribly. Not long afterwards, soldiers returned to take the couple's other horse. This time, Jehan was at home, and when he attempted to stop them, he too was beaten. The record indicates that once Henriette discovered that both horses had been stolen, she felt that the couple had lost everything, something which she said repeatedly. Having become psychologically overwhelmed by the circumstances, Henriette hanged herself not long after the thefts had occurred.[90]

Although the details of each case reveal little about the lives of these individuals, they offer just enough insight to shed light on some of the factors, such as the consequences of war, that contributed to their tragic suicides. It is important to acknowledge the extraordinary circumstances they, and countless others like them, endured without the benefit of modern psychological support and treatment. Each of them deserves to be remembered, not least for what their deaths reveal about the often-hidden costs of conflict.

Therapies and Cures

> Away with you! Begone! Begone,
> Gray Melancholy, Grief, Despair!
>
> *Ales vous ant, ales, ales*[91]

The support and assistance afforded to individuals suffering with their mental health tended to vary significantly. As is often the case, those with status and financial means generally received the better-quality care.[92] At the other end of the social ladder, people with mild to moderate mental health challenges were frequently left in the care of their families.[93] A fourteenth-century French example involving a woman named Perrin, the wife of Pierre Mauravaule, is indicative of the familial care that could be expected. When her mental health deteriorated, the local lord ordered her husband to look after her so that no harm would come to others in the village.[94] In more difficult circumstances, the individual could still be left with loved ones even if it meant they had to be restrained. Such restrictions were often used, not as punishment, but to keep the individual from injuring themselves and those around them.[95] The *Miracles of King Henry VI* describes a man named Walter Barker from Luton, who was in the service of a knight.[96] In 1485, he was the victim of violence when he was attacked by three men while out walking alone. The incident left Barker psychologically scarred. Previously a peaceful man, he was increasingly driven to violence, even harming his wife. Ultimately, his friends and family had to restrain him, placing him in iron manacles in an attempt to ensure his safety and that of those around him.[97]

In Copland's poem from the mid-1530s, *The Highway to the Spital-House*, the author and the porter of the hospital or almshouse converse about individuals whose mental health challenges were so significant that their families could not care for them or opted not to do so. When the author asks what becomes of them, the porter replies, 'We have chambers purposely for them, or else they should be lodged in Bedlam'.[98] Established by a former sheriff of London in 1247, the Priory of St Mary of Bethlehem, more commonly referred to as Bedlam, is arguably the most renowned medieval hospital for those who suffered serious mental health issues.[99] Little is known about its first 100 years or so, but by the early fifteenth century it allocated a limited number of permanent beds to patients who were 'mentally incapacitated' and required long-term care.[100] Elsewhere, in the fourteenth century, St. George's Hospital of Elbląg, which belonged to the Teutonic Knights in the north of Poland, had a few rooms designated for those with severe mental health challenges.[101] In early fifteenth century Valencia, Hospital de los Inocentes, or the Hospital of the Innocents, was established to care for the mental health of its patients.[102] Similarly, other hospitals, such as Holy Trinity in Salisbury and Hôtel Dieu in Paris, were known to provide designated beds for individuals with comparable needs. However, the capacity of establishments like these was usually quite limited.[103] Many infirmaries and almshouses simply refused to accept patients struggling with such issues. In towns and cities across Europe, individuals suffering from serious psychological issues and without a stable place to live were frequently imprisoned, mistreated or exiled to other locations.[104]

While the above provides a rather broad overview, in no way does it address the various other situations and circumstances faced by individuals experiencing mental health challenges during this period. The example of the previously mentioned Charles, Duke of Orléans, illustrates this point. After the Battle of Agincourt, he was taken to England, where he remained a political prisoner for 25 years before returning to France.[105] Whether in England or at home, his trauma-related depression and anxiety seem to have at times been quite acute. However, among the substantial body of poetry he produced during these many decades are works that, whether consciously or not, seem to have served as a form of self-therapy. They became a way for the duke to try and help himself in an age when issues of mental health were not well understood.[106] One such work is the poem *Ales vous ant, ales, ales*, or *Away with You! Begone! Begone!* from which the epigraph for this section is taken:

Away with you! Begone! Begone,
Gray Melancholy, Grief, Despair!
How could you dream you could ensnare
Me always as you once have done'?
Your stern dominion I disown;
Reason shall master it, I swear.
Away with you! Begone! Begone,
Gray Melancholy, Grief, Despair!
If with your retinue anon
You would revisit me, forbear!
I pray God curse you and declare
Your claims all void from this day on.
Away with you! Begone! Begone,
Gray Melancholy, Grief, Despair![107]

Charles' deep depression is evident in these verses, but so too is his desire to be free of it, as suggested by his repeated command for it to 'begone'. Using art in this way was well ahead of its time. Today, both writing and reading poetry are recognized as effective tools in the fight to manage some symptoms of PTSD. Among its many benefits, writing poetry allows individuals to express their emotions without fear of judgement or threat, while reading such works can help them connect with and better understand the feelings they are experiencing.[108]

The therapeutic benefits of other art forms, including music, have also been acknowledged in the treatment of individuals with PTSD.[109] Music therapy has been shown to be particularly effective in alleviating symptoms such as depression, insomnia and anxiety.[110] During the period explored here, as in earlier centuries, it was also understood to be useful in healing both the mind and the body.[111] Henri de Mondeville recognized that sadness could gradually diminish a person's strength, echoing beliefs held centuries earlier by ancient practitioners such as Hippocrates and Galen.[112] The French surgeon suggested that music, played on a viol or ten-stringed psaltery, be used to help distract and entertain patients.[113] By the end of the fourteenth century, an illustrated manual on health, known as the *Tacuinum Sanitatis*, had gained substantial notoriety. It brought to light the connections between various aspects of daily life, such as diet, herbal remedies, seasonal changes and attire, and their influence on an individual's overall health and well-being. There are several fifteenth-century examples of these *Tacuina* that still exist, such as the Liechtenstein *Tacuinum Sanitatis*, which show how music was thought to benefit a person's health and emotions.[114] Paracelsus (1493–1541), a physician from what is now north-central Switzerland, believed that music was a cure for anyone troubled by melancholy or other difficulties of the mind.[115] It was not just those in the medical community who stood by its benefits. The Venetian composer and music theorist, Gioseffe Zarlino (1517–90), was of the belief that medicine could heal the body, but it was vocal and instrumental music that could remedy a weak and broken spirit.[116]

The memoirs of the fifteenth-century historian Philip de Commines, who was himself a seasoned knight, record the mental health struggles of Charles the Bold, Duke of Burgundy, following the battles at Granson (also Grandson) and Morat in March and June, respectively, of 1476.[117] He sank into deep depression and became increasingly irritable, neglecting his hygiene and appearance before eventually isolating himself from others for several weeks. The duke exhibited a volatile temper and a tendency toward violence, coupled with a poor appetite and excessive drinking.[118] What is remarkable about this part of de Commines' text is the therapeutic advice the knight offers in dealing with such problems of the mind. Speaking generally rather than directly to Charles the Bold, he suggests three methods of treating such issues, any or all of which could just as easily be found in the toolkit of a modern mental health practitioner. The first approach relates to religion, which is perhaps not surprising given its importance in this period. Commines encourages seeking God's forgiveness for any transgressions, along with asking for divine guidance in difficult circumstances.[119] Similarly, in her *Epistle of the Prison of Human Life*, Christine de Pizan urges the grieving Marie of Berry to place her trust in God and to draw strength from the Bible.[120] Modern therapists and mental health professionals regularly suggest a comparable approach for those patients who have religious beliefs, regardless of their specific faith. The trauma sufferer can be helped by seeking to rekindle or strengthen the relationship they had with their god and other members of their faith.[121]

The next method discussed by de Commines involves connecting with close friends and others with whom there is a strong bond:

> It is also well to unbosom ourselves freely to some intimate friends, not to keep our sorrows concealed, but to expatiate on every circumstance of them, without being ashamed or reserved; for this mitigates the rigour of our misfortunes, revives the heart, and restores their usual vigour and activity to our dejected spirits.[122]

Dr. Bessel van der Kolk, a psychiatrist and researcher who has worked in the area of PTSD for many decades, emphasises the significance of strong relationships for individuals who have experienced trauma. The support from trusted friends, family and groups can offer a vital source of emotional and physical safety, playing a crucial role in healing.[123]

Finally, de Commines advocates the value of exercise and work in the recovery process. Once again, modern mental health practitioners are strongly behind the benefits of physical activity in the treatment of many of their trauma patients.[124]

Whether or not Charles the Bold took any of this advice is difficult to know, but he continued to struggle with his mental health and never fully recovered.[125] Just a few months after his decline began, he was killed in early January 1477 at the Battle of Nancy.

Medicines derived from a range of natural substances were also utilized to address various mental health issues. Some were costly and difficult to source, like the richly coloured blue rock *lapis lazuli*, frequently referred to as ultramarine. The distinguished Florentine doctor Taddeo Alderotti (c. 1215–95) recommended it as a cure for melancholy.[126] Just how it was given to patients is less clear. Nevertheless, in Robert Burton's early seventeenth-century book *Anatomy of Melancholy*, lapis lazuli is also mentioned as a remedy for depression. The rock needed to be washed no less than fifty times and ground into a powder before being administered to the patient in pill form.[127]

There were, of course, a variety of plants and herbs prescribed by doctors and apothecaries that were much more affordable and accessible, some of which continue to be used in natural medicine. The following examples represent just a small selection of the many types of *flora* that were used to treat the symptoms of compromised mental health:

- *St John's wort* has been taken for centuries to treat various health issues, including depression.[128] In fact, in 1525, it was recognized by Paracelsus as being useful in the treatment of things such as insomnia, depression and anxiety. It is an herbal remedy that is still widely used for the same purposes, especially in Europe and North America.[129]
- *Peony* is employed in traditional Chinese medicine to treat depression and was utilized in the same way during the period reviewed in this book.[130] The late fourteenth-century poem *Pearl*, which tells the story of a father grieving the loss of his daughter named Pearl, uses peonies as a literary device to ease his sorrow, depicting them in full bloom across her grave.[131] Peonies were also believed to be effective against anxiety and nightmares.[132]
- *Feverfew* had a few uses, including the treatment of extreme anxiety.[133] It was also utilized to treat depression. William Turner's *A New Herball*, an English herbal published in three parts between 1551 and 1568, states that the plant makes a good remedy '. . . for them that are grieved with melancholy'.[134]
- *Spurge*, also called *lathyrism* or *catapuce*, was used to help with nightmares. It is a plant that can cause a powerful purging of the stomach.[135] It can be found in Chaucer's *Nun's Priest's Tale*, where it is recommended to help with bad dreams involving such things as

'. . . terror of arrows, of fire with red flames, of great beasts . . .'.[136] The seeds of the plant continue to be used in traditional Chinese medicine.[137]

- *Rosemary* is found in the English *Banckes's Herbal* from 1525, which lists many uses for the plant, including the placement of its leaves under the head of the bed so that '. . . thou shalt be delivered of all evil dreams'.[138]

In recent times, some progress has been made in the treatment of trauma-based psychological disorders such as PTSD; however, they continue to pose real challenges for most patients. This highlights the reality that contemporary psychiatry and medicine still have a considerable way to go in comprehending the human mind and its many complexities. Working within an entirely different medical framework, it is perhaps not surprising that practitioners in the period covered by this volume also found it difficult to unravel its mysteries.[139] Certainly, there were many old wives' tales and quack remedies that did little more than strip patients of their money.[140] However, as numerous examples above illustrate, both laypeople and those practising medicine occasionally recognized the benefits of some treatments and cures that have come to be regarded as sound therapeutic practice today.

CONCLUSION

> From the same wretched shop and magazine of cruelty, are all sorts of Mines, Countermines, pots of fire, trains, fiery Arrowes, Lances, Crossebowes, barrels, balls of fire, burning faggots, Granats, and all such fiery engines and Inventions, which closely stuffed with fuell and matter for fire, and cast by the defendants upon the bodies and Tents of the asiailants, easily take fire by the violence of their motion. Certainly a most miserable and pernicious kind of invention, whereby we often see a thousand of heedlesse men blown up with a mine by the force of Gunpowder . . .[1]

The first years of the late Middle Ages saw the introduction of rudimentary gunpowder weapons on the battlefields of Europe. The technology developed quickly, and by the mid-1500s, as the above passage from Ambroise Paré suggests, there was a huge assortment of these weapons, many of which could kill and maim on a large scale.[2] Horrifically, far more deadly weapons were to come in the decades and centuries that would follow this period. To make things worse, it is estimated that between the sixteenth and eighteenth centuries, the number, size and frequency of conflicts in Europe surged to a level beyond what had been recorded in the past. This caused the growth in size of many armies, with some expanding by ten times their original number.[3] This resulted in a corresponding increase in the quantity and complexity of the physical and mental injuries suffered by the soldiers and sailors who fought these wars. Additionally, diseases, such as bubonic plague and typhoid, alongside infected wounds, would continue to take the lives of countless warriors who often lived in cramped and unsanitary conditions. The number of medical practitioners associated with Europe's armed forces naturally increased in an attempt to address the needs of the sick and wounded.[4] New treatment methods would be introduced, while many other techniques from earlier centuries persisted or were reintroduced, all with varying degrees of success.

GLOSSARY OF CHRONICLERS, WRITERS AND SURGEONS

Abulcasis or Abu al-Qasim: Sometimes referred to as the 'father of modern surgery', Abulcasis was born after 936, near Córdoba, Spain. The works of this distinguished physician were relied on by late medieval surgeons like John Arderne, who combined two of Abulcasis' procedures with his own post-operative care technique to come up with a method that could successfully treat anal fistulas. Abulcasis died in 1013.

Alain Chartier: Born around 1385 to a property-owning family in Bayeux, France, Chartier went on to become a notary and secretary to the dauphin, the future King Charles VII of France. He is well known for his poems, such as the epic *Le livre des quatre dames*, or *The Book of the Four Ladies*, which describes the grief of four French women who lost loved ones at the Battle of Agincourt. He died at Avignon in March 1430.

Alessandro Benedetti: Born around 1450 in Padua, Benedetti later became a physician to the Venetian army. In the last years of the fifteenth century, during the Italian Wars, he composed an important diary of his experiences, called *Diaria de bello Carolino* or *Diary of the Caroline War*. He died in October 1512.

***Amadís of Gaul*:** There are questions over the original authorship of this epic fourteenth-century tale from the Iberian Peninsula. In the early sixteenth century, Garci Rodriguez de Montalvo, a Castilian, extended and edited the work before popularizing it. The story focuses on the feats of the emotional, virtuous and battle-hardened knight, Amadís, the son of King Perión of Gaula and Elisena of England.

Ambroise Paré: Born in Bourg-Hersant, around 1510, Paré became a master barber-surgeon by the age of 31 advancing to the title of surgeon in his early 50s. He served the French army for nearly 30 years during a very turbulent period in French history. In times of peace, Paré worked in Paris, where he cared for the sick and injured. He introduced or reintroduced many important and effective treatments for things such as gunshot wounds and amputations, regularly saying of his cases, 'I dressed him, and God healed him'. Paré died on 20 December 1590.

***Amtliche Berner Chronik*:** This official *Chronicle of Bern* was commissioned by the city of Bern in 1474. It would take Diebold Schilling ten years to complete the work in three volumes, which include more than 600 large illustrations. The third volume, which is the most richly decorated of the group, describes the Burgundian Wars (1474–7).

Arnald of Villanova: The place of his birth is not known for certain, but he was born sometime around 1240. He studied medicine at Montpellier and later became the master at the school of medicine in Paris. He wrote several of his medical texts in Catalan. Arnald of Villanova died in 1311.

Avicenna or Ibn Sina: Known as the 'Prince of Physicians' by his countrymen, this Persian doctor was born around 980 and would write his first book on medicine by the time he was 21. He went on to pen more than forty works on a variety of subjects before he died in 1037. Many medieval European doctors, like Theodoric, relied on the ideas of Avicenna for their own texts.

Bruno da Longoburgo: Born around 1200 and later known as Bruno the Arabist, the medical texts of this mid-thirteenth-century surgeon were heavily influenced by earlier Islamic doctors like Avicenna and Abulcasis, as his alias implies. Around 1252, Bruno produced a major work called *Chirurgia Magna* and later a shorter version of basically the same text known as *Chirurgia Parva*. He died in 1286.

Christine de Pizan: Born in Venice about 1364, Christine and her family went to live in France while she was just a child, after her father, Tommaso da Pizan (also Thomas de Pizan), became physician and astrologer at the court of King Charles V. Later, the deaths of both her father and husband meant that she needed to make a living to support her mother and three young children. To do so, she began writing, at first producing poems of love, but would later go on to detail many other subjects, including war, feminism and Joan of Arc. She died around the year 1431.

Galen: Born in Greece about 129, Galen would begin studying medicine as a teenager. He moved to Rome in 162, where he climbed the ladder of the medical profession, becoming a physician to Roman emperors Commodus and Septimius Severus. He wrote several medical texts that would continue to be significant for many centuries to come. Galen died around the year 216.

Geoffroi de Charny: A notable knight of the fourteenth century, de Charny was born around 1306. In addition to diplomatic duties, fighting in tournaments and battles, he was also a writer. As well as *Demandes*, he composed *Livre Charny* that outlines much of his life. Recent research suggests that the *Book of Chivalry*, long thought to have been written by de Charny, may well have been composed by his son Geoffroi II de Charny (d. 1398). Fighting on the French side, de Charny was killed at the Battle of Poitiers in 1356.

Giovanni de Vigo: Also referred to as Jean de Vigo, he was born in 1450. Among his comprehensive group of medical texts, this Genoese surgeon is known for his misapprehension that gunpowder wounds were poisoned, as well as for his work during the syphilis epidemic of the late fifteenth and early sixteenth centuries. Vigo died in 1525.

Guy de Chauliac: Born around 1300, de Chauliac would eventually become both a surgeon and a physician. He managed to survive the Black Death, discovering that there was more than one type of the terrible disease. Chauliac also kept the pope alive while the plague raged across Europe. He wrote extensively on medicine, producing a surgical text of his own, along with other works, before he died on 25 July 1368. His medical texts remained influential for hundreds of years after his death.

Hans von Gersdorff: Born around 1455, von Gersdorff would go on to become a military surgeon. He published his *Feldbuch der Wundarzney*, or *Field Book of Wound Medicine*, in Strasbourg in 1517. Hans von Gersdorff died in 1529.

Heinrich von Pfolspeundt: A fifteenth-century soldier and barber-surgeon who flourished around 1460, von Pfolspeundt (also Pfolsprundt) probably came from the area that is now central Germany. A member of the Teutonic Order of Knights, he wrote a surgical text following the Siege of Marienburg in 1460. It is the first known work to mention a treatment for gunshot wounds. The date of von Pfolspeundt's death is not known.

Henri de Mondeville: Born around the year 1260, de Mondeville would go on to study medicine, likely at Montpellier and Paris. Later in Bologna, he became a student of Theodoric and would come to believe in his 'dry healing' method, which advocated that pus was not necessary in the proper healing of wounds. Mondeville served as a surgeon to the French army, as well as to the royal families of King Philip IV and King Louis X of France. Mondeville's surgical text was written between 1310 and 1320, the year of his death.

Hieronymus Brunschwig: Born about 1450, Brunschwig showed an interest in surgery from a very young age. He became an apprentice to a surgeon to learn his skills. In 1497, he published his *Buch der Cirurgia*, or *Book of Surgery*, the first text of its kind to take advantage of the printing press. Brunschwig died sometime around 1512.

Honoré Bonet: Born about 1340 in Provence, Bonet would later join the Benedictine order and become the prior of Salon (Selonnet). He wrote a comprehensive treatise on war and its rules in the late fourteenth century called *L'arbre des batailles*, or *The Tree of Battles*. It became a well-known work during the later Middle Ages, being relied on by military leaders and other writers like Christine de Pizan. Bonet died sometime around 1410.

Jean Froissart: Born in the mid-1330s in Valenciennes, Froissart would later travel extensively around Europe, where he often spent time at the royal courts. He began writing his famous chronicles of the first decades of the Hundred Years War around 1369. Jean Froissart died circa 1410.

Jehan Yperman: Born around 1260, Yperman would later be taught by the famous surgeon Lanfranchi of Milan in Paris. Yperman became chief surgeon to the Flemish armies around Ypres. Also considered the father of

Flemish surgery, he wrote his surgical text in a dialect of medieval Flemish called Thiois rather than Latin. He died sometime around 1330.

John Arderne: Sometimes called the father of English surgery, Arderne was born in 1307 and may have studied medicine at Montpellier. He was an army surgeon under Henry Plantagenet, 1st Duke of Lancaster and Earl of Derby. Arderne survived the Black Death and subsequent outbreaks of the plague. The date of his death is somewhat unclear, but it was likely on or before 1380.

John Bradmore: While not much is known of Bradmore's life, both he and his brother Nicholas were surgeons working in and around London in the late fourteenth and early fifteenth centuries. He became a royal surgeon and is noted for having saved the young Prince of Wales, the future King Henry V of England, after he was struck in the face by an arrow at the Battle of Shrewsbury. John Bradmore died c. 1413.

John Mirfield: Little is known about when or where John Mirfield was born, but London or Yorkshire are the more likely answers to the second question. He lived during the latter half of the fourteenth century, staying for many years at the Augustinian Priory at St Bartholomew's Close in Smithfield, London, where he would become a priest in 1395. While not formally educated in the field of medicine, he had a great interest in the subject. In his text *Breviarium Bartholomei*, he collected the contemporary medical knowledge of the late fourteenth century, which was largely made up of the works of earlier surgeons like William of Saliceto and Henri de Mondeville. John Mirfield died in 1407.

Lanfranchi of Milan: Likely born in Milan during the first half of the thirteenth century, Lanfranchi was a student of William of Saliceto and probably had contact with Theodoric at some point, as well. He became a Master Surgeon in Milan before fleeing to Lyon in 1290. From there he would go to Paris to teach. Among his students was Jehan Yperman. He also wrote his *Chirurgia Magna* in Paris around 1295, a text that became widely regarded by the medical community. Lanfranchi died in 1315.

***Le Morte D'Arthur*:** This adaptation of the adventures of King Arthur and his knights has traditionally been attributed to Sir Thomas Malory of

Newbold Revell, who flourished in the second half of the fifteenth century. While it seems likely that he was the author, the writer's identity has never been established for certain. The most famous version of the book was published by William Caxton in 1485.

Leech/Leche: Derived from the Old English word læce or the Old Danish word læke meaning physician or healer, the word was still in use throughout the period covered in this volume.

***Palmerin of England*:** Palmerin of England was written in the middle of the sixteenth century by Francisco de Moraes Cabral, a Portuguese diplomat. The Palmerin cycle is a group of stories that deal with the life and adventures of Palmerin d'Oliva, emperor of Constantinople and his descendants, including Palmerin of England, the focus of this, the sixth tale.

Philip de Commines or Commynes: A knight, historian and statesman, Philip was born around 1447 in Commines, in the area of what is now the French-Belgian border. He was raised in the Burgundian court and chronicled the events that occurred during much of his lifetime in eight volumes. The first six, which deal with the reign of Louis XI, were written between 1488 and 1494. The remaining two that focus on Charles VIII were penned between 1497 and 1501. He died in October 1511, but his books were not published until 1524.

Roger Frugard of Parma: Also called Roger of Parma or just Roger Frugard, he was born in 1140. Credited with one of the most seminal works of medieval medicine, Roger's surgical text was put together by his students, led by Guido II of Arezzo, between 1170 and 1180. It is arranged from head to toe, with much of the focus being on the treatment of wounds and ailments. It was instantly successful at Salerno and was soon being copied, translated and spread across Europe. Roger died sometime around 1195.

Roland of Parma: Roland of Parma produced his surgical text after 1240, before it was finally published around 1250. Most of his work was taken directly from Roger Frugard's groundbreaking text, although he did manage to add a few of his own experiences and observations. Other surgeons, like Theodoric and his father, were extremely critical of Roland and his work because it fell so close to Roger's surgery.

***Spiezer Chronik*:** Commissioned by Rudolph von Erlach, the *Spiezer Chronik*, or *Spiez Chronicle*, is another work by Diebold Schilling, this one being completed in the mid-1480s. Named after the chronicler's long-time home city of Spiez, it describes the early history of Bern from the city's founding through to the mid-fifteenth century. Unlike Schilling's *Amtliche Berner Chronik*, the *Spiezer Chronik* does not include the Burgundian wars.

Theodoric: The son of surgeon Hugo de Lucca, Theodoric was born in 1205. He would later produce his own surgical text around 1265, a combination of ancient, Islamic and contemporary medical knowledge. Theodoric also relied heavily on his father's experiences as a surgeon, in addition to his own. He and his father were proponents of the 'dry' or pus-free healing method. Theodoric died in 1296.

***Tirant lo Blanc*:** Known as *Tirant the White* in English, this late fifteenth-century chivalric epic was mostly written by a Valencian knight called Joanot Martorell and completed by his close friend Martí Joan de Galba after Martorell's death. It relates the adventures of a knight named Tirant as he travels across Europe and the Middle East.

William of Saliceto: Born around 1210, William was one of the most highly regarded surgeons of his time. His surgical text was written about 1275 and remained an important work long after it had been completed. Individual cases involving the wounded, including many soldiers, are catalogued throughout the volume, providing insight into the world of medicine in the late thirteenth century. William also taught such noted surgeons as Lanfranchi of Milan. He died in 1277.

NOTES

Preface

1. Tho Johnson (trans.), *The workes of that famous chirurgion Ambrose Parëy - Translated out of Latine and compared with the French* (London, Printed by Richard Cotes and Willi Du-gard, 1649), p. 675.

Chapter 1: Medicine from the Late Middle Ages to the Early Sixteenth Century

1. Henry Thomas Riley (ed.), *Chronica Monasterii S. Albani, Registra Quorundam Abbatum Monasterii S. Albani, qui Sæculo XVmo. floruere Vol. I., Registrum Abbatiæ Johannis Whethamstede, Abbatis Monasterii Sancti Albani* (London, Longman & Co., and Trübner & Co., 1872), p. 168, '. . . pugnaverant per pauculum spatium temporis sic atrociter in invicem, ut hic videres jacere unum excusso cerebro illic alteram brachio praeciso, ibi tertium confosso gutture, inibi quartum perforato pectore, totamque plateam ulterias repletam occisorum cadaveribus . . .'.
2. Brian Burfield, *Medieval Military Medicine - from the Vikings to the High Middle Ages* (Barnsley, Pen & Sword Military, 2022), p. 1. This passage is reminiscent of the epigraph taken from the earlier poem *The Song of the Crusade Against the Albigensians*, which begins the preceding volume.
3. Michael Livingston and Kelly DeVries (ed.), *The Battle of Crécy - A Casebook* (Liverpool, Liverpool University Press, 2015), pp. 111, 355.
4. Jim Bradbury, *The Medieval Archer* (Woodbridge, The Boydell Press, 1985), pp. 75, 146–50, for the increase in the power of some bows and crossbows by the late medieval period.
5. Jonathan Davies, *The Medieval Cannon 1326-1494* (Oxford, Osprey Publishing Ltd., 2019), pp. 4–7.
6. Ralph A. Griffiths, 'The Interaction of War and Plague in the Later Middle Ages', *Wales and Medicine, An Historical Survey from Papers Given at the Ninth British Congress on the History of Medicine* (Llandysul, J.D. Lewis and Sons Ltd., 1973), pp. 127–8. See also, Terry Jones, *Medieval Lives* (London, BBC Books, 2004), pp. 32–4.

7. James B. Colton (trans.), *John of Mirfield (d. 1407) Surgery, A Translation of his Breviarium Bartholomei, part IX* (New York, Hafner Publishing Company, 1969), p. 230.
8. G. E. Gask, 'The Medical Staff of King Edward the Third', *Proceedings of the Royal Society of Medicine*, 1 May 1926, p. 1.
9. Edward Maunde Thompson (ed.), *Chronicon Galfridi le Baker de Swynebroke* (Oxford, Clarendon Press, 1889), pp. 81–5, 92, 98–100, 143–53, for details of battles including Crécy and Poitiers, along with information regarding the Black Death. See also, D. F. Jamison, *The Life and Times of Bertrand de Guesclin, A History of the Fourteenth Century, In Two Volumes* (Charleston, John Russell, 1864), Vol. II, pp. 4–6, for the specific example of a fourteenth-century tournament in Lisbon in which an English knight called Matthew Gournay is injured.
10. Sir Percival Horton-Smith Hartley and Harold Richard Aldridge, *Johannes de Mirfield of St Bartholomew's, Smithfield - His Life and Works* (Cambridge, Cambridge University Press, 1936), p. 24.
11. Colton (trans.), *John of Mirfield*, Introduction, p. ix. Mirfield lived for many years at the Augustinian Priory of St Bartholomew in Smithfield, London, but his real interest lay across the road at the Hospital of St Bartholomew.
12. R. Theodore Beck, *The Cutting Edge - Early History of the Surgeons of London* (London, Lund Humphries, 1974), p. 39. Mirfield's work provides '. . . a great encyclopaedia of true contemporary medical knowledge'. See also, Colton (trans.), *John of Mirfield*, Introduction, p. x. As Mirfield readily confesses, most the treatments and cures offered in his *Breviarum Bartholomew* belong to others.
13. Burfield, *Medieval Military Medicine*, pp. 6–7, 10.
14. Carole Rawcliffe, *Medicine & Society in Later Medieval England* (Stroud, Alan Sutton Publishing Limited, 1995), p. 74. Throughout history, military surgeons have often been at the leading edge of advances in medicine.
15. Anne Curry, *The Battle of Agincourt - Sources and Interpretations* (Suffolk, The Boydell Press, 2009), pp. 286–7.
16. Colton (trans.), *John of Mirfield*, pp. 55, 65, 84, 130, 132. Mirfield's text includes many references to the use of rose oil and rose honey for the treatment of wounds. See also, British Library Board, Sloane MS 2272, *Anatomia Membrorum*, f. 137r: the English surgeon John Bradmore used rose honey for the same purpose after the Battle of Shrewsbury, 'Quaequidem tente intincte fuerunt in melle rose' 'Indeed, they were dipped in rose honey', and Dr Leonard D. Rosenman (trans.), *The Surgery of Master Jehan Yperman* (Xlibris Corporation, 2002), p. 299, for an earlier example.

17. Livingston and DeVries (ed.), *The Battle of Crécy*, pp. 45, ll. 403–406. See also, ibid., p. 341, note on ll. 404–05.
18. Eberhard Demm: 'Censorship', in: 1914-1918-online. International Encyclopedia of the First World War, ed. by Ute Daniel, Peter Gatrell, Oliver Janz, Heather Jones, Jennifer Keene, Alan Kramer, and Bill Nasson, issued by Freie Universität Berlin, Berlin 2017-03-29, p. 11.
19. Rachel Koopmans, *Wonderful to Relate, Miracle Stories and Miracle Collecting in High Medieval England* (Philadelphia, University of Pennsylvania Press, 2011), pp. 7–8, 201–05. See also, Irina Metzler, 'Indiscriminate Healing Miracles in Decline: How Social Realities Affect Religious Perception', *Contextualizing Miracles in the Christian West, 1100-1500* (Oxford, The Society for the Study of Medieval Languages and Literature, 2014), pp. 155–6.
20. Burfield, *Medieval Military Medicine*, pp. 21–8.
21. Father Ronald Knox and Shane Leslie (trans.), *The Miracles of King Henry VI - Being an account and Translation of Twenty-three Miracles taken from the Manuscript in the British Museum (Royal 13c.viii)* (Cambridge, Cambridge University Press, 1923), p. 77, no. 37.
22. Ibid., p. 78.
23. Ibid.
24. Ibid., p. 81.
25. Ibid., p. 82.
26. Ibid., pp. 82–3.
27. Burfield, *Medieval Military Medicine*, p. 27, for more on wax and other votive offerings.
28. Knox and Leslie (trans.), *The Miracles of King Henry VI*, p. 83.
29. Burfield, *Medieval Military Medicine*, p. 27, regarding the process of proving that a miracle had occurred.
30. Knox and Leslie (trans.), *The Miracles of King Henry VI*, p. 84. See also, Burfield, *Medieval Military Medicine*, p. 77, for more on the display of healed injuries at medieval shrines.
31. Dr Leonard D. Rosenman (trans.), *The Chirurgia of Roger Frugard* (Xlibris Corporation, 2002), p. 118.
32. Rosenman (trans.), *The Surgery of Master Jehan Yperman*, pp. 186–7 and Dr Leonard D. Rosenman (trans.), *The Major Surgery of Guy de Chauliac, An English Translation* (Xlibris Corporation, 2005), p. 343, for the surgical procedure to repair perforated intestines. See also, Burfield, *Medieval Military Medicine*, pp. 23–8, regarding other potential factors that may have played a role in such miracle accounts.

33. Ronald C. Finucane, *Miracles and Pilgrims – Popular Beliefs in Medieval England* (New York, St Martin's Press, 1995), pp. 66–7.
34. Sue Black, *Written in Bone, Hidden Stories in What We Leave Behind* (London, Transworld Publishers, 2020), pp. 10–11.
35. R. Colleter, C. P. Bataille, H. Dabernat, D. Pichot, P. Hamon, S. Duchesne, F. Labaune-Jean, S. Jean, G. Le Cloirec, S. Milano, M. Tros, S. Steinbrenner, M. Marchal, C. Guilbeau-Frugier, N. Telmon, É. Crubézy, and K. Jaouen, 'The last battle of Anne of Brittany: Solving mass grave through an interdisciplinary approach (paleopathology, biological anthropology, history, multiple isotopes and radiocarbon dating)', *PLoS One* 2021 May 5; 16 [5], pp. 1, 10–11.
36. Ibid., p. 17.
37. Percy MacKaye (trans.), *The Canterbury Tales of Geoffrey Chaucer - A Modern Rendering into Prose of the Prologue and Ten Tales* (New York, Duffield & Company, 1914), p. 10, from the Prologue.
38. Nancy Siraisi, *Medieval and Early Renaissance Medicine, An Introduction to Knowledge and Practice* (University of Chicago Press, 1990), pp. 104–06. See also, Jones, *Medieval Lives*, p. 135. Different parts of the body were thought to have been responsible for creating these humours, the liver produced black bile, while the gall bladder made yellow bile, blood emanated from the heart and lastly phlegm was made in the brain.
39. Dr Leonard D. Rosenman (trans.), *The Surgery of Lanfranchi of Milan* (Xlibris, 2003), p. 33. See also, MacKaye (trans.), *The Canterbury Tales*, p. 10.
40. Johnson (trans.), *The workes of that famous chirurgion Ambrose Paréy*, p. 320, from the first book written by Ambroise Paré: 'Wounds of the head are cured with far more difficulty at Paris, than at Avigvion, where notwithstanding on the contrary, the Wounds of the legs are cured with more trouble, than at Paris; the cause is, the air is cold and moist at Paris; which constitution seeing it is hurtfull to the brain and head, it cannot, but must be offensive to the Wounds of these parts.'
41. Rosenman (trans.), *The Surgery of Lanfranchi of Milan*, p. 36.
42. Johnson (trans.), *The workes of that famous chirurgion Ambrose Paréy*, p. 370.
43. Nancy Siraisi, *Taddeo Alderotti and his Pupils – Two Generations of Italian Medical Learning* (Princeton University Press, 1981), p. 139. See also, Rosenman (trans.), *The Surgery of Master Jehan Yperman*, p. 75, and Siraisi, *Medieval and Early Renaissance Medicine*, p. 68.
44. MacKaye (trans.), *The Canterbury Tales*, pp. 9–10.
45. Siraisi, *Medieval and Early Renaissance Medicine*, p. 68. See also, Lynn Thorndike, *University Records and Life in the Middle Ages* (New York,

Columbia University Press, 1944), pp. 336, 362, and Rosenman (trans.), *The Surgery of Lanfranchi of Milan*, p. 36. Lanfranchi taught at Paris.

46. Thorndike, *University Records and Life in the Middle Ages*, pp. 281–2.
47. D'Arcy Power (ed.), *Treatises of Fistula in Ano, Hæmorrhoids, and Clysters, by John Arderne, from an early fifteenth-century manuscript translation* (London, Kegan Paul, Trench, Trübner & Co., 1910), p. 16.
48. Ibid., pp. 17–20. See also, Wellcome Collection, *An English folding almanac in Latin*, MS.8932, c. 1415-1420, f. 5.
49. Rosenman (trans.), *The Surgery of Master Jehan Yperman*, pp. 74–5.
50. Ibid., p. 75.
51. Walter William Skeat (trans.), *The Vision of Piers Plowman, by William Langland Done Into Modern English* (London, Alexander Moring Ltd., 1905), p. 35, ll. 223–4.
52. Toni Mount, *Everyday Life in Medieval London, from the Anglo-Saxons to the Tudors* (Stroud, Amberley Publishing, 2014), pp. 161, 166–8. See also, Siraisi, *Medieval and Early Renaissance Medicine*, p. 20; Power (ed.), *Treatises of Fistula in Ano*, Introduction, p. xix, and Francis R. Packard, *Life and Times of Ambroise Pare [1510-1590]. With a New Translation of his Apology and an Account of his Journeys in Divers Places* (New York, Paul B. Hoeber, 1921), p. 15.
53. Siraisi, *Medieval and Early Renaissance Medicine*, p. 18.
54. Packard, *Life and Times of Ambroise Pare*, pp. 15–16, regarding rivalries. See also, Rawcliffe, *Medicine & Society*, p. 133, for competition between surgeons and barber-surgeons, and Power (ed.), *Treatises of Fistula in Ano*, p. 71, regarding one of John Arderne's treatments for haemorrhoids: 'The treatment by incision should be kept secret lest the barbers get to know of it, to the detriment of the Master Surgeons'.
55. Sydney Young, *The Annals of the Barber-Surgeons of London, Compiled from Their Records and Other Sources* (London, Blades, East & Blades, 1890), p. 66.
56. Henry E. Sigerist, *Hieronymus Brunschwig and his Work* (New York, Ben Abramson Publisher, 1946), pp. 37–9.
57. J. F. Malgaigne, *Surgery and Ambroise Paré, translated by Wallace B. Hamby* (Norman, University of Oklahoma Press, 1965), pp. 168–70. See also, Packard, *Life and Times of Ambroise Pare*, p. 16.
58. Edouard Nicaise, *La Grande Chirurgie de Guy de Chauliac, Chirurgien, Maistre en Médicine de l'Université de Montpellier, Composée en l'an 1363* (Paris, Félix Alcan, 1890), Introduction, p. liv, 'Du temps de Guy, les barbiers faisaient d'autres opérations, et il blâme les médecins chirurgiens de dédaigner

les petites opérations, même l'arrachement des dents. Au xv siècle, les barbiers de Montpellier, à leur tour, trouvent cette opération indigne d'eux et l'abandonnent à des arracheurs de dents . . .'. 'In Guy de Chauliac's time, barbers did other procedures like tooth-pulling, and he blames surgeons for refusing to do these minor operations. In the fifteenth century, the job was passed from the barbers of Montpellier to tooth-pullers . . .'. See also, James K. Mustain, 'A Rural Medical Practitioner in Fifteenth-Century England', *Bulletin of the History of Medicine*, vol. 46, no. 5, 1972, pp. 470–1, 476, and Rawcliffe, *Medicine & Society*, p. 72.

59. Katherine Park, 'Stones, Bones and Hernias', *Medicine from the Black Death to the French Disease* (Aldershot, Ashgate Publishing Limited, 1998), pp. 117, 128, n. 45.
60. Rawcliffe, *Medicine & Society*, p. 108. See also, Packard, *Life and Times of Ambroise Pare*, p. 15.
61. Mustain, 'A Rural Medical Practitioner in Fifteenth-Century England.', p. 469. See also, Rawcliffe, *Medicine & Society*, p. 108.
62. Packard, *Life and Times of Ambroise Pare*, p. 15. See also, Rawcliffe, *Medicine & Society*, p. 108.
63. MacKaye (trans.), *The Canterbury Tales*, p. 10.
64. Ian Mortimer, *1415 Henry V's Year of Glory* (London, Vintage Books, 2010), p. 144.
65. Terry Jones, *Terry Jones' Medieval Lives*, BBC Video, 2008, Disc 2, The Philosopher. See also, MacKaye (trans.), *The Canterbury Tales*, p. 10. Chaucer sums up the work of his physician in this manner, 'He was verily a perfect practitioner. The cause known, and the root of his ill, straightway he gave the sick man his remedy'.
66. Rawcliffe, *Medicine & Society*, pp. 115–16. See also, Faye Getz, *Medicine in the English Middle Ages* (Princeton, Princeton University Press, 1998), p. 32.
67. Kevin Brown, *The Pox – The Life and Near Death of a Very Social Disease* (Stroud, Sutton Publishing, 2006), pp. 1–2.
68. Rosenman (trans.), *The Surgery of Master Jehan Yperman*, pp. 22–3. Jehan Yperman provides an example of a university-educated surgeon. See also, Reginald R. Sharpe (ed.), *Calendar of Letter-Books Preserved Among the Archives of the Corporation of the City of London at the Guildhall, Letter-Book D., Circa A.D. 1309-1314* (London, John Edward Francis, 1902), p. 47. Early in the reign of Edward II of England, Robert Newcomen is shown as apprentice to Henry the Surgeon for 10 years; Mount, *Everyday Life in Medieval London*, p. 168, and Packard, *Life and Times of Ambroise Pare*, p. 15.
69. Mount, *Everyday Life in Medieval London*, p. 168, See also, Siraisi, *Medieval and Early Renaissance Medicine*, p. 153, and Mortimer, *1415 Henry V's Year of Glory*, p. 144.

70. Henry Thomas Riley (trans.), *Memorials of London and London Life, in the XIIIth, XIVth and XVth Centuries: Being a Series of Extracts, Local, Social, and Political, from the Early Archives of the City of London A.D. 1276-1419* (London, Longmans, Green, and Co., 1868), p. 337.
71. Mount, *Everyday Life in Medieval London*, p. 168, See also, Mortimer, *1415 Henry V's Year of Glory*, p. 144.
72. Rosenman (trans.), *The Chirurgia of Roger Frugard*, p. 44.
73. Rawcliffe, *Medicine & Society*, pp. 143–4.
74. Jost Amman and Hans Sachs, *The Book of Trades (Ständebuch)* (New York, Dover Publications, Inc., 1973), p. 59, for original German language version of this poem and the image of the barber-surgeon.
75. Vern L. Bullough, 'Training of the Nonuniversity-Educated Medical Practitioners in the Later Middle Ages', *Journal of the History of Medicine and Allied Sciences*, vol. 14, no. 4, 1959, p. 453. See also, Rawcliffe, *Medicine & Society*, p. 132.
76. Packard, *Life and Times of Ambroise Pare*, pp. 15–16.
77. Rawcliffe, *Medicine & Society*, p. 133. See also, Bullough, 'Training of the Nonuniversity-Educated Medical Practitioners in the Later Middle Ages', pp. 453–4.
78. Packard, *Life and Times of Ambroise Pare*, pp. 16–17.
79. Rawcliffe, *Medicine & Society*, p. 132. See also, Sigerist, *Hieronymus Brunschwig and His Work*, p. 32. The Germanic surgeon Hieronymus Brunschwig wrote essays and treatises in his native language for the benefit of German speaking barber-surgeons.
80. Rawcliffe, *Medicine & Society*, p. 133.
81. Siraisi, *Medieval and Early Renaissance Medicine*, pp. 22–3. Caner eventually lost his licence to practice.
82. D. Lottin, *Recherches Historiques sur la Ville d'Orléans, Tome Premier* (Orléans, D'Alexandre Jacob, 1836), p. 175, '. . . et qu'il serait établi une apothicairerie garnie de drogues pour les pauvres, avec un médecin et un chirurgien experts pour les visiter'. '. . . and an apothecary was to be established, stocked with drugs for the poor, plus the expert help of a doctor and surgeon to visit them'.
83. Mount, *Everyday Life in Medieval London*, p. 161. See also, Rawcliffe, *Medicine & Society*, p. 165.
84. Rosenman (trans.), *The Surgery of Master Jehan Yperman*, pp. 31, 'All grocer-apothecaries must agree to own the book called the Antidotary of Nicolas, a complete true copy'. See also, Rawcliffe, *Medicine & Society*, p. 165, and Riley (trans.), *Memorials of London and London Life*, p. 274. Apothecaries did not always get their diagnoses right. A case in London from

1354, against John le Spicer, explains how he ended up causing his client, Thomas de Shene, more harm than good to the right side of his jaw.

85. Sir Thomas Urquhart and Peter Motteux (trans.), *Rabelais, Gargantua and Pantagruel, Translated Into English, Volume I* (London, David Nutt, 1900), p. 93.
86. Rawcliffe, *Medicine & Society*, p. 151. See also, Mount, *Everyday Life in Medieval London*, p. 162.
87. Rosenman (trans.), *The Surgery of Master Jehan Yperman*, pp. 62, 79, 182, Dr Leonard D. Rosenman (trans.), *The Surgery of Master Henri de Mondeville, In Two Volumes* (Xlibris Corporation, 1996), Volume II, pp. 949, 991, and Johnson (trans.), *The workes of that famous chirurgion Ambrose Paréy*, p. 310.
88. Siraisi, *Medieval and Early Renaissance Medicine*, pp. 146–7. See also, MacKaye (trans.), *The Canterbury Tales*, p. 10. Chaucer writes about the physician, 'He had his apothecaries full ready to send him his drugs and sirups, for each of them made the other to gain . . .'.
89. Felix J. H. Skene (ed.), *Liber Pluscardensis, Two Volumes* (Edinburgh, William Paterson, 1877), Vol. II, p. 225, '. . . while the king was severely wounded by two arrows . . .'. See also, Michael A. Penman, *David II, 1329-71* (Edinburgh, John Donald, 2005), p. 139.
90. Thomas Beaumont James and John Simons (ed.), *The Poems of Laurence Minot 1333-1352* (Exeter, University of Exeter, 1989), p. 97. The near-contemporary poem, *On the Battle of Neville's Cross*, by an unknown author, notes, 'David Bruce will not forget this battle. He was wounded, defeated and captured.' The original Latin version is in the British Library, Royal 13 A XVIII.
91. C. H. Talbot and E. A. Hammond, *The Medical Practitioners in Medieval England, A Biographical Register* (London, Wellcome Historical Medical Library, 1965), pp. 94, 386.
92. Ibid., pp. 310–12. See also, E. W. M. Balfour-Melville, *Miscellany of the Scottish History Society, Ninth Volume* (Edinburgh, T. and A. Constable Ltd, 1958), p. 3.
93. Penman, *David II, 1329-71*, p. 189, regarding John Adam and Master Jordan. See also, Balfour-Melville, *Miscellany of the Scottish History Society, Ninth Volume*, p. 4, for le Leche and Master Jordan, and Talbot and Hammond, *The Medical Practitioners in Medieval England*, pp. 198–9, for more on Master Jordan of Canterbury.
94. Johnson (trans.), *The workes of that famous chirurgion Ambrose Paréy*, p. 39.
95. James Hamilton Wylie, and William Templeton Waugh, *The Reign of Henry the Fifth, in 3 Volumes* (Cambridge, The University Press, 1914–1919),

Vol. III, p. 280. See also, Rawcliffe, *Medicine & Society*, pp. 121, 187, and Thorndike, *University Records and Life in the Middle Ages*, p. 299.

96. Riley (trans.), *Memorials of London and London Life*, pp. 464–5. In court, Clerk falsely claimed that the charm written on the parchment read, 'Soul of Christ, sanctify me; body of Christ, save me; blood of Christ, drench me; as thou art good Christ, wash me'.
97. Ibid., pp. 465–6.
98. Ibid., p. 466, a urinal was a glass flask used by medieval physicians to examine, smell and even taste a patient's urine, a practice known as Uroscopy. Such a flask was used in medieval images to indicate that an individual was a physician, See also, Rawcliffe, *Medicine & Society*, pp. 46–50, for more about Uroscopy.
99. George Eyre-Todd (ed.), *Mediaeval Scottish Poetry* (Glasgow, William Hodge & Co., 1892), p. 199.'To be a leiche he fenyt him thair', 'He feigned to be a physician there'.
100. Ibid., p. 200. The poem notes that, 'In leichecraft he was homecyd', or 'In leechcraft he was homicide'.
101. Ibid., pp. 155–6, for more on Damian.
102. Dr Leonard D. Rosenman (trans.), *The Surgery of Henri de Mondeville, In Two Volumes* (Xlibris Corporation, 1996), Vol. 1, p. 204.
103. Edouard Nicaise, *Chirurgie de Maitre Henri de Mondeville, Chirurgien de Philippe le Bel, Roi de France* (Félix Alcan, Paris, 1893), p. 102, '. . . c'était là un miracle divin, et une vengeance, de ce qu'il voulait guérir les maladies des Saints, dont le traitement doit être réservé aux seuls chirurgiens divins'.
104. Johnson (trans.), *The workes of that famous chirurgion Ambrose Paréy*, pp. 38–40.
105. Ibid., p. 39.
106. Ibid., pp. 39–40.
107. Packard, *Life and Times of Ambroise Pare*, p. 29.
108. Henry Noble MacCracken (ed.), *The Minor Poems of John Lydgate* (London, Kegan Paul, Trench, Trübner & Co., Ltd.), 1911, p. 16, verse 10.
109. Debra L. Stoudt, 'Medieval German Women and the Power of Healing', *Women Healers & Physicians, Climbing a Long Hill* (Lexington, The University Press of Kentucky, 1997), pp. 32–3. See also, Isabella Gagliardi, 'La disparition progressive des femmes médecins du Moyen Âge, une histoire oubliée', *La Conversation*, 3 January 2023, p. 4, 'La disparation progressive des femmes médecins est à mettre en relation avec les interdictions ecclésiastiques . . .', 'The gradual disappearance of female doctors is linked to prohibitions put in place by the church . . .'.
110. Siraisi, *Medieval and Early Renaissance Medicine*, p. 27.

111. Kate-Campbell Hurd-Mead, *A History of Women in Medicine from the Earliest Times to the Beginning of the Nineteenth Century* (Haddam, Conn., The Haddam Press, 1938), p. 273. See also, Stoudt, 'Medieval German Women and the Power of Healing', p. 14.
112. Stoudt, 'Medieval German Women and the Power of Healing', p. 14.
113. Hurd-Mead, *A History of Women in Medicine*, p. 311.
114. Colonel Charles L. Heizmann, 'Military Sanitation in the Sixteenth, Seventeenth and Eighteenth Centuries', *The Annals of Medicine, Volume I* (New York, Paul B. Hoeber, 1917), p. 282.
115. April Harper, 'The Image of the Female Healer in Western Vernacular Literature of the Middle Ages', *Social History of Medicine* 24, Issue 1, 2011, p. 118.
116. Robert Southey (trans.), *Amadís of Gaul, by Vasco Lobeira - In Four Volumes* (London, T.N. Longman and O. Rees, 1803), Vol. II, p. 54. The brothers are called Galaor and Florestan. See also, ibid., Vol. II, p. 72, the text later goes on to say, 'Don Galaor and Florestan remained in the castle of Corisanda till their wounds were well healed.', and ibid., pp. Vol. I, pp. 149–50, 195, Vol. II, 256, 260, for more regarding female healers.
117. Edith Rickert (trans.), *Early English Romances in Verse: Done into Modern English by Edith Rickert: Romances of Friendship* (London, Chatto and Windus, 1908), p. 170. See also, ibid., pp. 143–5.
118. Robert Southey (trans.), *Palmerin of England, by Francisco de Moraes - In Four Volumes* (London, Longman, Hurst, Rees, and Orme, 1807), Vol. I, p. 223. See also, ibid., Vol. I, p. 305 and Vol. III, 40, 47, 394.
119. David H. Rosenthal (trans.), *Tirant Lo Blanc, by Joanot Martorell & Martí Joan de Galba* (Baltimore, The Johns Hopkins University Press, 1996), p. 75. *Tirant Lo Blanc* was written for the most part by Joanot Martorell, but upon his death it was completed by Martí Joan de Galba.
120. Burfield, *Medieval Military Medicine*, pp. 34–7, for similar works from the centuries that precede the late medieval period.
121. Johnson (trans.), *The workes of that famous chirurgion Ambrose Paréy*, p. 283, from Paré's description of the metal trepanation tools he designed and created.
122. Wellcome Collection, *Alchemical and Medical Miscellany*, MS.117, pp. 207, 240. This manuscript was transcribed in 1462, by a Bartholomaeus Marcellus.
123. Burfield, *Medieval Military Medicine*, pp. 37–9.
124. C. H. Talbot, *Medicine in Medieval England* (London, Oldbourne Book Co. Ltd, 1967), pp. 195–6. See also, Getz, *Medicine in the English Middle Ages*, p. 8.
125. Wylie and Waugh, *The Reign of Henry the Fifth*, Vol. I, p. 498.

126. Ibid.
127. Getz, *Medicine in the English Middle Ages*, p. 8. Hexham was hanged for his crimes. See also, Talbot, *Medicine in Medieval England*, pp. 195–6, for other practitioners of medicine who were also moneyers.
128. Rawcliffe, *Medicine and Society*, p. 75. See also, Getz, *Medicine in the English Middle Ages*, p. 8, and Talbot, *Medicine in Medieval England*, p. 195.
129. Talbot and Hammond, *The Medical Practitioners in Medieval England*, p. 124.
130. *Calendar of the Patent Rolls, Preserved in the Public Record Office, Henry V, Vol. II, A.D. 1416-1422* (London, published for His Majesty's Stationery Office by Wyman & Sons, 1911), p. 31.
131. Johnson (trans.), *The workes of that famous chirurgion Ambrose Paréy*, pp. 576–7, 581, 586.

Chapter 2: Surgeons, Conflicts and Tournaments

1. Johnson (trans.), *The workes of that famous chirurgion Ambrose Paréy*, p. 1.
2. Rosenman (trans.), *The Surgery of Henri de Mondeville*, Vol. I, p. 63.
3. Burfield, *Medieval Military Medicine*, pp. 109–10.
4. Nicaise, *Chirurgie de Maitre Henri de Mondeville*, Préface, p. xxv, 'C'est ainsi qu'il accompagna plusieurs fois les armées, soit avec le Roi, soit avec le comte de Valois . . .'. 'He managed to accompany the armies several times, either with the King or with the Count of Valois . . .'.
5. Rosenman (trans.), *The Surgery of Henri de Mondeville*, Vol. I, pp. 55–6.
6. Nicaise, *Chirurgie de Maitre Henri de Mondeville*, pp. 187–8. 'Il en fut ainsi pour le traitement des plaies selon la méthode de Théodoric. Maître Jean Pitard et moi, qui avons les premiers apporté cette méthode en France, et l'avons employee les premiers à Paris, dans le traitement des blessures et dans plusieurs campagnes de guerre, contre la volonté et l'avis de tous, en particulier des médecins. — Nous avons enduré bien des dédains et des paroles honteuses de la part du peuple; et de la part de nos confrères, les chirurgiens, bien des menaces et des perils . . . Mais le Sérénissime prince Charles, comte de Valois, nous est venue en aide ainsi que quelques autres, qui nous avaient vu paravane dans les camps, soigner des plaies suivant cette méthode.'
7. Malgaigne, *Surgery and Ambroise Paré*, pp. 40–1, for more on Pitard.
8. Rosenman (trans.), *The Surgery of Henri de Mondeville*, Vol. I, p. 54. See also, Fielding H. Garrison, *An Introduction to the History of Medicine* (Philadelphia, W. B. Sauders Company, 1929), pp. 157–8.

9. Rosenman (trans.), *The Surgery of Henri de Mondeville*, Vol. I, p. 64.
10. Nicaise, *Chirurgie de Maitre Henri de Mondeville*, Introduction, p. xxvi, 'Je ne suis pas destiné à vivre longtemps, étant asthmatique, toussailleux, phtisique et en consomption'.
11. Rosenman (trans.), *The Surgery of Henri de Mondeville*, Vol. I, p. 67.
12. Rosenman (trans.), *The Surgery of Master Jehan Yperman*, p. 12. See also, Daniel de Moulin, *A History of Surgery, with emphasis on the Netherlands* (Dordrecht, Martinus Nijoff Publishers, 1988), p. 60.
13. Rosenman (trans.), *The Surgery of Master Jehan Yperman*, p. 23. See also, Thorndike, *University Records and Life in the Middle Ages* pp. 124–5. In the final few years of the thirteenth century, when Yperman was in Paris, war between Flanders and France meant that the French capital was not always terribly welcoming to those Flemish students who attended the university. In 1296, the French King, Philip IV, had to issue an edict protecting Flemish students, keeping them '. . . under our protection in the universities of Paris and Orléans . . .'.
14. Dr Jacques Vrebos, *The Legacy of Jehan Yperman to Plastic Surgery* (Brussels, by the Author, 1997), p. 4. Belle hospital was founded in 1276.
15. Rosenman (trans.), *The Surgery of Master Jehan Yperman*, p. 30. See also M. C. Broeckx, *La Chirurgie de Maître Jehan Yperman Chirurgien Belge (XIIIe - XIVe Siècle), Publiée pour la Première fois d'après la copie flamande de Cambridge* (Antwerp, J. de Koninck, 1866), pp. 28–9, and Moulin, *A History of Surgery*, p. 60, Moulin suggests a date of 1310 for Yperman's surgery, but 1328 seems much closer to the mark, based on actual dates within the surgeon's text.
16. Rosenman (trans.), *The Surgery of Master Jehan Yperman*, p. 13, Rosenman notes that there are a few parts of the original surgery in Picardese-French and Latin. See also, Vrebos, *The Legacy of Jehan Yperman to Plastic Surgery*, p. 2.
17. Rosenman (trans.), *The Surgery of Master Jehan Yperman*, p. 27.
18. Ibid., pp. 57, 73. See also, ibid., p. 23, for Rosenman's notes on Yperman being taught by Lanfranchi.
19. Ibid., pp. 54, 80, 221, 248, for various examples of these three surgeons. See also, Moulin, *A History of Surgery*, p. 60, and Vrebos, *The Legacy of Jehan Yperman to Plastic Surgery*, pp. 6–7. Vrebos notes that Yperman lived not far from the community of Templar Knights in Ypres, who were themselves military advisors to the local armies. He suggests they may well have shared their knowledge of Muslim, Hebrew and Greek medicine useful in the treatment of the wounds of war and those illnesses that plagued the armies of the time.

20. Moulin, *A History of Surgery*, p. 60. See also, Broeckx, *La Chirurgie de Maitre Jehan Yperman*, pp. 86, 94, 132, for examples.
21. Rosenman (trans.), *The Surgery of Master Jehan Yperman*, p. 87.
22. Janis L. Pallister (trans.), *Ambroise Paré on Monsters and Marvels* (Chicago, The University of Chicago Press, 1983), pp. 39–40.
23. Rosenman (trans.), *The Surgery of Master Jehan Yperman*, p. 87.
24. Burfield, *Medieval Military Medicine*, pp. 9–10.
25. Malgaigne, *Surgery and Ambroise Paré*, p. 53. See also, Beck, *The Cutting Edge*, p. 25.
26. Malgaigne, *Surgery and Ambroise Paré*, pp. 53–4.
27. Beck, *The Cutting Edge*, p. 25.
28. Malgaigne, *Surgery and Ambroise Paré*, p. 51.
29. Ibid., p. 53.
30. Nicaise, *La grande chirurgie de Guy de Chauliac*, Préface, p. iv, 'La Chirurgie de Guy de Chauliac est le premier livre didactique de cette science, et elle a servi à son enseignement jusqu'au xviii siècle'. See also, Rosenman (trans.), *The Major Surgery of Guy de Chauliac*, English Translator's Preface, p. c, and Malgaigne, *Surgery and Ambroise Paré*, pp. 57–8.
31. Rosenman (trans.), *The Major Surgery of Guy de Chauliac*, p. 250.
32. H. Haeser und A. Middeldorpf, *Buch der Bündth-Ertznei von Heinrich von Pfolsprundt, Bruder des deutschen Ordens, 1460* (Berlin, Druck und Verlag von Georg Reimer, 1868), Vorwort (Foreward), pp. xiii, 'Der Verfasser unserer Schrift nennt sich selbst "Heinrich von Pfolsprundt, Bruder des deutschen Ordens." In Betreff aller übrigen persönlichen Verhältnisse Sind wit lediglich auf Vermuthungen beschränkt . . .'.
33. Ibid., Vorwort, p. xv, 'Eine fernere Frage richtet sich auf die Quellen, aus denen Pfolsprundt seine Kenntnisse schöpfte. Der Inhalt seiner Schrift spricht, wie unten näher gezeigt werden wird, unzweifelhaft dafür, dass Pfolsprundt seinen ersten chirurgischen Unterricht in der Barbierstube erhielt, dass er aber auf vielfachen Wanderungen „in deutschen und welschen Landen* die Unterweisung erfahrener „Meister' genoss. Mehrere von diesen werden . . . genaunt, nämlich „Johann von Birer' (auch Bires, Biris, Birris) . . .'. See also, ibid., Vorwort, pp. xvi, 8, 25.
34. Frederick Charles Woodhouse, *The Military Religious Orders of the Middle Ages, The Hospitallers, The Templars, The Teutonic Knights, and Others* (London, Society for Promoting Christian Knowledge, 1879), pp. 287–9. The Thirteen Years' War was fought between the Teutonic Order of Knights and an alliance of Poland and the Prussian Confederation. It included the Siege of Marienburg (1457–60).
35. Haeser und Middeldorpf, *Buch der Bündth-Ertznei*, Vorwort, p. xv, '. . . die des Jahres 1460, in welchem Pfolsprundt sein werk verfasste'.

36. Garrison, *An Introduction to the History of Medicine*, p. 201, while it is clear that von Gersdorff was an army surgeon, there is debate about whether Brunschwig, while a surgeon, held a similar position with a military influence. See also, Fielding H. Garrison, *Notes on the History of Military Medicine* (Washington, Association of Military Surgeons, 1922), p. 110, and Sigerist, *Hieronymus Brunschwig and His Work*, p. 23.
37. Haeser und Middeldorpf, *Buch der Bündth-Ertznei*, Vorwort, p. xix, 'Er erwähnt ausser Birer und den übrigen "Meistern" nicht einen einzigen älteren oder neueren arzt, namentlich nicht einen einzigen chirurgischen schriftsteller; jedenfalls aus dem einfachen grunde, weil er selbst sie nicht kannte.' See also, Campbell and Colton (trans), *The Surgery of Theodoric*, Vol. I, pp. 80, 138; Rosenman (trans.), *The Surgery of Master Jehan Yperman*, pp., and Malgaigne, *Surgery and Ambroise Paré*, pp. 390–4, for examples of ancient and medieval medical practitioners commonly mentioned within other surgeries.
38. Haeser und Middeldorpf, *Heinrich von Pfolsprundt, 1460*, Vorwort, p. xix, 'Er besitzt sogar nicht die mindeste anatomische kenntniss . . .'. 'He does not have even the slightest knowledge of anatomy . . .'. While von Pfolspeundt was clearly not well versed in this area, this statement is something of an exaggeration on the part of Haeser and Middledorpf.
39. Ibid., 'Fast komisch freilich sind die sofort folgenden Vorschriften, vor dem Besuche Verwundeter nicht Zwiebeln zu essen und keinen verdächtigen Beischlaf zu üben, wegen der Gefahr, durch die hieraus entspringende Vergiftung'.
40. Sigerist, *Hieronymus Brunschwig and His Work*, pp. 11–12. See also, Moulin, *A History of Surgery*, p. 78.
41. Haeser und Middeldorpf, *Buch der Bündth-Ertznei*, Vorwort, p. xix, '. . . dass er in Fällen, denen er selbst nicht gewachsen ist, den Kranken „ williglich ' an andere erfahrene Meister verweise'.
42. Packard, *Life and Times of Ambroise Pare*, p. 19.
43. Ibid., p. 11. Packard notes that Paré may well have studied under his brother.
44. Ibid., pp. 19–20.
45. Ambroyse Paré, *La Méthode de traicter les playes faictes par hacquebutes et aultres bastons à feu et de celles qui sont faictes par flèches, dardz et semblables, aussy des combustions spécialement faictes par la pouldre à canon composée par Ambroyse Paré* (Paris, V. Gaulterot, 1545). This lengthy title of Ambroise Paré's first text translates as, 'The method of treating the wounds caused by arquebus and other fire weapons and those which are made by arrows, darts and the like, also combustion made by gunpowder composed by Ambroise Paré'.

46. Stephen Paget (trans.), *Ambroise Paré and His Times, 1510-1590* (New York, G.P. Putnam's Sons, 1897), pp. 31, 49, 52.
47. Nicaise, *Chirurgie de Maitre Henri de Mondeville*, p. 172, 'Si en effet les assistants ne sont pas soigneux et consciencieux . . . cela crée des différences et des difficultés dans l'œuvre de chirurgie.'
48. Power (ed.), *Treatises of Fistula in Ano*, p. 112, n. 9/20. See also, ibid., p. 22, 'felaw of þe lech' or 'fellow of the leech', and Dr Leonard D. Rosenman (trans.), *The Surgery of William of Saliceto* (Xlibris Corporation, 1998), p. 36 fn. 31, surgeons of lesser means and fame sometimes used the patient's friends and family as assistants.
49. Rosenman (trans.), *The Surgery of Master Jehan Yperman*, p. 25.
50. Siraisi, *Medieval and Early Renaissance Medicine*, pp. 30, 75. See also, Rawcliffe, *Medicine & Society*, p. 165, and Sigerist, *Hieronymus Brunschwig and his Work*, p. 23.
51. Packard, *Life and Times of Ambroise Paré*, p. 98, Claude Viart was with Paré for 20 years, eventually becoming a master surgeon himself. See also, Siraisi, *Taddeo Alderotti and his Pupils*, p. 112, Alessandra Giliani, may have worked with the surgeon and professor Mondino de Luzzi (c.1270–c.1326). However, the actual existence of Giliani is still a matter up for debate.
52. Rosenman (trans.), *The Surgery of William of Saliceto*, pp. 36–7.
53. Rosenman (trans.), *The Surgery of Master Henri de Mondeville*, Volume I, p. 194. See also, ibid., p. 285.
54. Nicaise, *La Grande Chirurgie de Guy de Chauliac*, p. 19. These were reiterated by de Chauliac, 'Les conditions des assistants sont quatre, qu'ils soient paisibles, gracieux, ou agreables, fidelles et discrets' or 'The four conditions of the assistants are peaceful, gracious or pleasant, faithful and discreet'.
55. Eldridge Campbell and James Colton (trans), *The Surgery of Theodoric, c. 1267– Volumes I and II* (New York, Appleton-Century Crofts, Inc., 1955), Vol. I, pp. 172, 193, 197, 217.
56. Rosenman (trans.), *The Surgery of Master Jehan Yperman*, p. 199. See also, ibid., pp. 195, 260, for other bone related injuries requiring an assistant(s) to correct the problem, and Rosenman (trans.), *The Surgery of Lanfranchi of Milan*, pp. 211, 216–17, for similar.
57. Colton (trans.), *John of Mirfield*, p. 204, Mirfield documented a method of stopping the flow of blood in weapons injuries, which relied heavily on the assistant being up close to the wound. See also, Rosenman, *The Surgery of Henri de Mondeville, Vol. II*, p. 734, de Mondeville recommends that a few assistants, who knew what to expect, be on hand during amputations, and Power (ed.), *Treatises of Fistula in Ano*, p. 22, for the role of the leech's mate during surgery to treat a fistula-in-ano.

58. Nicaise, *Chirurgie de Maitre Henri de Mondeville*, p. 243, '. . . il tirera fortement les cheveux des tempes du malade et lui parlera haut comme s'il le querellait, il l'appellera plusieurs fois de son nom dans l'oreille, et le frappera de ci et de là, lui donnera un souflet, lui frictionnera les extrémités, provoquera l'éternuement ou le vomissement avec une plume ou avec le doigt, secs ou trempés d'huile . . .'.
59. Ibid., '. . . il lui mettra des aromates sous les narines.' '. . . he (the surgeon) can try spices under the assistant's nostrils'.
60. Ibid., p. 112.
61. Ibid., p. 110, 'Non pas! Le maître ne le voudrait pas; mais vous agiriez mieux à son égard en lui offrant des coupes, ou autre chose de ce genre, bien que je sois certain que lui n'en garderait rien'.
62. Ibid., p. 110.
63. George Eyre-Todd (trans.), *The Bruce, being the Metrical History of Robert the Bruce King of the Scots, Compiled A.D. 1375, by Master John Barbour Archdeacon of Aberdeen* (London, Gowans & Gray Limited, 1907), p. 85.
64. Burfield, *Medieval Military Medicine*, pp. 12, 29.
65. Irina Metzler, *Disability in Medieval Europe – Thinking about physical impairment during the high Middle Ages, c. 1100–1400* (Abingdon, Routledge, 2006), p. 118. See also, Rosenman (trans.), *The Surgery of Master Jehan Yperman*, p. 25.
66. Broeckx, *La Chirurgie de Maître Jehan Yperman*, p. 11.
67. Talbot and Hammond, *The Medical Practitioners in Medieval England*, p. 328.
68. Joseph Bain (ed.), *Calendar of Documents Relating to Scotland, Preserved in Her Majesty's Public Record Office, London, Volume III, A.D. 1307-1357* (Edinburgh, H.M. General House, 1887), pp. 142–3 (reference from, Talbot and Hammond, *The Medical Practitioners in Medieval England*, p. 328, fn. 2), see entry 766 for extracts of the 'Medicinalia' and shipping route of Stephen the surgeon's supplies for Edward II's campaign. Among the drugs and medicines were 6lbs of apostolicon, worth 12*s*, and 2lbs of mastic, valued at 4*s*, both of which were used in the treatment of wounds.
69. William R. E. Smart, 'On The Medical Services of the Navy and Army from the Accession of Henry VIII to the Restoration', *The British Medical Journal*, 7 Feb. 1874, p. 168. When this article was written the manuscript mentioned was contained in the library of the Doria Palace in Genoa.
70. G.E. Gask, 'The Medical Services of Henry the Fifth's Campaign of the Somme in 1415', *Proceedings of the Royal Society of Medicine*, 1 May 1923, p. 3.

71. Ibid. See also, Talbot and Hammond, *The Medical Practitioners in Medieval England*, pp. 256, 296, 327, 367, for examples, men like Philip Brycheford and Robert Hynkeley were with Morestede, while Stephen Lambe and Walter Hales were among those reporting to Bredewardyn. Many of the eighteen surgeons came from London.
72. Travers Twiss (ed.), *Monumenta Juridica, The Black Book of the Admiralty, in 4 Volumes* (London, Longman, 1871) Vol. I, p. 282.'The Statutes and Ordinaunces to be Keped in Time of Werre'. See footnotes 1 and 2 for more on the origins of these ordinances.
73. Ibid., Vol. 1, p. 285, '. . . no maner of man robbe no viteler, marchaunte, leche, surgeone, barbour . . . upon the same peyne.' 'Peyne' here represents pain of death.
74. Francis Grose, *Military Antiquities Respecting a History of the English Army, from the Conquest to Present Times - Two Volumes* (London, T. Egerton Whitehall & G. Kearsley, 1801), Vol. I, pp. 239–40, for the names of the twelve surgeons.
75. Claude Bernard Petitot, 'S'ensuyt l'estat de la maison du duc Charles de Bourgongne, dict le hardy, composé par le memse auteur l'an 1474', *Collection Complète des Mémoires Relatifs a l'histoire de France, Tome X* (Paris, Foucault, Libraire, 1825), p. 493, 'Et pour ceste cause a ordonné le duc en chascune compaignie de cent lances un chirurgien . . .'.
76. Dorothy M. Schullian (trans.), *Diaria de bello Carolino (Diary of the Caroline War)* (New York, Frederick Ungar Publishing Co., 1967), p. 7.
77. James Watt, 'Surgeons of the Mary Rose, The practice of surgery in Tudor England', *The Mariner's Mirror - The International Journal of the Society for Nautical Research*, Vol. 69, No. 1, February 1983, p. 5.
78. Heizmann, 'Military Sanitation in the Sixteenth, Seventeenth and Eighteenth Centuries', p. 282. See also, William H. Prescott, *History of the Reign of Ferdinand and Isabella, The Catholic of Spain, In Three Volumes* (London, Richard Bentley, 1849), Vol. I, pp. 483–4, for Isabella.
79. Sir Edward Strachey (ed.), *Le Morte d'Arthur - Sir Thomas Malory's Book of King Arthur and of his Noble Knights of the Round Table - The Text of Caxton* (London, MacMillan and Co., Limited, 1919), p. 106. While it does seem likely that Sir Thomas Malory of Newbold Revell was the author of *Le Morte d'Arthur*, the writer's identity is not known for certain.
80. Schullian (trans.), *Diaria de bello Carolino*, p. 109.
81. Michael Mallett, *Mercenaries and Their Masters - Warfare in Renaissance Italy* (New Jersey, Rowman and Littlefield, 1974), pp. 199–200. See also, Stephen Paget (trans.), 'Journeys in Diverse Places, by Ambroise Paré',

*The Harvard Classics, Scientific Papers, Physiology * Medicine * Surgery * Geology*, Volume 38, p. 8; Garrison, *Notes on the History of Military Medicine*, p. 99, and Samuel Rush Meyrick, *A critical inquiry into antient armour: as it existed in Europe, but particularly in England, from the Norman conquest to the reign of King Charles II, with a glossary of military terms of the middle ages; In Three Volumes* (London, Robert Jennings, 1824), Vol. II, p. 26. Some knights could rely on the assistance of their squires when they became injured. The English knight, Lord James Audeley, who was wounded in the face and body at the Battle of Poitiers, was rescued by four of his squires. When he began to faint on the field of combat, they made good his escape, removed his armour, bound his wounds and provided him with refreshment.

82. Juliana Hill Cotton, 'Benedetto Reguardati of Nursia (1398-1469)', *Medical History*, Volume XIII 1969, pp. 175–6.
83. Henricus Denifle, *Chartularium Universitatis Parisiensis - Sub Auspiciis Consilii Generalis Facultatum Parisiensium - Tomus II* (Paris, Ex Typis Fratrum Delalain, 1889), p. 256, no. 812, '. . . militem, cirurgicum, discretis viris decano . . .'. In the late summer and autumn of 1322, John of Padua was involved in a case in Paris against a man called James Felicia, who had been practicing medicine illegally.
84. Thorndike, *University Records and Life in the Middle Ages*, pp. 341–2, from Launoy, *Regii Navarrae gymnasii Parisiensis historia*, 1667, I, pp. 157–8.
85. Strachey (ed.), *Le Morte Arthur*, p. 423.
86. Ibid., p. 418.
87. Timothy Lewis (ed.), *A Welsh Leech Book or Llyfr o Feddyginiaeth* (Liverpool, D. Salisbury Hughes), 1924, Introduction, p. xi, See also, Paget (trans.), 'Journeys in Diverse Places, by Ambroise Paré', p. 8, and Burfield, *Medieval Military Medicine*, pp. 30–4.
88. Schullian (trans.), *Diaria de bello Carolino*, p. 109, p. 97.
89. Siraisi, *Medieval and Early Renaissance Medicine*, p. 176.
90. Colton (trans.), *John of Mirfield*, p. 207. See also, MacKaye (trans.), *The Canterbury Tales*, p. 58, for similar in the *Knight's Tale*, '. . . some had salves and some had charms . . .'.
91. Colton (trans.), *John of Mirfield*, p. 207. See also, Rawcliffe, *Medicine & Society*, p. 95, most patients believed in such charms. In fact, they were not just the domain of uneducated soldiers, as some professionals also used them.
92. Colton (trans.), *John of Mirfield*, p. 207, pp. 207–08.
93. Revd Oswald Cockayne, *Leechdoms, Wortcunning and Starcraft of Early England, Volumes I–III* (London, Longman, Green, Longman, Roberts

and Green, 1864–6), Vol. II, p. 113, from *Bald's Leechbook*, '. . . sing over it nine times a litany, and nine times the Pater noster, and nine times this incantation.'. See also, ibid., pp. 117, 119, 293, for other examples.

94. Colton (trans.), *John of Mirfield*, p. 207.
95. Livingston and DeVries (ed.), *The Battle of Crécy*, p. 73. *Poem of the Eight Coats-of-Arms* is the only surviving poem of Jean de Batery (also Bateri).
96. Metzler, *Disability in Medieval Europe*, p. 120. See also, Edith Rickert (trans.), *Early English Romances in Verse: Done into Modern English by Edith Rickert: Romances of Love* (London, Chatto and Windus, 1908), p. 140, as described in *Sir Degrevant* these events could go on for many days, ever increasing the risk to life and limb, 'For each of fourteen days, there was a jousting of serried knights . . .'.
97. Ian Wilson, *The Book of Geoffroi de Charny, with the Livre Charny edited and translated by Nigel Bryant* (Woodbridge, The Boydell Press, 2021), p. 111.
98. Richard W. Kaeuper and Elspeth Kennedy (trans.), *The Book of Chivalry of Geoffroi de Charny: Text, Context, and Translation* (Philadelphia, University of Pennsylvania Press, 1996), p. 87, Section 4.
99. Wilson, *The Book of Geoffroi de Charny*, pp. 149–52.
100. Kaeuper and Kennedy (trans.), *The Book of Chivalry of Geoffroi de Charny*, p. 87, Section 4.
101. Christopher Gravett, *Knights at Tournament* (Oxford, Osprey Publishing Ltd. 1988), pp. 22–4.
102. Rickert (trans.), *Early English Romances in Verse: Romances of Love*, pp. 126–7.
103. Gravett, *Knights at Tournament*, pp. 50–1. See also, Time Team (DVD), *Castle Howard and Other Digs*, Disc 2, Episode 2, *Joust Dig It* (Videotext Communications Ltd., in association with The Picture House Television Co. Ltd., 2003), for more on Henry VIII's grand tiltyard at Greenwich, London.
104. James Tait (ed.), *Chronica Johannis de Reading et Anonymi Cantuariensis, 1346-1367* (Manchester, University of Manchester Press, 1914), p. 130, 'Ubi dominus Henricus, dux Lancastriae, congressu lancearum enormiter laesus, ad actus armorum postea minus valuit.' 'Henry, duke Lancaster, was seriously injured with a lance while jousting and afterward he was less able to perform acts of arms'.
105. Ibid., pp. 273–4, 'laesus fuit in crure'.
106. Viscount Harold Arthur Dillon and William St. John Hope (ed.), *Pageant of the Birth Life and Death of Richard Beauchamp Earl of Warwick K.G., 1389-1439* (London, Longmans Green and Co., 1914), pp. 67–8, the original

manuscript, known as Cottonian MS. Julius E. IV., is held in London's British Library. See also, ibid, pp. 27–8, 57–62 for more illustrations and descriptions of various of jousts and battles on foot.

107. M. L. Bellaguet, *Chronique du Religieux de Saint-Denys, Contenant le Regne de Charles VI, de 1380 a 1422, Publiée en Latin pour la Premiere Fois et Traduite, Tome Premier* (Paris, Imprimerie de Crapelet, 1839), 'Ils portèrent à messire Boucicault et à Renaud de Roye de rudes coups qui les forcèrent à garder le lit pendant neuf jours; mais grâce aux soins empressés des médecins que le roi avait envoyés et mis à leur disposition avec d'autres serviteurs de sa cour, ils se rétablirent complétement'.
108. Thomas Johnes (trans.), *The Chronicles of Enguerrand de Monstrelet; containing an account of the cruel civil wars between the houses of Orleans and Burgundy; of the possession of Paris and Normandy by the English; their expulsion thence; and of other memorable events that happened in the kingdom of France, as well as in other countries. Beginning at the year MCCCC., where that of Sir John Froissart finishes, and ending at the year MCCCCLXVII, and continued by others to the year MDXVI, In Two Volumes* (Henry G. Bohn, London, 1853), Vol. I, p. 569
109. Ibid.
110. Ibid.
111. Rosenthal (trans.), *Tirant Lo Blanc*, p. 75. See also, Southey (trans.), *Amadís of Gaul*, Vol. II, p. 34.
112. Johnson (trans.), *The workes of that famous chirurgion Ambrose Paréy*, p. 273.
113. Ibid.
114. K. Markatos, M. Karamanou, K. Arkoudi and G. Androutsos, 'Henry II of France (1519-1559) and His Death From Meningoencephalitis Following Cranial Trauma', *World Neurosurg*. 2017 Oct; 106: pp. 442–5. See also, Kian Eftekhari, Christina H. Choe, M. Reza Vagefi and Lauren A. Eckstein, 'The last ride of Henry II of France: Orbital injury and a king's demise', *Survey of Opthalmology*, Volume 60, Issue 3, May–June 2015, pp. 274–8.
115. Wilson, *The Book of Geoffroi de Charny*, p. 111.

Chapter 3: Discovery and Rediscovery

1. Julius Zupitza (ed.), *The Romance of Guy of Warwick, Part II* (London, N. Trübner & Co.,1887), p. 279, ll. 4861–2.
2. Sigerist, *Hieronymus Brunschwig and His Work*, p. 22. See also, Beck, *The Cutting Edge*, p. 14; Robert S. Gottfried, 'English Medical Practitioners,

1340-1530', *Bulletin of the History of Medicine*, vol. 58, no. 2, 1984, pp. 170–1, and Thomas Dormandy, *The Worst of Evils, The Fight Against Pain* (Yale University Press, New Haven, 2006), p. 103.

3. Nicaise, *Chirurgie de Maitre Henri de Mondeville*, p. 236.'. . . puisque ce qui est nouveau, demande nouvel avis ; aussi faut-il au chirurgien un prompt génie naturel'.
4. Power (ed.), *Treatises of Fistula in Ano*, p. 110. See also, Rosenman (trans.), *The Surgery of Henri de Mondeville*, Vol. II, p. 656, 'Perseverance will find its reward'.
5. Rosenman (trans.), *The Surgery of Henri de Mondeville*, Vol. I, pp. 218–19. See also, Hartley and Aldridge, *Johannes de Mirfield of St Bartholomew's*, p. 51.
6. Nicaise, *Chirurgie de Maitre Henri de Mondeville*, p. 346, 'S'il est utile ou nécessaire de faire l'essai d'un nouveau moyen, on le fera d'abord sur des pauvres; car s'il réussit mal, le chirurgien pourra s'excuser plus facilement', 'When it is useful or necessary to attempt a new method, try it first on a poor person, because if things go wrong they will not be able to do anything against the surgeon'. See also, Rosenman (trans.), *The Surgery of Henri de Mondeville*, Vol. I, pp. 462, 463 fn. 328.
7. Malgaigne, *Surgery and Ambroise Paré*, p. 151.
8. Ibid., p. 152.
9. Ibid.
10. Rosenman (trans.), *The Surgery of Master Jehan Yperman*, p. 186, for more on how the intestines were returned inside the abdominal cavity.
11. Malgaigne, *Surgery and Ambroise Paré*, p. 152. See also, ibid., pp. 46, 185–6, 237, 250, 271, 308, for other examples of experimentation and dissection by Ambroise Paré and others.
12. Colton (trans.), *John of Mirfield*, p. 8.
13. Rickert (trans.), *Early English Romances in Verse: Romances of Friendship*, pp. 144, 162.
14. S. Salehi, K. Koeck and T. Scheibel, 'Spider Silk for Tissue Engineering Applications'.*Molecules* 2020 Feb 8; 25 [3:] 737, p. 1 and Rosenman (trans.), *The Major Surgery of Guy de Chauliac*, p. 306.
15. Rosenman (trans.), *The Surgery of William of Saliceto*, pp. 221 no. 31, 253, no. 438, Dr Rosenman indicates that spider silk does not appear in the texts of Theodoric, William of Saliceto or Lanfranchi of Milan.
16. Rosenman (trans.), *The Surgery of Henri de Mondeville*, Vol. II, p. 778 and Rosenman (trans.), *The Surgery of Master Jehan Yperman*, p. 54.
17. Rosenman (trans.), *The Major Surgery of Guy de Chauliac*, p. 306.

18. Colton (trans.), *John of Mirfield*, p. 8.
19. Johnson (trans.), *The workes of that famous chirurgion Ambrose Paréy*, p. 747. This comes from a section of Paré's text titled 'Living Creatures, Plants and Minerals'.
20. Salehi et al., 'Spider Silk for Tissue Engineering Applications', pp. 1, 12. See also, D. Harvey, P. Bardelang, S. L. Goodacre, A. Cockayne and N. R. Thomas, 'Antibiotic Spider Silk: Site-Specific Functionalization of Recombinant Spider Silk Using "Click" Chemistry', *Advanced Materials*, Volume 29, Issue 10, March 2017, p. 1, and Simon Fruergaard, Marie Braad Lund, Andreas Schramm, Thomas Vosegaard and Trine Bilde, 'The myth of antibiotic spider silk', *iScience*, 2021, p. 1.
21. Harvey, et al, 'Antibiotic Spider Silk', pp. 1, 4.
22. Colton (trans.), *John of Mirfield*, p. 8.
23. Harvey, et al., 'Antibiotic Spider Silk', p. 1.
24. Nicaise, *Chirurgie de Maitre Henri de Mondeville*, p. 231, '. . . il fallut inventer un nouvel engin'.
25. Clive Ponting, *Gunpowder, An Explosive History: From the Alchemists of China to the Battlefields of Europe* (London, Pimlico, 2006), p. 147. See also, Philippe Contamine, *War in the Middle Ages (La guerre au moyen âge) - Translated by Michael Jones* (New York, Barnes and Noble Books, 1984), pp. 199–200.
26. Rosenman (trans.), *The Surgery of Master Henri de Mondeville*, Vol. I, pp. 356–7. See also, Oliver Jessop, 'A New Artefact Typology for the Study of Medieval Arrowheads', *Medieval Archaeology*, Vol. XL (1996), pp. 194–5, for diagrams and classification of several types of late medieval arrowheads.
27. Rosenman (trans.), *The Surgery of Master Henri de Mondeville*, Vol. I, p. 356. See also, Sir N. Harris Nicolas, *The Controversy Between Sir Richard Scrope and Sir Robert Grosvenor in the Court of Chivalry, 1385-1390, Vol. II* (London, Samuel Bentley, 1832), pp. 15–16.
28. Nicaise, *Chirurgie de Maitre Henri de Mondeville*, p. 230, 'Mais si nous enlevons la flèche, peut-être l'infirme sera-t-il sauvé'.
29. Rawcliffe, *Medicine & Society*, p. 76.
30. Haeser und Middeldorpf, *Buch der Bündth-Ertznei*, Vorwort, p. xxviii, 'Die Hauptvorschrift Pfolsprundt's bei der Verwundung durch Pfeile besteht darin, dieselben (nach vorheriger Beseitigung des über die Haut hervorragenden Holzschaftes durch Säge oder Messer), zwölf bis vierzehn Tage stecken zu lassen . . .', 'Von Pfolspeundt's main instruction around arrow wounds is to leave them in place for 12 to 14 days (after removing the wooden shaft with a knife or saw above the skin level)'. See also, Burfield, *Medieval Military Medicine*, pp. 47, 156, n. 32, for examples of this practice from earlier centuries.

31. Rosenman (trans.), *The Surgery of Master Henri de Mondeville*, Vol. I, p. 357, the process is not unlike a child's loose tooth being attached to a piece of string and then tied to a doorknob. When the door is closed, the tooth is pulled out. See also, Burfield, *Medieval Military Medicine*, p. 156, n. 37.
32. Rosenman (trans.), *The Surgery of Master Henri de Mondeville*, Vol. I, pp. 360–1.
33. Nicaise, *Chirurgie de Maitre Henri de Mondeville*, p. 235, 'Il est parfois nécessaire que le chirurgien invente de sa propre industrie, d'autres instruments que ceux-là, suivant les besoins . . .'.
34. Ibid., p. 231, n. 1. Nicase refers to this as a 'fer de garrot', or 'un trait d'arbalète', i.e. a crossbow bolt.
35. Rosenman (trans.), *The Surgery of Master Henri de Mondeville*, Vol. I, p. 351, n. 239.
36. Ibid., p. 351, n. 241.
37. Nicaise (trans.), *Chirurgie de Maitre Henri de Mondeville*, p. 231.
38. Southey (trans.), *Amadís of Gaul*, Vol. III, p. 231.
39. Sigerist, *Hieronymus Brunschwig and His Work*, p. 21.
40. Oskar Cameron Gruner (trans.), *The Canon of Medicine of Avicenna, Volume I* (New York, AMS Press, 1973), p. 413. See also, Sigerist, *Hieronymus Brunschwig and His Work*, p. 21, for other earlier examples.
41. Sigerist, *Hieronymus Brunschwig and His Work*, p. 21.
42. Campbell and Colton (trans.), *The Surgery of Theodoric*, Vol. II, pp. 212–13. See also, Burfield, *Medieval Military Medicine*, p. 55.
43. Campbell and Colton (trans.), *The Surgery of Theodoric*, Vol. II, p. 213. See also, Pierre Huard and Mirko Dražen Grmek, *Mille Ans De Chirurgie, En Occident: V – XV Siècles* (Paris, Les Éditions Roger Dacosta, 1966), p. 67, '. . . les éponges anesthésiques avaient la grosseur d'un abricot . . .', '. . . the anaesthetic sponges were the size of an apricot . . .'.
44. Campbell and Colton (trans.), *The Surgery of Theodoric*, Vol. II, p. 213. See also, Huard and Grmek, *Mille Ans De Chirurgie*, p. 67, Huard and Grmek have suggested that the narcotic benefits were absorbed through the oral and nasal mucous membranes, 'Il y avait ainsi non pas inhalation mais résorption des alcaloïdes végétaux par les muqueuses buccale et nasale'.
45. Campbell and Colton (trans.), *The Surgery of Theodoric*, Vol. II, p. 213.
46. Southey (trans.), *Amadís of Gaul*, Vol. III, p. 199.
47. Beck, *The Cutting Edge*, p. 13. See also, P. Juvin and J. M. Desmonts, 'The ancestors of inhalational anesthesia: the Soporific Sponges (XIth-XVIIth centuries): how a universally recommended medical technique was abruptly discarded', *Anesthesiology* 2000 Jul; 93 [1], p. 267.
48. Power (ed.), *Treatises of Fistula in Ano*, p. 101, 'swyneȝ grese' (swine's grease).

49. Ibid.
50. Rosenman (trans.), *The Major Surgery of Guy de Chauliac*, p. 477.
51. Ibid. See also, Strachey (ed.), *Le Morte d'Arthur*, p. 272. Intriguingly, in Malory's *Le Morte d'Arthur*, the queen and healer, Morgan le Fay, makes use of a strong liquid in her treatment of the injured knight Alisander, something that kept him asleep for three days and nights, and Brian Moffat and Other Participants in SHARP, *SHARP Practice 4, Fourth Report on Researches into the Medieval Hospital at Soutra, Lothian/Borders Region Scotland* (Edinburgh, SHARP, 1992), Section 65a.
52. Haeser und Middeldorpf, *Buch der Bündth-Ertznei*, Vorwort, pp. xli-xlii., 'Von allen den zahlreichen Heilmitteln Pfolsprundt's hat nur eins wahrhaft geschichtliches Interesse: die Anwendung narkotischer Inhalationen, um bei schmerzhaften Operationen oder bei Schlaflosigkeit Schlaf herbeizuführen', 'Of all Pfolspundt's many remedies, just one has any true historical interest: the use of narcotic inhalations, which induce sleep for painful operations or insomnia'. See also, ibid., p. 21.
53. Sigerist, *Hieronymus Brunschwig and His Work*, p. 21. See also, Garrison, *Notes on the History of Military Medicine*, p. 111, and Robert S. Holzman, 'The Legacy of Atropos, the Fate Who Cut the Thread of Life', *Anesthesiology*, 1998, 89, p. 244, for von Gersdorff.
54. Johnson (trans.), *The workes of that famous chirurgion Ambrose Paréy*, p. 278. See also, Moulin, *A History of Surgery*, p. 87.
55. Wellcome Collection, *Jackson, Jane*, MS.373, ff. 99r-99v, there are a few later examples of the use of this type of sedative, such as from this 1642 English manuscript of Jane Jackson.
56. Huard and Grmek, *Mille Ans De Chirurgie*, p. 67.
57. Campbell and Colton (trans.), *The Surgery of Theodoric*, Vol. I, p. 118.'. . . since it is impossible to apportion the medication accurately in accordance with the condition of the wounded, many patients receive somniferous medicine and sink into the sleep of death'.
58. Sigerist, *Hieronymus Brunschwig and His Work*, pp. 21–2. See also, Moffat and Other Participants, *SHARP Practice 4*, Section 65a, regarding 'cure or kill' treatment.
59. Moffat and Other Participants, *SHARP Practice 4,* Section 65a. See also, Brian Moffat, *SHARP Practice 6, The Sixth Report on Researches into the Medieval Hospital at Soutra Scottish Borders/Lothian, Scotland* (Pathhead, SHARP, 1998), p. 12, for other caches of seeds discovered at Soutra Aisle.
60. Moffat, *SHARP Practice 6*, p. 12.
61. Piers D. Mitchell, 'Anatomy and surgery in Europe and the Middle East during the Middle Ages', *Anatomy and Surgery from Antiquity to the Renaissance* (Amsterdam, Adolf Hakkert, 2016), p. 320.

62. Piers D. Mitchell, *Medicine in the Crusades – Warfare, Wounds and the Medieval Surgeon* (Cambridge University Press, 2004), p. 202.
63. Power (ed.), *Treatises of Fistula in Ano*, p. 32, 'I saw a man of Northampton that had three holes in the left buttock and three in the testicles'.
64. Ibid., p. 1.
65. Ibid., p. 107, n. 1/8, '. . . he was probably operated upon not later than 1358'. See also, ibid., p. 1.
66. Ibid., Forewords, p. xv, regarding those in civic and religious positions in medieval society.
67. Ibid., pp. 2, 109, for those in military service. See also, Ruth Putnam, *Charles the Bold, Last Duke of Burgundy, 1433-1477* (London, G.P. Putnam's Sons, 1908), p. 449, Charles the Bold, Duke of Burgundy (1433–77), is another who suffered from this problem. One of the marks searchers used to identify his naked body after the Battle of Nancy was a fistula near his groin.
68. Power (ed.), *Treatises of Fistula in Ano*, Forewords, p. xv, as Power mentions, chronic constipation is another possible cause.
69. Dr Leonard D. Rosenman (trans.), *The Surgery of Bruno da Longoburgo – An Italian Surgeon of the Thirteenth Century, by Mario Tabanelli* (Pittsburgh, Dorrance Publishing Co., Inc., 2003), p. 82. The thirteenth-century surgeon, Bruno da Longoburgo, notes that occasionally worms pass through these openings.
70. Power (ed.), *Treatises of Fistula in Ano*, p. 2.
71. Rosenman (trans.), *The Surgery of William of Saliceto*, p. 66, fn. 75. See also, Rosenman (trans.), *The Surgery of Bruno da Longoburgo*, pp. 82–3, and Campbell and Colton (trans), *The Surgery of Theodoric*, Vol. II, pp. 114–18.
72. Paul Pifteau (trans.), *Chirurgie de Guillaume de Sâlicet, Achevée en 1275* (Toulouse, Imprimerie Saint-Cyprien, 1898), p. 138, '. . . n'est certes pas guérie facilement, et il vaut mieux et il est plus honorable pour le médecin de l'abandonner'.
73. Ibid., p. 139, 'Mais crois-moi, de cette maniere il peut etre mal procede, comme je l'ai vu en mon temps, dans la cure de ces cas', 'But believe me when I tell you that I have seen this method go wrong so many times during my career'.
74. Power (ed.), *Treatises of Fistula in Ano*, Forewords, p. xvii. See also, ibid. p. 3. Arderne notes that he was the only one in England who could perform the surgery to treat an anal fistula. He says that there was one amongst the retinue of Edward III of England's son, the Black Prince, but according to Arderne he was a fraud.
75. Rawcliffe, *Medicine & Society*, p. 74. See also, Power (ed.), *Treatises of Fistula in Ano*, Forewords, p. xvii.

76. Power (ed.), *Treatises of Fistula in Ano*, Forewords, pp. xii & 10.
77. Ibid., Forewords, p. xviii. See also, Siraisi, *Medieval & Early Renaissance Medicine*, p. 185.
78. Siraisi, *Medieval and Early Renaissance Medicine*, p. 172, regarding medieval patients being restrained during surgery. See also, Rawcliffe, *Medicine and Society*, pp. 76–7, and Colton (trans.), *John of Mirfield*, p. 94, for an example of such an operation on the hand, where a board was tied to a patient's hand so that their fingers could not move.
79. Power (ed.), *Treatises of Fistula in Ano*, Forewords, pp. xvii–xviii. Power's text can be a little difficult to follow. See also, Rosenman (trans.), *The Surgery of Bruno da Longoburgo*, pp. 82–3, for the separate procedures in more straightforward language.
80. Power (ed.), *Treatises of Fistula in Ano*, Forewords, p. xviii. See also, Rawcliffe, *Medicine & Society*, p. 74, and Rosenman (trans.), *The Surgery of Bruno da Longoburgo*, p. 83. An example from the surgery of Bruno shows the caustic therapies used by other surgeons, '. . . apply astringent medicines in the tract until by corrosion . . .'.
81. Power (ed.), *Treatises of Fistula in Ano*, Forewords, p. xviii.
82. NHS Website – Treatment, Anal Fistula, www.nhs.uk/conditions/anal-fistula/treatment/.
83. Power (ed.), *Treatises of Fistula in Ano*, p. 22.
84. Ibid., p. 101.
85. Charles Lethbridge Kingsford (ed.), *Chronicles of London* (Oxford, Clarendon Press, 1905), p. 63.
86. *Calendar of the Patent Rolls, Preserved in the Public Record Office, Henry IV. Vol. II. A.D. 1401-1405* (London, printed for His Majesty's Stationery Office by Mackie and Co Ltd., 1905), p. 294.
87. British Library Board, Harley MS 1736, *Tracts on Surgery, etc*, f. 48v. See also, Henry Thomas Riley (ed.), *Chronica Monasterii S. Albani. Thomæ Walsingham Quondam, Monachi S. Albani, Historia Anglicana, Vol. II, A.D. 1381-1422* (London, Longman, Green, Longman, Roberts, and Green, 1864), p. 258, '. . . Princepsque, Regis primogentius, pertentans proeliandi primitias, ictu sagittae vulneratus in facie'.'. . . and the prince, the king's firstborn, trying the first fruits of battle, was wounded in the face by an arrow'.
88. Kingsford (ed.), *The First English Life of Henry the Fifth*, p. 9, 'Bringe me therefore wounded as I ame amongest the first and the formost of our partie, that not only by words but also by deeds I may enforce the courage of our men, as it becommeth a Prince for to doe'.
89. British Library Board, Harley MS 1736, *Tracts on Surgery, etc*, f. 48v. See also, British Library Board, Sloane MS 2272, *Anatomia Membrorum*, f. 137r,

'Castello de Kyllyngworth' and Wylie and Waugh, *The Reign of Henry the Fifth,* Volume I, p. 190, 'It was at Kenilworth that he had been nursed after receiving his "shallow scratch" at Shrewsbury . . .'.

90. British Library Board, Harley MS 1736, *Tracts on Surgery, etc*, ff. 48r-48v, '. . . after the schafte wase takyn owt and the hede ther of a bod styll in the hyndyr parte of a bone of the hede after the mesur of vj ynche . . .'. The term 'vj' here represents 6 inches.
91. S. J. Lang, 'John Bradmore and his book Philomena', *Soc Hist Med.* 1992 Apr;5 [1], pp. 124–5.
92. Ibid., p. 123.
93. British Library Board, Sloane MS 2272, *Anatomia Membrorum*, f. 137r, 'In primis tentas paruas feci et uulneri imposui de medulla sanibus ueteris et bene siccate et bene sute in panno lineo mundo ad longitudinem vulneris. Quaequidem tente intincte fuerunt in melle rose'. 'At first, I made small tents to apply to the wound, using the pith of elder, well dried to which I attached clean linen cloth so that I could reach the length of the wound. Indeed, they were dipped in rose honey'. See also, Rosenman (trans.), *The Surgery of Master Jehan Yperman*, p. 130, Yperman used smaller versions of these tents, also cut from elder, to dilate abscesses in the corner of the eye so that treatment could be administered.
94. British Library Board, Harley MS 1736, *Tracts on Surgery, etc*, f. 48v, and British Library Board, Sloane MS 2272, *Anatomia Membrorum*, 137r.
95. British Library Board, Sloane MS 2272, *Anatomia Membrorum*, f. 137r.
96. Ibid., '. . . uno squirtillo inpleto cum vino albo . . .'.
97. Ibid., 'unguento fusco'. See also, Sheila J. Lang, *The 'Philomena' of John Bradmore and its Middle English Derivative: A Perspective on Surgery in Late Medieval England (Thesis)* (St Andrews, University of St Andrews, 1998), p. 70, for more on the 'brown ointment'.
98. Kevin Goodman, 'The Strange Case of Henry V's Wandering Wound', *Ramparts: Magazine of the Friends of Dudley Castle*, Summer 2015, p. 3.
99. Ibid., p. 4.
100. T. K. Cobb, 'Wrong site surgery – where are we and what is the next step?', *Hand* (N Y). 2012 Jun; 7[2], pp. 229–30. There are up to forty operations a week in the US alone that are done on the wrong side of the body.
101. Edward Barrington de Fonblanque, *Annals of the House of Percy, from the Conquest to the Opening of the Nineteenth Century, In Two Volumes* (London, Richard Clay & Sons, 1887), Volume 1, p. 226, fn. 1, proof, if proof be needed, of the potential severity of such an injury comes from the other side of lines at the Battle of Shrewsbury. Henry Percy, known as 'Hotspur', was likely struck in the face and killed by an arrow as he was '. . . raising his

vizor to wipe his brow'. See also, Eyre-Todd (trans.), *The Bruce*, pp. 173–4, for similar.

102. Livingston and DeVries (ed.), *The Battle of Crécy*, p. 85, from the Italian *Chronicle of the Este Family*, one of the earliest chronicle sources for the Battle of Crécy. See also, ibid., p. 348.
103. John Adair, 'The Newsletter of Gerhard von Wesel, 17 April 1471', *Journal of the Society for Army Historical Research*, vol. 46, no. 186, 1968, p. 69.
104. Paolo Santoni-Rugiu and Philip J. Sykes, *A History of Plastic Surgery* (Berlin, Springer, 2007), pp. 174–7. See also, Manfredi Greco MD, Antonio Greto Ciriaco and Marco Vonella, MD and Tiziana Vitagliano, 'The Primacy of the Vianeo Family in the Invention of Nasal Reconstruction Technique', *Annals of Plastic Surgery* 64[6], June 2010, pp. 702–03, and Malgaigne, *Surgery and Ambroise Paré*, pp. 94–6.
105. Haeser und Middeldorpf, *Buch der Bündth-Ertznei*, Vorwort, p. xxxviii, the text does not mention the name of the Italian doctor from whom he learnt this procedure, but it does say he '. . . leuten mit derselben geholfen und dadurch viel Geld verdient hatte', '. . . had helped many people with it and so earned a great deal of money'. See also, Santoni-Rugiu and Sykes, *A History of Plastic Surgery*, p. 176, and Metzler, *Disability in Medieval Europe*, pp. 102–03.
106. A. K. Gupta, 'The Pioneer of Plastic Surgery – "Sushruta"', *Dev Sanskriti Interdisciplinary International Journal*, Vol. 6, July 2015, pp. 40–1. The Indian physician Sushruta, who flourished around the sixth century BC, is acknowledged as the pioneer of this type of reconstructive surgery.
107. Metzler, *Disability in Medieval Europe*, pp. 103. See also, Heinrich Schipperges, *Die Kranken im Mittelalter* (München, c.H. Beck, 1990), p. 162 (from Metzler) for the details of Abulcasis' procedure.
108. Gupta, 'The Pioneer of Plastic Surgery', pp. 40–1. This earlier practice involved using a flap of skin from the area of the cheek beside the nose as the donor tissue. While it may have been more 'comfortable' during the initial phase of the procedure, it would have been far more disfiguring in the long run.
109. Haeser und Middeldorpf, *Buch der Bündth-Ertznei*, Vorwort, p. xxxvii, 'Zuerst soll aus Pergament oder Leder ein Modell der zu . . .', 'First, a model of parchment or leather should be made . . .'. See also ibid., pp. 29–31, where this procedure is set out in the manuscript. Like other treatments in von Pfolspeundt's text, its description is made much clearer in the considerable foreword to the manuscript.
110. Ibid., 'Die beschreibung dieses theils des verfahrens ist ziemlich dunkel.' 'The description of this part of the procedure is rather obscure'.

111. Ibid., Vorwort, p. xxxviii, 'Pfolsprundt fügt schliesslich hinzu, dass auch bei bereits eingetretener vernarbung der nasenwunde die rhinoplastik ausführbar sey . . .'. 'Finally, von Pfolspeundt notes that rhinoplasty can still be performed if the nasal wound has already scarred . . .'.
112. Ibid., Vorwort, pp. xxxvii and xxxviii '. . . einlegen von zwei mit flachs umwickelten federkielen in die nasenhöhle bewirkt. Schliesslich wird die nase durch äusserlich aufgelegte säckchen in die gehörige form gebracht'.'. . . insert two quills wrapped up with flax into the nasal cavity. Finally, the nose is brought into the right shape by externally placed bags.
113. Ibid., p. 21, 'Dy erfte künft, wie man einen schlaffen macht. Wye man eynen schlaffen macht, den man schneiden wolde, ader fünft gerne schloffenn machen, der krangk were, vnd nicht schloffen künde'. See also, ibid., Vorwort, p. xli.
114. Johnson (trans.), *The workes of that famous chirurgion Ambrose Paréy*, p. 578. The evidence offered by both von Pfolspeundt and Paré backs up claims that this procedure was being used in Italy prior to 1460.
115. Ibid.
116. Ibid. See also, Schipperges, *Die Kranken im Mittelalter*, p. 162. Abulcasis added, 'Um die Heilung zu fördern, soll man einem solchen Kranken gekochte Butter zum Trinken geben; er soll auch ein Abführmittel bekommen'. 'To promote proper healing, boiled butter can be given to the patient to drink, as well as a laxative'.
117. Johnson (trans.), *The workes of that famous chirurgion Ambrose Paréy*, p. 578.

Chapter 4: Fire and Gunpowder

1. A.V. Judges (ed.), *The Elizabethan Underworld - A Collection of Tudor and Stuart Tracts and Ballads, telling of the lives and misdoings of vagabonds, thieves, rogues and cozeners, and giving some account of the operation of the criminal law* (London, Routledge & Kegan Paul Ltd., 1965), p. 98, from *A Caveat or Warning for Common Cursitors, Vulgarly Called Vagabonds*, by Thomas Harman, 1566.
2. J.W. Thomas (trans.), *Medieval German Lyric Verse - In English Translation* (Chapel Hill, The University of North Carolina Press, 1968), p. 237. See also, Johnes (trans.), *The Chronicles of Enguerrand de Monstrelet*, Vol. I, p. 312, for another such incident (5 September 1414) caused by an intentionally set fire, which led to numerous injuries and deaths, along with considerable damage to war equipment.
3. Eyre-Todd (trans.), *The Bruce*, p. 302, '. . . that had a strong covering without and many armed men within'. See also, John Norris, *Medieval Siege Warfare* (Stroud, Tempus Publishing Limited, 2007), p. 71.

4. Eyre-Todd (trans.), *The Bruce*, p. 302.
5. Ibid., p. 304.
6. Norris, *Medieval Siege Warfare*, pp. 212–13.
7. Norbert Ohler, *Krieg und Frieden im Mittelalter* (Hamburg, Nikol Verlagsgesellschaft mbH & Co, 1997), p. 261, 'Auch schüttete er aus vorragenden "Pechnasen" heiße Flüssigkeit auf die Feinde . . .' 'He poured hot liquid onto the enemies from overhanging projections . . .'. Also noted is the use of bees, lowered toward the enemy in baskets before being shaken. The irritation caused the bees to attack the soldiers, even crawling inside their armour. See also, Zürich, Zentralbibliothek, Ms. Rh. hist. 33b: War technology (Illuminated Manuscript) f. 133r, and Bern, Burgerbibliothek, Mss.h.h.I.3: Diebold Schilling, *Amtliche Berner Chronik*, vol. 3, p. 38.
8. Wylie and Waugh, *The Reign of Henry the Fifth*, Vol. II, pp. 37–8. See also, Sumner Willard (trans.) and Charity Cannon Willard (ed.), *The Book of Deeds of Arms and of Chivalry, Christine de Pizan* (Pennsylvania, The Pennsylvania University Press, 1999), p. 108.
9. Rosenthal (trans.), *Tirant Lo Blanc*, p. 141.
10. J. R. Partington, *A History of Greek Fire and Gunpowder* (Baltimore, Johns Hopkins University Press, 1999), pp. 30–1. Partington believes that Greek fire was made using a petroleum base. See also, Norris, *Medieval Siege Warfare*, p. 172; Willard (trans.) and Cannon Willard (ed.), *The Book of Deeds of Arms and of Chivalry*, p. 141 fn. 113, and Burfield, *Medieval Military Medicine*, pp. 80–1.
11. J. A. Giles (trans.), *Roger of Wendover – Flowers of History, In Two Volumes* (London, Henry G. Bohn, 1849), Vol. II, p. 409. See also, Willard (trans.) and Cannon Willard (ed.), *The Book of Deeds of Arms and of Chivalry*, p. 141.
12. Partington, *A History of Greek Fire and Gunpowder*, p. 103, Battle of St Omer. See also, Power (ed,), *Treatises of Fistula in Ano*, Forewords, p. xiii, siege of Algeçiras, and Norris, *Medieval Siege Warfare*, p. 213, siege of Breuteil.
13. Riley (ed.), *Chronica Monasterii S. Albani. Thomæ Walsingham Quondam, Vol. II*, pp. 98–9.
14. Norris, *Medieval Siege Warfare*, p. 173. See also, Willard (trans.) and Cannon Willard (ed.), *The Book of Deeds of Arms and of Chivalry*, p. 141, fn. 113.
15. Burfield, *Medieval Military Medicine*, p. 81, for sources where engineers and specialists were involved in the procurement and use of Greek fire. See also, Partington, *A History of Greek Fire and Gunpowder*, p. 27, for a Hungarian engineer using Greek fire at Constantinople in 1453.
16. Eyre-Todd (trans.), *The Bruce*, p. 293.

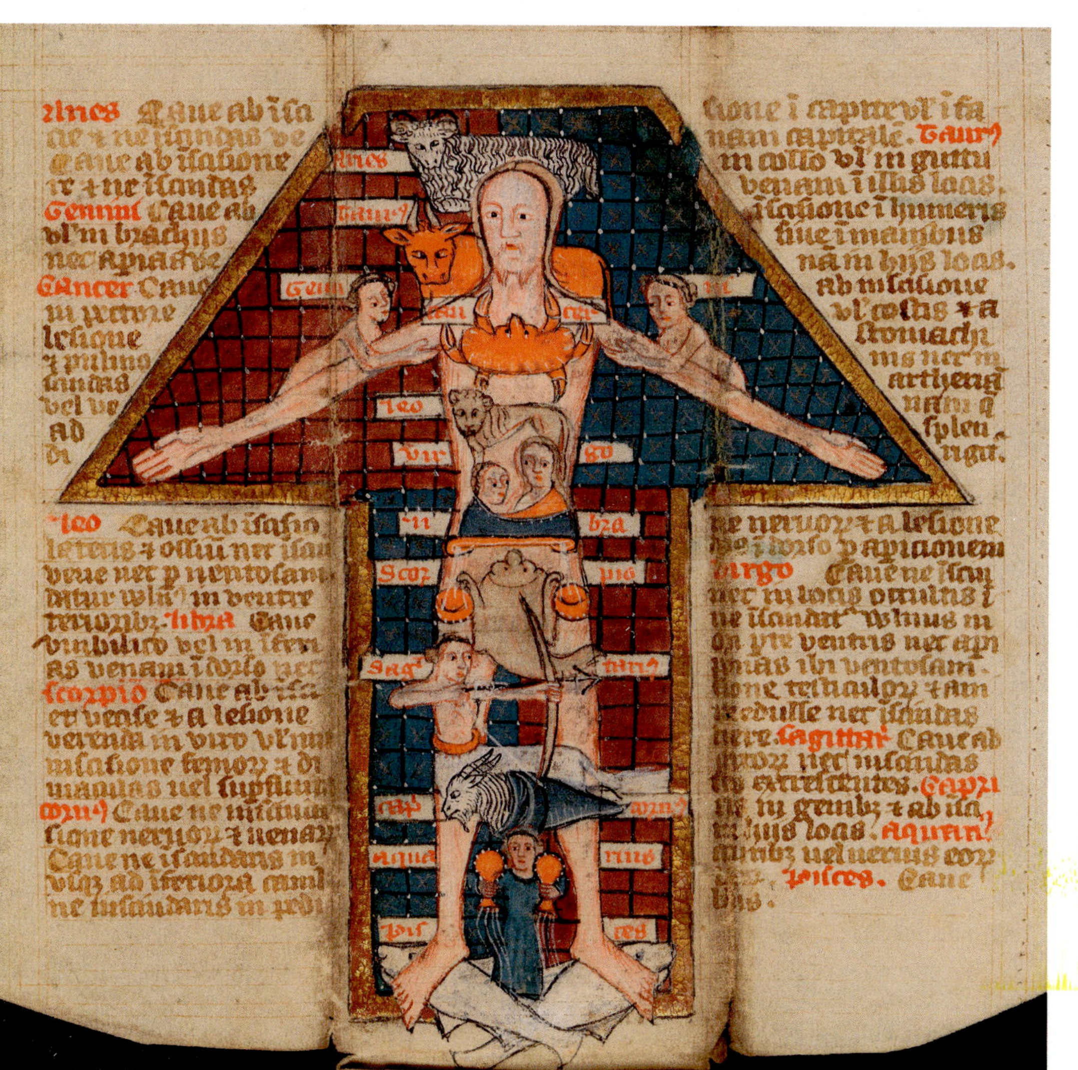

1. Zodiac Man. (From an English folding almanac in Latin, Date: c. 1415–20, MS.8932, f. 5. Courtesy of the Wellcome Collection)

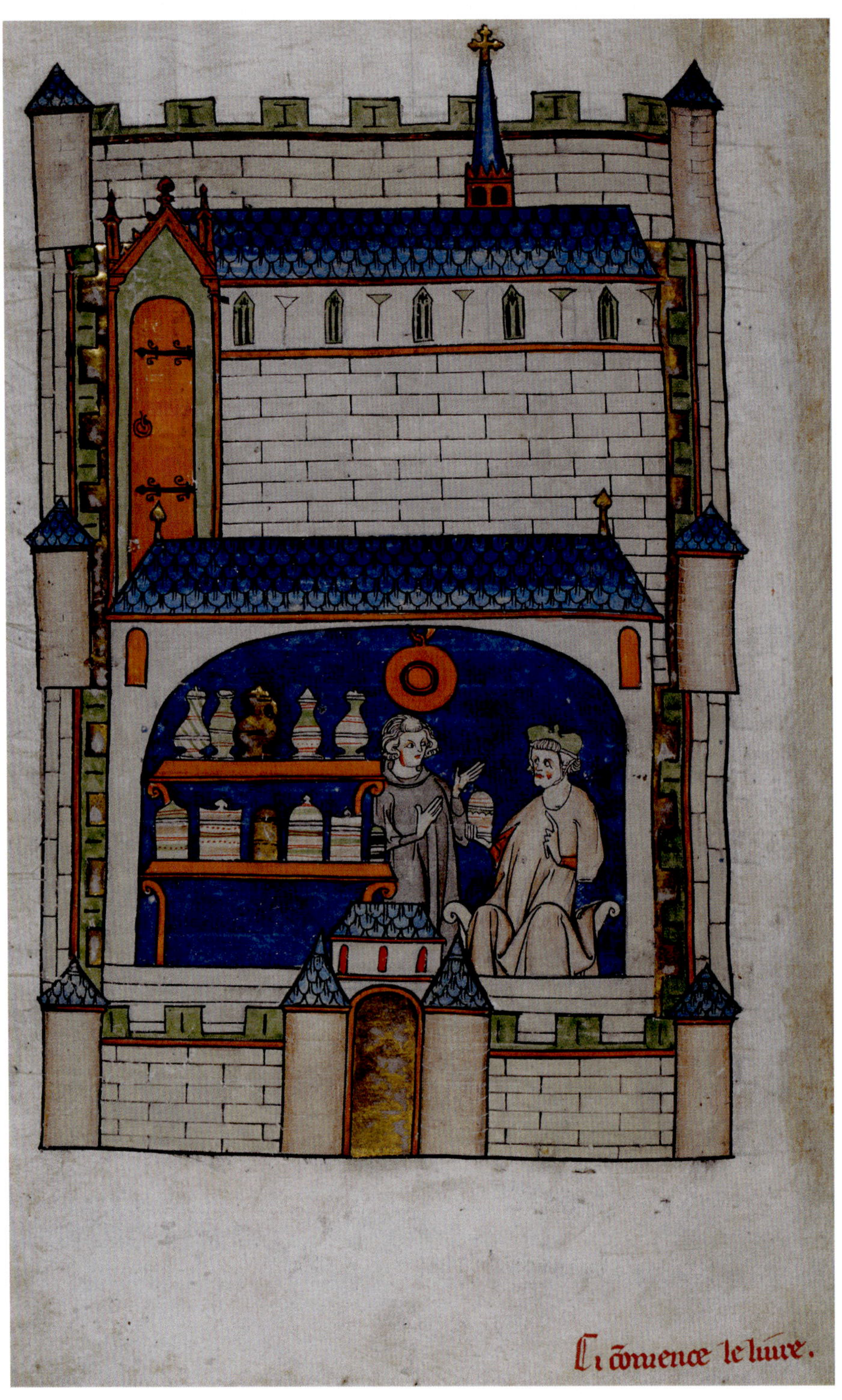

2. An apothecary's shop, showing jars and boxes of medicines on the shelves, and a flat dish for mixing ingredients. (Frugardi, Roger, of Parma, France (near Amiens); 1300–10, Courtesy of the British Library archive, Sloane 1977, f. 49v)

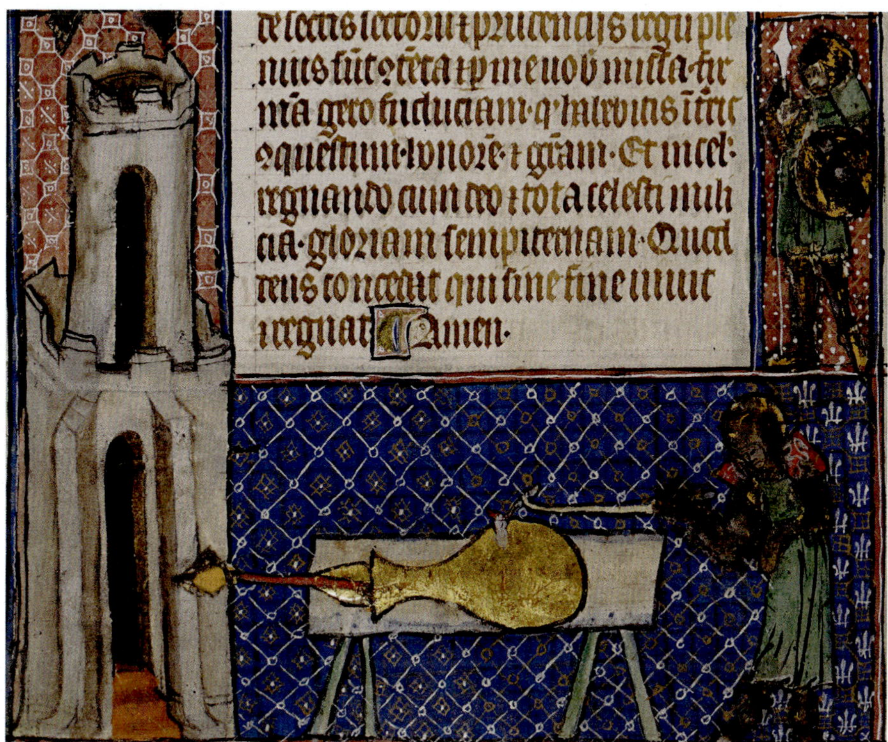

Above: **3.** From an English manuscript, attributed to Walter of Milemete, dating from 1326–7, depicting one of the earliest European images of a cannon. (De Nobilitatibus Sapientii Et Prudentiis Regum Manuscript, Courtesy of the Governing Body of Christ Church, Oxford, MS 92 fol. 70v)

Right: **4.** Depiction of the dreadful consequences of a cannon misfire or accident – fifteenth century. (Courtesy of Zürich, Zentralbibliothek, Ms. Rh. hist. 33b: War technology (Illuminated Manuscript), f. 102r)

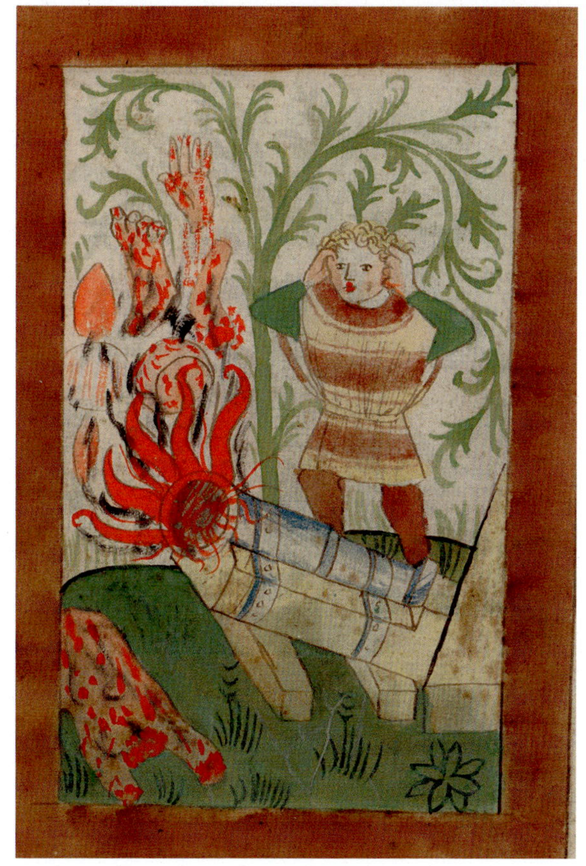

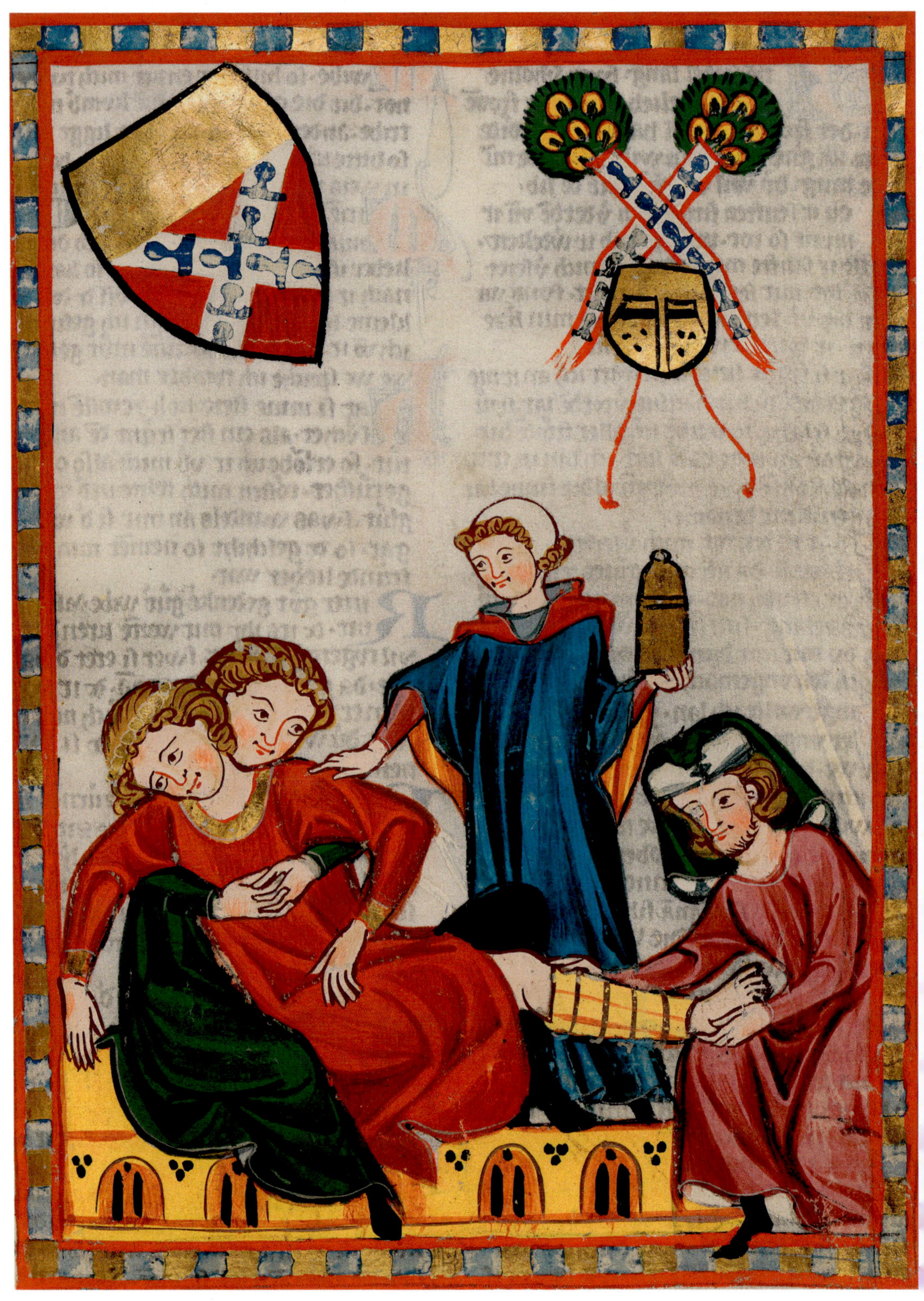

5. Treatment for a knight who has suffered a broken leg – fourteenth century. (Courtesy of Universitätsbibliothek Heidelberg, Große Heidelberger Liederhandschrift (Codex Manesse), 1340, Cod. Pal. germ. 848, f. 158r)

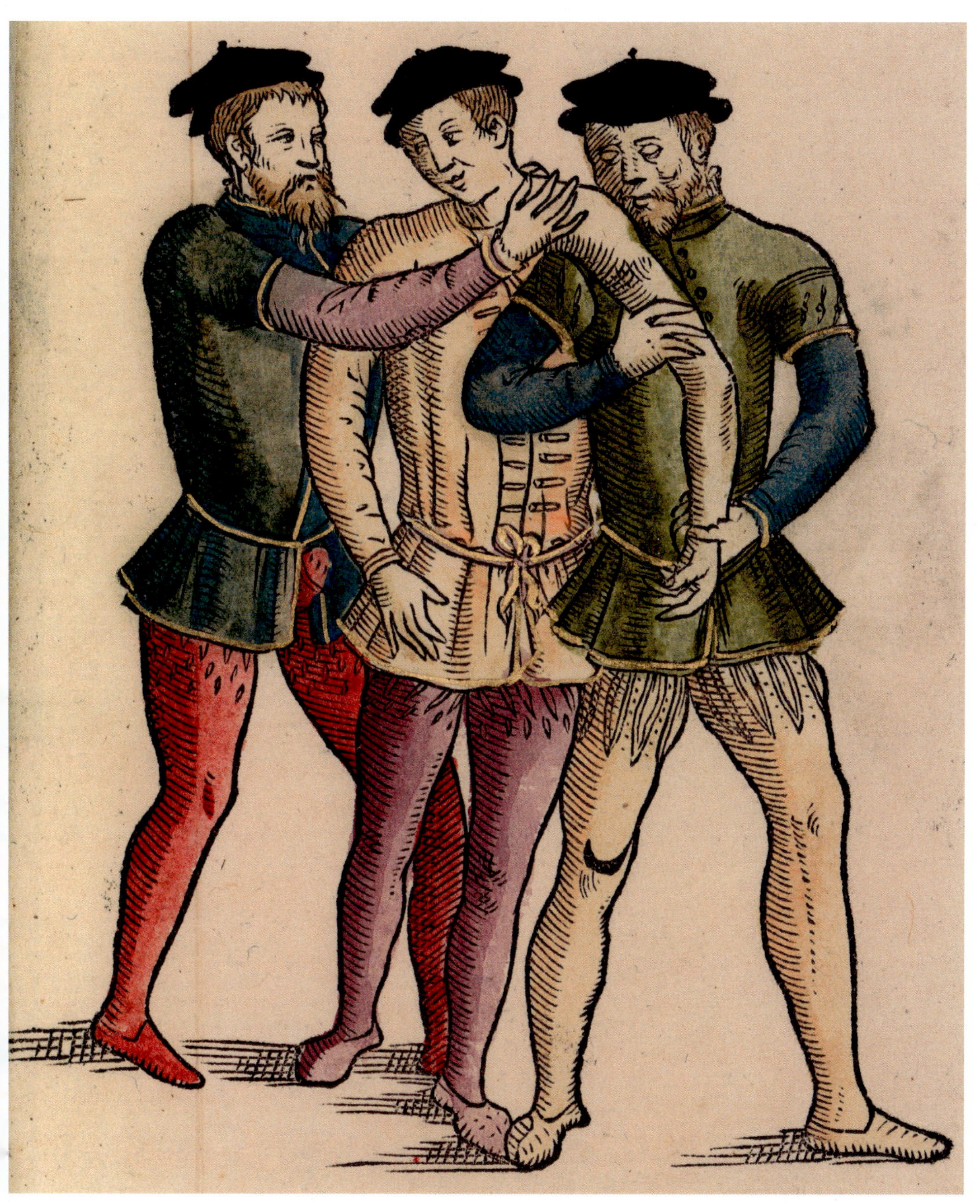

6. The dislocated shoulder of a patient is reduced by a surgeon holding and shaking the patient as the assistant pulls the arm downwards. (1564 – *Instrumenta chyrurgiae et icones anathomicae* / [Ambroise Paré], p. 267. Courtesy of the Wellcome Collection)

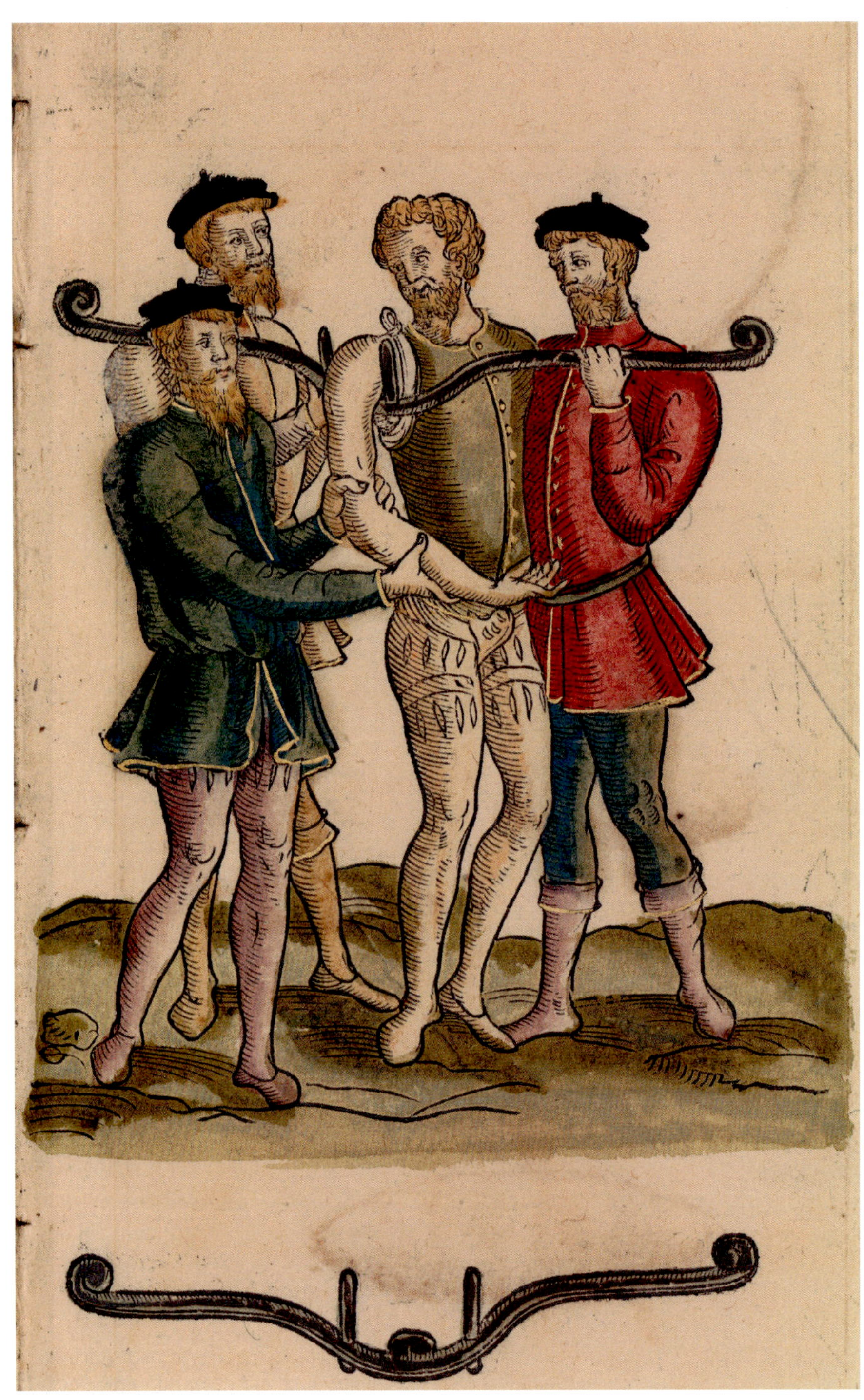

7. A surgeon reduces a dislocated shoulder with the help of two assistants holding a bar under the patient's armpit. (1564 – *Instrumenta chyrurgiae et icones anathomicae* / [Ambroise Paré], p. 303. Courtesy of the Wellcome Collection)

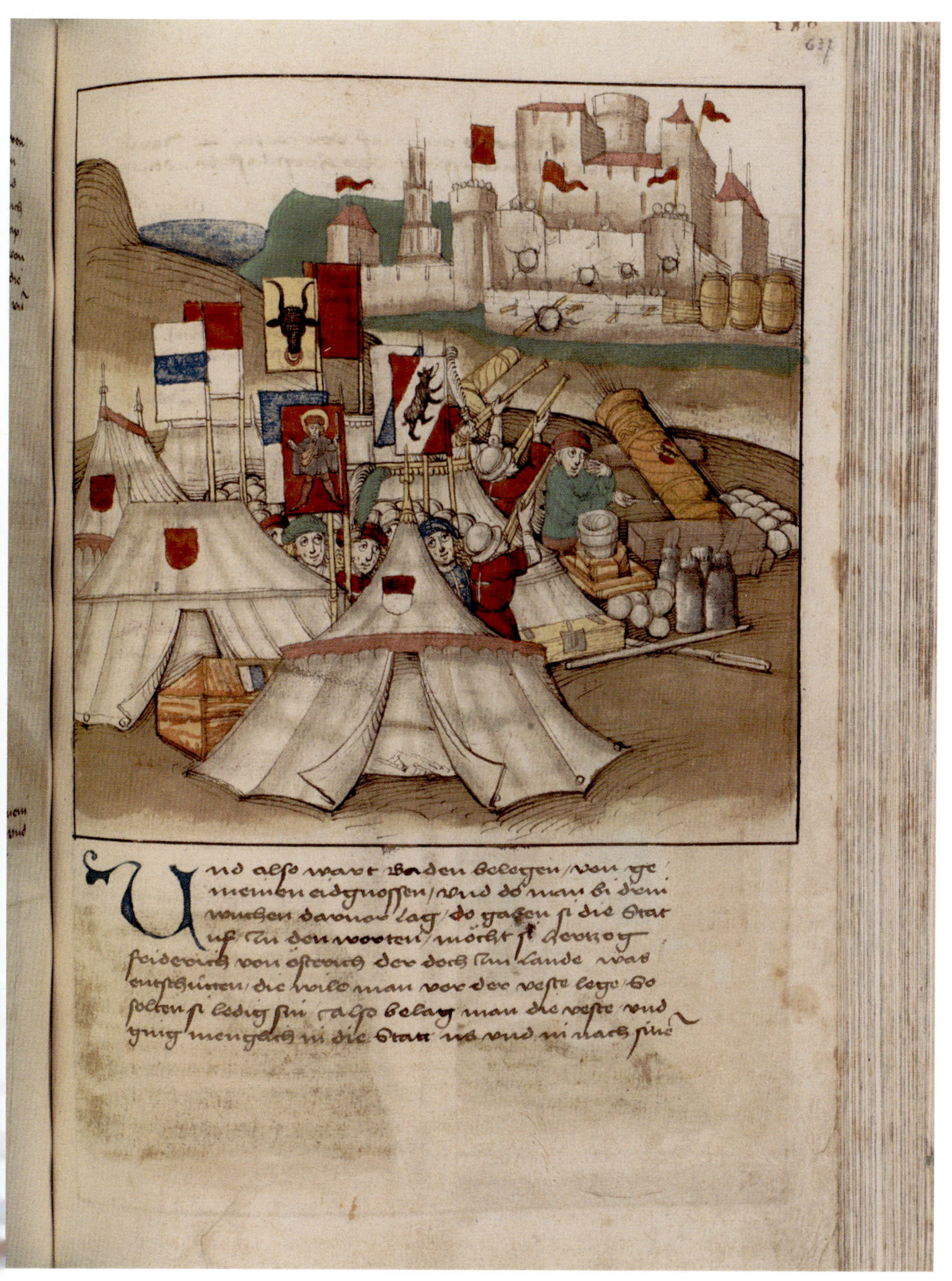

Und also wart Baden belegen von ge
meinen eidgnossen/ und do man bi dem
wuchen darvor lag/ do gaben si die Stat
uf Zu den worten/ möcht si hertzog
fridrich von österrich der doch Zun lande was
entschütten/ die wolt man vor der veste lege So
solten si ledig sin/ also belag man die veste und
gyng mengklich in die Statt us und in nach sine

8. A cannoneer, wearing green, attempts to shield his left ear from the blast of the cannon as it is ignited – fifteenth century. (Diebold Schilling, *Spiezer Chronik*, Courtesy of Burgerbibliothek Bern, Mss.h.h.I.16, p. 637)

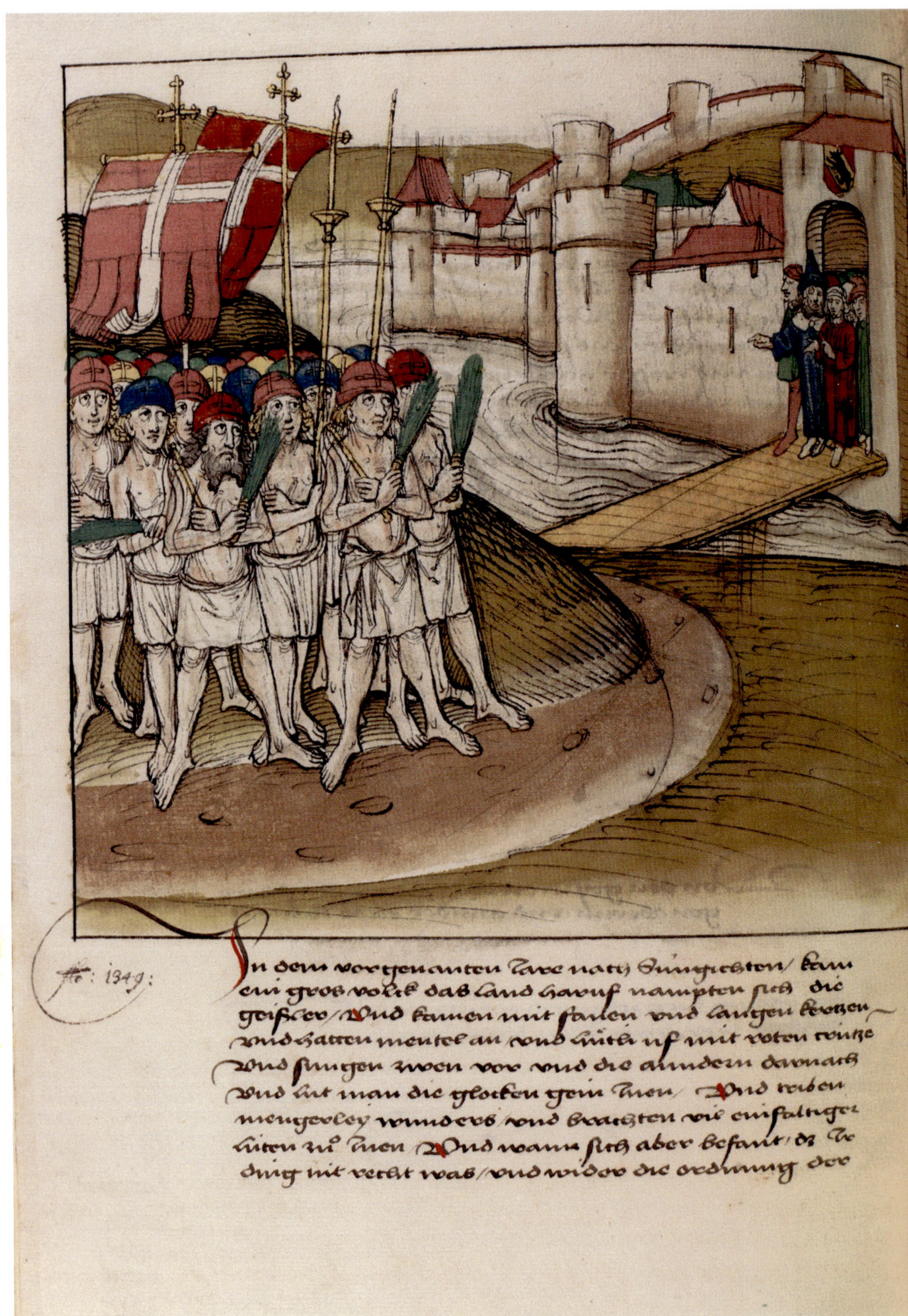

9. Flagellants arrive at Bern in 1349 during the Black Death – fifteenth century. (Diebold Schilling, *Spiezer Chronik*, Courtesy of Burgerbibliothek Bern, Mss.h.h.I.16, p. 336)

17. Willard (trans.) and Cannon Willard (ed.), *The Book of Deeds of Arms and of Chivalry*, p. 141, '. . . a certain fire, which some call Greek fire . . . no Christian soldier should make use of such inhumane weapons . . .'.
18. Camille Favre et Léon Lecestre (ed.) *Le Jouvencel par Jean de Bueil, Suivi du commentaire de Guillaume Tringant, Tome Sécond* (Paris, Renouard H. Laurens successeur, 1887), pp. 57–8, '. . . chrestien n'est loisible de user de telles inhumanitez qui meismement sont contre tout droit de guerre . . . lequel aucuns appellent feu grec'.'. . . a Christian is not permitted to use such inhumanities which are even against all rights of war . . . which some call Greek fire'. See also John Payne (trans.), *Poems of François Villon* (Boston, John W. Luce & Company, 1917), p. 179. Another reference to Greek fire from the mid-fifteenth century can be found in a poem by François Villon called *Ballade joyeuse des Taverniers*, or *A Merry Ballad of Vintners*. It contains a litany of punishments that would befall any taverner who should be foolish enough to water down the wine they sold. Among the potential penalties: 'Singe their perukes with Greek fire', perukes, i.e. wigs.
19. Shaun F. D. Hughes (trans.), 'The Saga of Án Bow-Bender', *Medieval Outlaws, Ten Tales in Modern English* (Stroud, Sutton Publishing, 1998), p. 199, 'The retainers leaped to and snatched him from the fire, and Björn was badly burned'.
20. Ibid.
21. Rosenman (trans.), *The Surgery of Master Jehan Yperman*, pp. 235, 311, an ointment made from warm wine and cow faeces mixed with egg yolk comes from the treatise called *Experimentator*.
22. Ibid., p. 235.
23. Ibid., p. 236.
24. Rosenman (trans.), *The Major Surgery of Guy de Chaulic*, p. 473 and Rosenman (trans.), *The Surgery of Henri de Mondeville*, Vol. II, pp. 806.
25. Rosenman (trans.), *The Major Surgery of Guy de Chauliac*, p. 473.
26. Rosenman (trans.), *The Surgery of Henri de Mondeville*, Vol. II, p. 807.
27. Nicaise, *La Grande Chirurgie de Guy de Chauliac*, p. 431, 'La seconde intention est accomplie, en ouvrant les vessies avec ciseaux, ou quelque dechiquetoir'.
28. Rosenman (trans.), *The Major Surgery of Guy de Chauliac*, p. 473.
29. Johnson (trans.), *The workes of that famous chirurgion Ambrose Paréy*, p. 334. A second therapy recommended by Paré was a pain-relieving ointment used by the women who treated burn patients in the Hôtel Dieu hospital in Paris during the sixteenth century. It was made by mixing the yolks of eight freshly-laid eggs with lard, rosewater and a narcotic such as henbane.

30. Ibid., p. 310.
31. Ibid. See also Burfield, *Medieval Military Medicine*, pp. 54, 158, for earlier uses of onions, leeks and salt to treat burns and wounds.
32. Johnson (trans.), *The workes of that famous chirurgion Ambrose Paréy*, p. 310.
33. Packard, *Life and Times of Ambroise Paré*, p. 29.
34. Hartley and Aldridge, *Johannes de Mirfield of St Bartholomew's*, pp. 90–1, from Part XIII, Distinction 4, Chapter 12 of de Mirfield's text. See also, Colton (trans.), *John of Mirfield*, Introduction, p. xiv.
35. Willard (trans.) and Cannon Willard (ed.), *The Book of Deeds of Arms and of Chivalry*, p. 109.
36. Davies, *The Medieval Cannon*, pp. 4–7. See also, Partington, *A History of Greek Fire and Gunpowder*, Preface, p. 106, gunpowder was known in Europe from the thirteenth century, and quite famously, had originated in China at least two or three centuries prior to that.
37. John Bourchier (Lord Berners) (trans.) and G.C. Macaulay (ed.), *The Chronicles of Froissart* (London, MacMillan and Co., Limited, 1904), p. 246, among the many others noted in this chapter.
38. Guillaume Dupuytren, *Traité, théorique et pratique, des blessures par armes de guerre, rédigé d'après les leçons cliniques de m. le baron Dupuytren, Tome Premier* (Paris, J.B. Baillière, 1834), Préface, p. xxxiv, 'C'est dans le quinzième siècle seulement que les plaies par armes à feu commencèrent à être considérées comme devant nécessairement entrer dans les manuels de chirurgie', 'It was only during the fifteenth century that gunshot wounds started to be considered as necessary in surgical manuals.'
39. Rosenman (trans.), *The Surgery of Master Jehan Yperman*, p. 162, fn. 143. Rosenman questions what Yperman meant by 'firearms', suggesting that he might have been referring to shrapnel wounds. Despite being brief, it represents one of the earliest references to injuries caused by gunpowder weapons found in any sort of European text, medical or otherwise.
40. Malgaigne, *Surgery and Ambroise Paré*, p. 62.
41. Partington, *A History of Greek Fire and Gunpowder*, pp. 323–4. See also, Hartley and Aldridge, *Johannes de Mirfield of St Bartholomew's*, pp. 90–1.
42. Hartley and Aldridge, *Johannes de Mirfield of St Bartholomew's*, p. 45. In their 'Introductory', the authors note the recipe for gunpowder being 'somewhat out of place in a work devoted to the Healing Art . . .'.
43. Garrison, *An Introduction to the History of Medicine*, p. 201.
44. Johnson (trans.), *The workes of that famous chirurgion Ambrose Paréy*, p. 767.
45. Davies, *The Medieval Cannon*, p. 9.

46. Axel E. W. Müller, *Gunpowder Technology in the Fifteenth Century, A Study, Edition and Translation of the Firework Book* (Woodbridge, The Boydell Press, 2024), p. 89. See also, Cyril Stanley Smith, and Martha Teach Gnudi (trans.), *The Pirotechnia of Vannoccio Biringuccio, The Classic Sixteenth-Century Treatise on Metals and Metallurgy* (New York, Dover Publications, Inc. 1990), pp. 422–8, 433–5.
47. Davies, *The Medieval Cannon*, pp. 4–7. See also, Partington, *A History of Greek Fire and Gunpowder*, Preface, p. 106.
48. Ponting, *Gunpowder, An Explosive History*, pp. 108–09. See also, Jonathon Sumption, *The Hundred Years War - Trial by Battle* (Philadelphia, University of Pennsylvania Press, 1991), p. 528; Partington, *A History of Greek Fire and Gunpowder*, p. 314, and Davies, *The Medieval Cannon*, p. 9.
49. Partington, *A History of Greek Fire and Gunpowder*, pp. 314–15.
50. Desmond Seward, *A Brief History of the Hundred Years War, The English in France, 1337-1453* (London, Robinson, 2003), p. 258, regarding the 'corning' of gunpowder, a method of processing which had the unexpected benefit of making it more powerful. See also, Davies, *The Medieval Cannon*, p. 11, and Partington, *A History of Greek Fire and Gunpowder*, p. xxvii.
51. Seward, *A Brief History of the Hundred Years War*, p. 55. See also, Frank Bottomley, *The Castle Explorer's Guide* (New York, Avenel Books, 1979), pp. 24–5.
52. Ponting, *Gunpowder, An Explosive History*, p. 115. See also, Andrew R. Scoble (ed.), *The Memoirs of Philip de Commines, Lord of Argenton: Histories of Louis XI. and Charles VIII. Kings of France, and of Charles the Bold, Duke of Burgundy. To which is added, The Scandalous Chronicle or Secret History of Louis XI., by Jean de Troyes - Two Volumes* (London, Henry G. Bohn, 1855–6), Vol. I, p. 29. In 1465, at the Battle of Montlhéry, 'A barrel of their powder was accidentally blown up where the king had been, which set fire to several waggons that were placed along the hedge'; and Johnes (trans.), *The Chronicles of Enguerrand de Monstrelet*, Vol. II, p. 363.
53. Petitot, 'S'ensuyt l'estat de la maison du duc Charles de Bourgongne, dict le hardy, composé par le memse auteur l'an 1474', p. 493.
54. Garrison, *An Introduction to the Historien of Medicine*, p. 201.
55. Johnson (trans.), *The workes of that famous chirurgion Ambrose Paréy*, p. 310. See also, ibid., p. 767, for another serious case.
56. Ibid., p. 310.
57. Ibid., p. 334.
58. Ibid., p. 335. See also, Malgaigne, *Surgery and Ambroise Paré*, p. 111. The Florentine anatomist and physician Antonio Benivieni (c.1440–1507) treated

a young girl whose forearm became attached to her upper arm by scar tissue after she was badly scalded. First, he dissected the scar, which released her forearm from the upper arm. The girl was still unable to fully extend her arm, so Benvieni gave her a small weight to carry around in her hand. She continued to increase the length of time that she held it until her arm could be fully extended.

59. Johnson (trans.), *The workes of that famous chirurgion Ambrose Parëy*, p. 335.
60. Patricia Skinner, 'Looking for Burn Victims or Survivors in Medieval Europe', *Trauma in Medieval Society* (Leiden, Brill, 2018), pp. 98–9.
61. Johnson (trans.), *The workes of that famous chirurgion Ambrose Parëy*, p. 767.
62. Trevor Russell Smith and Michael Livingston (ed.), *Of Knyghthode and Bataile* (Michigan, Medieval Institute Publications, 2021), p. 108, line 2854.
63. Ponting, *Gunpowder, An Explosive History*, p. 107.
64. Ibid. See also, Davies, *The Medieval Cannon*, pp. 4–5.
65. Davies, *The Medieval Cannon*, p. 10.
66. Brigadier O.F.G. Hogg, *English Artillery, 1326-1716, Being the History of Artillery in this Country Prior to the Formation of the Royal Regiment of Artillery* (London, Royal Artillery Institution, 1963), p. 49. See also, Bourchier (trans.) and Macaulay (ed.), *The Chronicles of Froissart*, p. 289, and Davies, *The Medieval Cannon*, p. 11.
67. Davies, *The Medieval Cannon*, pp. 27–8. See also, Ponting, *Gunpowder, An Explosive History*, pp. 26–7.
68. Hogg, *English Artillery*, pp. 49–50. See also, Schullian (trans.), *Diaria de bello Carolino*, p. 101, 'Iron, bronze and lead balls sped hissing aloft . . .'
69. Contamine, *War in the Middle Ages*, p. 199.
70. Ibid. See also, Ponting, *Gunpowder, An Explosive History*, p. 110.
71. Contamine, *War in the Middle Ages*, p. 199.
72. Schullian (trans.), *Diaria de bello Carolino*, p. 101. This continued to be the case for some time to come, as the Battle of Fornovo in July 1495 shows.
73. Ponting, *Gunpowder, An Explosive History*, pp. 109, 147, 157–62. See also, ibid., p. 118. The first known sinking of a ship by gunfire was not until 1499; Johnes (trans.), *The Chronicles of Enguerrand de Monstrelet*, Vol. II, p. 402, and John Scoffern, *Projectile Weapons of War and Explosive Compounds* (London, Cooke & Whitley, 1852), pp. 13–17.
74. Seward, *A Brief History of the Hundred Years War*, p. 227. See also, Ponting, *Gunpowder, An Explosive History*, p. 115.
75. Contamine, *War in the Middle Ages*, p. 200.

76. Ibid.
77. Mortimer, *1415 Henry V's Year of Glory*, p. 338. See also, Hogg, *English Artillery*, p. 205, and, Geoffrey Hindley, *Medieval Sieges and Siegecraft* (New York, Skyhorse Publishing, 2009), pp. 66–7.
78. Riley (ed.), *Chronica Monasterii S. Albani. Thomæ Walsingham Quondam, Vol. II,* p. 308.
79. Sir William Hardy and Edward Hardy (trans.), *A Collection of the Chronicles and Ancient Histories of Great Britain, Now Called England - by John de Wavrin, Lord of Forestel - from A.D. 1399 to A.D. 1422* (London, Eyre and Spottiswoode, 1887), pp. 370–1.
80. Louis Claude Douët-D'Arcq, *Choice de Pièces Inédites Relatives au Règne De Charles VI, Tome Second* (Paris, Jules Renouard et Cio, 1864), p. 86, '. . . il est griefment malade et mutillé en l'une de ses jambes d'un coup de canon en manière qu'il ne se peut aidier . . .', '. . . he is grievously unwell and one of his legs is mutilated by cannon shot and nothing can be done . . .'.
81. Geoffrey Hilton (trans.), *The Deeds of Henry V Told by John Streeche* (Kenilworth, published by the Author, 2014), p. 51. See also, Seward, *A Brief History of the Hundred Years War*, p. 258. During the Siege of Cherbourg (1450), four cannons exploded.
82. J. G. MacKay (ed.), *The Historie and Cronicles of Scotland - from the Slauchter of King James the First to the Ane thousande fyve hundreith thrie scoir fyftein zeir - Written and Collected by Robert Lindsay of Pitscottie, Three Volumes* (Edinburgh, William Blackwood and Sons, 1899), Vol. I, p. 143, '. . . king did stand neir hand by the gunneris quhen the artaillzerie was dischargand . . . ane peace of ane misframit gune that brak in the schutting, be the quhilk he was strickin to the ground and dieit haistelie thairof . . .'. See also, ibid., p. 148, for a poem about the death of James II at the siege of Roxburgh Castle, which describes the explosion of the cannon that killed him, and Rev. John Silvester Davies, *An English Chronicle of the Reigns of Richard II., Henry IV., Henry V., and Henry VI. - Written before the year 1471* (London, The Camden Society, 1856), p. 99.
83. Zürich, Zentralbibliothek, Ms. Rh. hist. 33b: War technology (Illuminated Manuscript), f. 163r. See also, Davies, *The Medieval Cannon*, p. 26.
84. Henry W. L. Himes, *Gunpowder and Ammunition Their Order and Progress* (London, Longmans, Green and Co., 1904), pp. 206–07, fn. 1. In 1479, near Paris, a cannon burst, killing fourteen and wounding another fifteen or sixteen.
85. Colonel B. Noland Carter and Lieutenant Colonel Michael E. DeBakey, 'Current Observations on War Wounds of the Chest', *The Journal of Thoracic*

Surgery, August 1944, Vol. 13, No. 4, p. 276. While these medieval blasts did not have the impact of a high explosive shell of the First World War, they still would have caused devastating injuries to those standing close enough to the explosion when the weapon failed.

86. Johnson (trans.), *The workes of that famous chirurgion Ambrose Paréy*, p. 315.
87. Ponting, *Gunpowder, An Explosive History*, pp. 115–17.
88. Andrew Lang (trans.), *The Miracles of Madame Saint Katherine of Fierbois* (London, David Nutt, 1897), p. 148.
89. Ibid., p. 149. The entry notes that the miracle had been, '. . . affirmed to be true, in presence of Messire Georges Guiot, priest, Brother Pierre Queroan, warders of this chapel, Guillaume Guierrier, and several others'.
90. Ibid., p. 148.
91. Vallet de Viriville (ed.), *Chronique de Charles VII, roi de France, Par Jean Chartier, Nouvelle Édition Revue Sur Les Manuscrits, Suivie de divers Fragmens inédits, Trois Tomes* (Paris, P. Jannet, 1858), Tome II, p. 317, '. . . et entra le boulet en sa jambe entre les deux os . . .', '. . . the ball entered his leg between the two bones . . .'.
92. Ibid., '. . . lequel fut incontinent retiré , et fut si bien pensé î par les médecins et chirurgiens, que le péril du feu en fut mis hors', '. . . which was removed immediately and was so well thought through by the doctors and surgeons that the need for cauterization was eliminated'. See also, Viriville (ed.), *Chronique de Charles VII, roi de France*, Tome III, p. 28, for another injury related to a culverin. Mr. Jehan Justinian had to seek unspecified medical treatment after being hit.
93. Garrison, *An Introduction to the History of Medicine*, p. 201, fn. 3, for the more modern German language of the text from which this is translated, 'Auch machstu solchs suchel wol von eissen machenn . . . mith dem hebstu die kleine gelodt oder kugel hiraus, die von buchsenn hinein geschossenn sein, und auch was sunst in den wunden ist'. See also, Haeser und Middeldorpf, *Buch der Bündth-Ertznei*, p. 60, for original language, and Garrison, *Notes on the History of Military Medicine*, p. 110.
94. Rosenman (trans.), *The Chirurgia of Roger Frugard*, p. 47. See also, Dr Leonard D. Rosenman (trans.), *The Surgery of Roland of Parma* (Xlibris Corporation, 2001), p. 42, and Burfield, *Medieval Military Medicine*, pp. 43, for the example of Mathfred.
95. Schullian (trans.), *Diaria de bello Carolino*, p. 175.
96. Haeser und Middeldorpf, *Buch der Bündth-Ertznei*, p. 135. See also, Garrison, *Notes on the History of Military Medicine*, p. 110.
97. Garrison, *Notes on the History of Military Medicine*, p. 110. See also, Sigerist, *Hieronymus Brunschwig and His Work*, p. 22.

98. Schullian (trans.), *Diaria de bello Carolino*, p. 175.
99. Sigerist, *Hieronymus Brunschwig and His Work*, pp. 22–3. See also, T. Clifford Allbutt, *The Historical Relations of Medicine and Surgery to the End of the Sixteenth Century* (London, MacMillan and Co., Limited, 1905), p. 84. Allbutt suggests that both Brunschwig and Gersdorff believed, '. . . that these wounds were envenomed burns; so that the chief aim of the surgeon should be to destroy the dead flesh and to neutralise the venom'; Moulin, *A History of Surgery*, p. 79, Moulin is less certain about Gersdorff's belief in a poisoned wound; and Malgaigne, *Surgery and Ambroise Paré*, p. 206.
100. Sigerist, *Hieronymus Brunschwig and His Work*, p. 23. See also, Rawcliffe, *Medicine & Society in Later Medieval England*, pp. 152–3; Alixe Bovey, *Tacuinum Sanitatis, An Early Renaissance Guide to Health* (London, Sam Fogg, 2005), p. 54, no. 16, treacle being dispensed by an apothecary, and Johnson (trans.), *The workes of that famous chirurgion Ambrose Parey*, p. 555, 'Treacle, which hath for an ingredient the flesh of Vipers . . .'.
101. Siraisi, *Medieval & Early Renaissance Medicine*, pp. 118–19. See also, Carole Rawcliffe, *Leprosy in Medieval England* (Suffolk, The Boydell Press, 2009), p. 220.
102. Malgaigne, *Surgery and Ambroise Paré*, p. 182, Malgaigne refers to the method as 'deplorable'.
103. Johnson (trans.), *The workes of that famous chirurgion Ambrose Parey*, p. 309, 'Now I have read in *John de Vigo* that wounds made by Gunshot were venenate or poisoned, and by that reason . . . for their cure, it was expedient to burn or cauterize them with oil of Elders scalding hot, with a little Treacle mixed therewith.'
104. Packard, *Life and Times of Ambroise Paré*, p. 158, fn. 20. Paré notes the year of this campaign as 1536, but it was in fact 1537.
105. Johnson (trans.), *The workes of that famous chirurgion Ambrose Parey*, p. 309.
106. Ibid.
107. Ibid.
108. Ibid.
109. Malgaigne, *Surgery and Ambroise Paré*, pp. 239–40.
110. Johnson (trans.), *The workes of that famous chirurgion Ambrose Parey*, p. 783.
111. Packard, *Life and Times of Ambroise Paré*, p. 174. Paré suggests this occurred in 1543, but it was 1542.
112. Burfield, *Medieval Military Medicine*, p. 47. The idea of the patient standing in the same position they had been in just prior to the injury harkens back to Roger Frugard's twelfth-century surgery. When treating a patient who had suffered

an arrow wound, he suggested that it was best to discover which direction the arrow had entered from to help establish where it may have ended up.

113. Ibid., p. 46. The *Eyrbyggja Saga*, written in the thirteenth century, describes a similar event. Snorri, a temple priest and healer, removed a small arrowhead from a warrior by first locating it with his hands at the base of the soldier's throat.
114. Johnson (trans.), *The workes of that famous chirurgion Ambrose Parèy*, p. 316. See also, Packard, *Life and Times of Ambroise Paré*, pp. 174–5.
115. Johnson (trans.), *The workes of that famous chirurgion Ambrose Parèy*, p. 308. Even at this point in the early history of gunpowder, there was already a huge number of weapons that relied on its force, some of which are spelled out by Paré.
116. Ibid., p. 776.
117. Thérouanne, in northern France, was the location of the headquarters of the First Division of the Portuguese Army during the First World War.
118. Osbert Sitwell, *Argonaut and Juggernaut* (London, Chatto & Windus, 1919), p. 122. The poet and writer Osbert Sitwell saw active service during the First World War until he suffered blood poisoning in 1916.

Chapter 5: Bones, Teeth and Skulls

1. MacKaye (trans.), *The Canterbury Tales*, p. 56, from the *Knight's Tale*.
2. Southey (trans.), *Amadís of Gaul*, Vol. III, p. 270. Rather confusingly, Amadís is already disguised as the Knight of the Green Sword by this point in the tale. See ibid., Vol. II, p. 239.
3. Ibid., Vol. III, pp. 289–90.
4. Ibid., Vol. III, p. 294.
5. Wilson, *The Book of Geoffroi de Charny*, p. 119. See also, Kaeuper and Kennedy, *The Book of Geoffroi de Charny*, pp. 175, 177, Section 40, likely written by de Carney's son, Geoffroi II de Charny, 'For, whoever might want to consider the hardships, pains, discomforts, fears, perils, broken bones and wounds which the good knights who uphold the order of knighthood as thy should endure and have to suffer frequently . . .'.
6. Smith and Livingston (ed.), *Of Knyghthode and Bataile*, pp. 34, 123, regarding line 457.
7. Marian T. Park, Giancarlo Mignucci-Jiménez, Lena Mary Houlihan and Mark C. Preul, 'Management of injuries on the 16th-century battlefield: Ambroise Paré's contributions to neurosurgery and functional recovery', *Neurosurgical Focus*, 2022 Sep; 53[3], p. 3.
8. Johnson (trans.), *The workes of that famous chirurgion Ambrose Parèy*, p. 766.

9. Ibid., p. 363.
10. Rosenman (trans.), *The Surgery of Master Jean Yperman*, pp. 260–2. See also, Rosenman (trans.), *The Major Surgery of Guy de Chauliac*, pp. 415, 421; Haeser and Middeldorpf, *Buch der Bündth-Ertznei*, pp. 68–79, and Johnson (trans.), *The workes of that famous chirurgion Ambrose Parey*, pp. 369–74.
11. Burfield, *Medieval Military Medicine*, pp. 60–3. See also, Tony Waldron, *Palaeopathology* (Cambridge, Cambridge University Press, 2009), pp. 148–9, in the archaeological record, ribs tend to rank among the most common types of healed fractures found in adult skeletons.
12. Rosenman (trans.), *The Surgery of Henri de Mondeville*, Vol. II, p. 539.
13. Southey (trans.), *Amadís of Gaul*, Vol. II, p. 204.
14. Strachey (ed.), *Le Morte d'Arthur*, p. 103.
15. Rosenthal (trans.), *Tirant Lo Blanc*, p. 330.
16. Rosenman (trans.), *The Surgery of Master Jehan Yperman*, p. 262.
17. Ibid., pp. 138 fn. 109, 267–8. See also, Power (ed.), *Treatises of Fistula in Ano*, p. 130 n. 74/26.
18. Rosenman (trans.), *The Major Surgery of Guy de Chauliac*, p. 417.
19. Ibid.
20. Ibid., pp. 417–18.
21. Ibid., p. 418. See also, Johnson (trans.), *The workes of that famous chirurgion Ambrose Parey*, p. 368. Paré wrote about the severity of the pain involved with broken ribs, calling it, '. . . a pricking pain, far more grievous then in a plurisie . . .'.
22. Rosenman (trans.), *The Major Surgery of Guy de Chauliac*, p. 418.
23. Johnson (trans.), *The workes of that famous chirurgion Ambrose Parey*, p. 368.
24. Ibid.
25. Ibid.
26. Smith and Livingston (ed.), *Of Knyghthode and Bataile*, p. 32, line 379, 'Th'entrails ar covert in steel and bonys'. See also, Southey (trans.), *Amadís of Gaul*, Vol. III, pp. 198–9, for an example.
27. Carter et al., 'Current Observations on War Wounds of the Chest', pp. 286–7.
28. Johnson (trans.), *The workes of that famous chirurgion Ambrose Parey*, pp. 777–8.
29. Richard Strange, *The Life and Gests of St. Thomas of Hereford – From the Original 1674 Printing* (London, Burns and Oates, 1879), p. 142.
30. Willard (trans.) and Cannon Willard (ed.), *The Book of Deeds of Arms and of Chivalry*, p. 1, and Smith and Livingston (ed.), *Of Knyghthode and Bataile*, p. 7. Writers like Christine de Pizan and the anonymous poet who wrote *Of Knyghthode and Bataile* relied heavily on the text of Vegetius for their works. See also, Kaeuper and Kennedy, *The Book of Chivalry of Geoffroi de Charny*,

pp. 85, 87, Sections 3 and 4. By contrast, Geoffroi II de Charny's late fourteenth-century knightly manual, *The Book of Chivalry*, depended much less on the Roman writer, if at all. The text of de Charny represents more of an ideal of a knight's life, which does include a strong focus on military exercise.

31. Flavius Vegetius Renatus, *De Re Militari – Concerning Military Affairs* (Leonaur, 2012), p. 68.
32. Willard (trans.) and Cannon Willard (ed.), *The Book of Deeds of Arms and of Chivalry*, p. 24. See also, Smith and Livingston (ed.), *Of Knyghthode and Bataile*, p. 49, ll. 887–8.
33. Mallett, *Mercenaries and Their Masters*, p. 199.
34. BBC, *History Cold Case*, Series One, Episode Three, *Stirling Man* (London, Shine TV Limited and Red Planet Pictures, 2011), see minutes 50–51 regarding identity. See also, BBC News article, *Stirling Castle knight revealed as English nobleman*, 21 May 2010.
35. BBC, *History Cold Case*, Series One, Episode Three, *Stirling Man*, see minutes 30–31.
36. Ibid., see minutes 26–27.
37. Bari Hooper, Stephanie Rickett, Andrew J. G. Rogerson and Susan Yaxley, 'The grave of Sir Hugh de Hastyngs, Elsing', *Norfolk Archaeology*, vol. 39 (1984/86), pp. 93–4.
38. Ibid., pp. 94–6.
39. Ian Mortimer, *The Time Traveller's Guide to Medieval England – A Handbook to Visitors to the Fourteenth Century* (London, The Bodley Head, 2008), pp. 262–3. See also, Martyn Whittock, *A Brief History of Life in the Middle Ages* (London, Constable & Robinson Ltd, 2009), p. 193.
40. Emily Sarah Jocelyn Mitchell, *War, Wounds, and Medicine: A Re-Examination of the Crew of the Mary Rose (Thesis)* (Southampton, University of Southampton, 2022), pp. 148–9. See also, Black, *Written in Bone*, pp. 206–07; BBC News, *Mary Rose skeletons studied by Swansea sports scientists*, 12 March 2012, and Paris, Bibliothèque nationale de France, Département des manuscrits, Français 2643, *Chroniques de Jehan Froissart*, ff. 165v, 207r. Medieval archers adopted an awkward stance that engaged as many muscles as possible in order to pull large, heavy war bows. This meant repeatedly contorting the back and side into unorthodox positions, as shown by these two illustrations, bottom left of image, f. 165v, and bottom right of image f. 207r.
41. Esther Cohen, *The Modulated Scream* (Chicago, The University of Chicago Press, 2009), p. 4.
42. Irina Metzler, 'Disability in the Middle Ages: Impairment at the Intersection of Historical Inquiry and Disability Studies', *History Compass*, Vol. 9, Issue 11, January 2001, p. 48.

43. Cohen, *The Modulated Scream*, pp. 93–4.
44. Rawcliffe, *Medicine & Society*, p. 135. See also, Gruner (trans.), *The Canon of Medicine of Avicenna, Volume I*, p. 238. Still popular in the fourteenth and fifteenth centuries, Avicenna had recommended a number of mineral baths that could be used for different applications, including sulphur baths, 'These soothe and warm the nerves and relieve pain', and Siraisi, *Medieval and Early Renaissance Medicine*, pp. 30, 137.
45. Mallett, *Mercenaries and Their Masters*, p. 199.
46. Irina Metzler, *A Social History of Disability in the Middle Ages – Cultural Considerations of Physical Impairment* (New York, Routledge, 2013), pp. 52–4, 235 n. 119. See also, Mitchell, *Medicine in the Crusades*, pp. 121–2, for an image and description of healed lumbar fractures from a Frankish male dated to the twelfth or thirteenth century. This was a common type of injury caused by a fall from height.
47. Strange, *The Life and Gests of St. Thomas of Hereford*, p. 142.
48. Ibid., p. 143.
49. Rosenman (trans.), *The Surgery of Lanfranchi of Milan*, p. 212. See also, Metzler, *Disability in Medieval Europe*, p. 306, n. 336. Dr Metzler suggests that Lanfranchi may have omitted a procedure for spinal injuries because they so often led to paralysis, something that was incurable anyway.
50. Campbell and Colton, *The Surgery of Theodoric*, Vol. I, p. 192.
51. Ibid.
52. Ibid.
53. Ibid.
54. Rosenman (trans.), *The Major Surgery of Guy de Chauliac*, p. 413.
55. Ibid.
56. Packard, *Life and Times of Ambroise Paré*, p. 182, for le Connestable as a French general.
57. Ibid., p. 257.
58. Johnes (trans.), *The Chronicles of Enguerrand de Monstrelet*, Vol. I, p. 508. The Lyonnel mentioned here is Lyonnel de Vandonne, unhorsed by l'Estandart de Mailly during a siege in 1423.
59. François Plaine (ed.), *Monuments du procès de canonisation du bienheureux Charles de Blois, duc de Bretagne, 1320-1364* (Saint-Brieuc: Imprimerie de R. Prud'homme, 1921), pp. 281–2. See also, Jonathon Sumption, *The Hundred Years War - Volume III, Divided Houses* (London, Faber and Faber Ltd., 2009), pp. 98–9, 762, for details of this siege and the date of February 1371, and Wilson, *The Book of Geoffroi de Charny*, p. 115, for similar in Geoffroi de Charny's *Livre*.

60. Plaine (ed.), *Monuments du procès de canonisation du bienheureux Charles de Blois*, p. 282, '. . . et brachium dextrum eciam fractum et deslocatam, et fuit pluribus lapidibus percussus ita fortiter quod in pluribus partibus corporis sui erat quasi totaliter denigratus, et in isto statu remansit in dova seu fossatis dicti castri, et tunc socii istius de dicta dova per super quoddam palicium ipsum extraxerunt . . . . . .' '. . . and his right arm was also broken and dislocated, and being struck with several stones so strongly many parts of his body were almost completely blackened, and in that state he remained in the ditch until his comrades pulled him to safety using a cloak . . .'.
61. Ibid., '. . . et in dicto loco de Claromonte fecit rupturas et dislocaciones predictas bituminari seu colari . . .' 'and in the said place of Clermont he had the aforesaid breaks and wounds treated with bitumen . . .'. See also, Sumption, *The Hundred Years War - Volume III*, pp. 762–3.
62. Plaine (ed.), *Monuments du procès de canonisation du bienheureux Charles de Blois*, p. 282, '. . . et dixerunt sibi cirurgici Parisii quod dicte rupture et dislocaciones erant in bono statu . . .' '. . . and the Parisian surgeons said to him that the injuries and damages were in good condition . . .'.
63. Johnson (trans.), *The workes of that famous chirurgion Ambrose Parèy*, p. 388. Paré notes, 'The shoulder is easily dislocated . . .'. See also, Waldron, *Palaeopathology*, p. 155, who also states that the shoulder is the one most frequently and easily dislocated joints of the body.
64. Bourchier (trans.) and Macaulay (ed.), *The Chronicles of Froissart*, p. 50, Sir Henry has his arm pulled out of the socket, and Schullian (trans.), *Diaria de bello Carolino*, p. 173, a leader of the Venetian infantry, Niccolò Savorgnan, suffered a dislocated shoulder when his horse became frightened and fell on top of him. See also, Strachey (ed.), *Le Morte d'Arthur*, pp. 73, 116, and Southey (trans.), *Palmerin of England*, Vol. I, pp. 185–6, 333, Vol. III, p. 388, for more of these types of injuries.
65. Jared A. Wolfe, Daniel L. Christensen, Timothy C. Mauntel, Brett D. Owens, Lance E. LeClere, and Jonathan F. Dickens, 'A History of Shoulder Instability in the Military: Where We Have Been and What We Have Learned', *Military Medicine*, Volume 183, Issue 5-6, May-June 2018, p. 158.
66. Ibid., p. 160.
67. Joseph and Frances Gies, *Life in a Medieval Castle* (New York, Harper & Row Publishers, 1981), p. 180. See also, Kaeuper and Kennedy, *The Book of Chivalry of Geoffroi de Charny*, pp. 85, 87, Sections 3 and 4.
68. Rosenman (trans.), *The Chirurgia of Roger Frugard*, p. 112. See also, Rosenman (trans.), *The Surgery of Roland of Parma*, pp. 75–6, and Rosenman (trans.), *The Surgery of William of Saliceto*, pp. 168–71.

69. K. Markatos, M. Karamanou, G. Tsouroufl is, G. Androutsos and A.F. Mavrogenis, 'Ambroise Paré (1510–1590): on the diagnosis and treatment of shoulder dislocations', *Int Orthop.* 2018 Jan; 42 [1], pp. 215–16.
70. Rosenman (trans.), *The Major Surgery of Guy de Chauliac*, p. 427. One of his methods is recognizable from previous centuries. The patient lay flat with a ball wedged into their armpit. The surgeon then pushed their heel against the ball while manipulating the arm back into place. See also, Burfield, *Medieval Military Medicine,* p. 66, for more on the earlier method.
71. Rosenman (trans.), *The Major Surgery of Guy de Chauliac*, p. 427.
72. Ibid.
73. Ibid.
74. Ibid., p. 428.
75. Haeser und Middeldorpf, *Buch der Bündth-Ertznei*, Vorwort, p. xxix, Wie grosse Schwierigkeiten die Einrichtung veralteter Luxationen machte, geht auch daraus hervor, dass Pfolsprundt dem Wundarzte den Rath ertheilt, vorher Messe zu hören', 'The difficulty in resetting an old dislocation can be seen in the fact that von Pfolspeundt recommends that the surgeon say mass first'.
76. Ibid., 'sie erfordern die sechs-bis zwölfmalige Wiederholung eines den ganzen Tag hindurch fortgesetzten Bades, erweichende Umschläge', 'they require bathing and softening compresses six to twelve times per day'.
77. Ibid., 'Das sehr undeutlich beschriebene Verfahren bei der Einrenkung scheint sich vorzüglich auf Luxationen nach aissen und hinten zu beziehen…Nach erfolgter Reposition wird zur Fixirung des Oberarm-Kopfes eine hollered in Charpie gehüllte Kugel in die Achselhöhle gebracht'., 'The very vaguely described procedure for realignment seems to refer primarily to outward and posterior dislocations . . . After the reduction has been completed, a wooden ball covered in charpie (lint) is placed in the armpit to keep the head of the upper arm fixed in position'.
78. Johnson (trans.), *The workes of that famous chirurgion Ambrose Parèy*, pp. 389–96.
79. Ibid., p. 390, 'Thus the shoulder, drawn downwards by the one which stands under the armhole, and moved and shaken by the other . . .'.
80. Ibid., pp. 389–90.
81. Ibid., p. 390, the bandage was to be, 'two els long'. An ell varied in length from country to country. In France it was approximately 1.37m or 54in, while in England, it was about 1.14m or 45in.
82. Ibid.
83. Ibid.

84. Rickert (trans.), *Early English Romances in Verse: Romances of Friendship*, p. 141, from *The Story of Grey-Steel*.
85. Rosenthal (trans.), *Tirant Lo Blanc*, p. 280.
86. Hooper et al., 'The Grave of Sir Hugh de Hastyngs, Elsing', p. 96. The damage included five teeth that were completely broken off and another that was partially fractured. A further tooth, the upper right second incisor, may also have been broken during the same incident, as it had to be extracted just weeks before his death in 1347. Sir Hugh's upper left second incisor is another that could have been extracted at the same time.
87. Burfield, *Medieval Military Medicine*, p. 68. See also, Hooper et al., 'The Grave of Sir Hugh de Hastyngs, Elsing', pp. 96–8. Also found within Sir Hugh's grave is evidence of either a wig or a hat. If it is a wig, it is especially indicative of a man concerned about his appearance.
88. Michel Hébert, 'L'armée provençale en 1374', *Annales du Midi, revue archéologique, historique et philologique de la France méridionale*, Tome 91, N°141, 1979, p. 8 [4]. Although the roll is now just a fragment, Michel Hébert was still able to examine many of the details of this late fourteenth-century group of fighting men in this well-regarded study from 1979.
89. Ibid., p. 22 [18], 'catégories fort simples : carens uno dente, carens aliquibus dentibus, et dentibus raris'.
90. Malin Holst and Jennifer Coughlan, 'Dental health and disease', *Blood Red Roses - The Archaeology of a Mass Grave from the Battle of Towton AD 1461* (Oxford, Oxbow Books, 2000), pp. 85–8.
91. Meyrick, *A critical inquiry into antient armour*, Vol. II, p. 64.
92. Ibid.
93. Burfield, *Medieval Military Medicine*, p. 68
94. Johnson (trans.), *The workes of that famous chirurgion Ambrose Paréy*, p. 578.
95. Don Walker, *Disease in London, 1st–19th centuries – An illustrated guide to diagnosis* (London, Museum of London Archaeology, 2012), p. 257.
96. BBC, *History Cold Case*, Series One, Episode Three, *Stirling Man*, see minutes 6–7.
97. Rosenman (trans.), *The Surgery of Master Jehan Yperman*, pp. 149–51, and Haeser und Middeldorpf, *Buch der Bündth-Ertznei*, Vorwort, xxxix.
98. Rosenman (trans.), *The Major Surgery of Guy de Chauliac*, p. 531.
99. Ibid., p. 533. Mastic and pyrethrum, an extract from the daisy flower, could be used to reduce the production of saliva.
100. Ibid., as recommended by Abulcasis. See also, Sir D'Arcy Power (trans.), *De Arte Phisicali et de Cirurgia of Master John Arderne, Surgeon of Newark Dated 1412* (New York, William Wood & Co., 1922), p. 21, fn. *, according

to Arderne, calamus draco, also known as dragon's blood, 'fastened the teeth'.

101. Johnson (trans.), *The workes of that famous chirurgion Ambrose Paréy*, p. 415, the mixture of vinegar and water was known as oxycrate at the time.
102. Scoble (ed.), *The Memoirs of Philip de Commines*, Vol. II, pp. 316–17.
103. A. Boucherie, S. Jørkov ML and M. Smith, 'Wounded to the bone: Digital microscopic analysis of traumas in a medieval mass grave assemblage (Sandbjerget, Denmark, AD 1300–1350)', *Int J Paleopathol.* 2017, Dec;19, p. 74. See also, Willard (trans.) and Cannon Willard (ed.), *The Book of Deeds of Arms and of Chivalry*, p. 31, and Burfield, *Medieval Military Medicine*, p. 59.
104. Boucherie et al., 'Wounded to the bone', p. 74. See also, Thom Richardson, 'Armour', *Blood Red Roses - The Archaeology of a Mass Grave from the Battle of Towton AD 1461* (Oxford, Oxbow Books, 2000), pp. 143–7; Mortimer, *1415 Henry V's Year of Glory*, p. 441, and Seward, *A Brief History of the Hundred Years War*, p. 52.
105. Bengt Thordeman, Poul Nörlund, and Bo. E. Ingelmark, *Armour from the Battle of Wisby 1361, Vol. I* (Stockholm, Almqvist & Wiksells Boktryckeri-A.-B., 1939), p. 180.
106. Boucherie et al, 'Wounded to the bone', pp. 74–6; A. Shannon Novak, 'Battle-related trauma', *Blood Red Roses - The Archaeology of a Mass Grave from the Battle of Towton AD 1461* (Oxford, Oxbow Books, 2000), pp. 94–101, and Anna Kjellström, 'A Sixteenth-Century Warrior Grave from Uppsala, Sweden: The Battle of Good Friday', *International Journal of Osteoarchaeology*, 15: 2005, pp. 32–6.
107. Walker, *Disease in London*, p. 94.
108. Guiseppe Brizzolara (ed.), *La Cronica de Cristoforo da Soldo, Raccolta Storici Italiani dal cinquecento al millecinquecento, Tomo XXI, Parte III* (Bologna, Nicola Zanichelli, 1900), p. 115, 'ne li quali fu ferito uno fiolo fu de Gatta mellata . . . e fu ferito de una cerbotana ne la testa passatoli lo elmeto et ficcholi la ballota de piombo nel cervello', 'Among those who were wounded was Gattamelata . . . and he was injured by a gunshot to the head; the lead ball passed through his helmet and went into his brain.'
109. Ibid., p. 116, the details of his treatment are very limited, '. . . fu mandato per molti medici i quali subito lo scodegò e trovoli un buso nella grappa Io grando come è uno grosso e trovoli nel cervello la ballota de piombo, la quala fu cavata', '. . . he was sent to many doctors who immediately inspected him and found the lump. They found and removed the lead ball in his brain.'
110. Ibid.
111. Kjellström, 'A Sixteenth-Century Warrior Grave from Uppsala', pp. 23–4.
112. Ibid., pp. 36–7.
113. Ibid., p. 39.

114. Rosenman (trans.), *The Surgery of Master Jehan Yperman*, p. 75. 'When granulation tissue appears, use fresh lint made from a cloth used in head-scarves.'
115. Ibid., pp. 75–6.
116. Ibid., p. 76.
117. Ibid., pp. 76–7. See also, Thordeman, Nörlund, and Ingelmark, *Armour from the Battle of Wisby 1361*, p. 196, fig. 192, for a similar healed head injury.
118. Rosenman (trans.), *The Surgery of Master Jehan Yperman*, p. 77. Yperman does not state which material he used to suture this soldier's scalp. His general instructions for closing these wounds state that it should be silk or linen. In cases where a less than pleasant scar was achieved, Yperman was insistent that the surgeon '. . . never commit the folly of re-incising'.
119. Park et al., 'Management of injuries on the 16th-century battlefield' p. 3.
120. Johnson (trans.), *The workes of that famous chirurgion Ambrose Paréy*, p. 272, 'But 1 being very desirous to know, what might be the true cause of his death, dividing his scull; observed that the second table was broken . . .'.
121. Ibid.
122. Ibid.
123. Ibid., p. 282, See also, Burfield, *Medieval Military Medicine*, pp. 26, 73–4.
124. Rosenman (trans.), *The Surgery of Master Jehan Yperman*, pp. 69–70, Rosenman (trans.), *The Surgery of Henri de Mondeville*, pp. 457-459, Rosenman (trans.), *The Major Surgery of Guy de Chauliac*, pp. 327–8, Johnson (trans.), *The workes of that famous chirurgion Ambrose Paréy*, pp. 285–7. See also, Haeser und Middeldorpf, *Buch der Bündth-Ertznei*, Vorwort, p. xviii. Von Pfolspeundt's surgery does not contain instructions for trepanation, '. . . keine Anweisung zu blutigen Operationen, namentlich nicht zur Trepanation . . .'.
125. Campbell and Colton, *The Surgery of Theodoric*, Vol. I, p. 124
126. Rosenman (trans.), *The Surgery of Master Jehan Yperman*, pp. 69–70.
127. Johnson (trans.), *The workes of that famous chirurgion Ambrose Paréy*, p. 286. See also, ibid., pp. 285, 287, Monsieur dela Bretesche and a footman of Monsieur de Goulaines, both of whom required trepanation to treat their issues.
128. Ibid., p. 781.
129. Ibid., p. 782.
130. Ibid., pp. 283–6. See also, Burfield, *Medieval Military Medicine*, p. 73, for a possible precursor to Paré's drill.

Chapter 6: Mutilated and Maimed

1. Strachey (ed.), *Le Morte d'Arthur*, p. 118.
2. Metzler, *A Social History of Disability in the Middle Ages*, pp. 39–40, 229–30, n 39, for more on the seriously wounded.

3. Thompson (ed.), *Chronicon Galfridi le Baker de Swynebroke*, p. 110, 'Dire nostros aggrediebantur, saxis evolantibus a turriculis malorum et pilis vibrantibus atque quarellis acriter et crebro nostros winerantes . . .', 'They [Castilians] attacked us ferociously from their turrets, causing terrible wounds to our men with their rocks, arrows and bolts . . .'.
4. Ibid., p. 111, 'Reportarunt enim sui capita saucia commissuris lineis involuta, brachia et tibias quarellis et telis terebrata, atque dentes evulsos, nasos quoque decisos, labra fissa, et oculos erutos . . .'.
5. Philip Yorke, *The Royal Tribes of Wales* (Wrexham, John Painter, 1799), p. 16. The Welsh nobleman John ap Maredudd (also Meredudd), a cousin of Sir Owen Tudor, received a wound to his face and for the remainder of his life he was known as Squier y Graith or The Squire with the Scar. See also, Strachey (ed.), *Le Morte d'Arthur*, p. 423, '. . . saw by a wound on his cheek that he was Sir Launcelot'; Thomas (trans.), *Medieval German Lyric Verse*, pp. 23, 25, and Wilson, *The Book of Geoffroi de Charny*, p. 121.
6. Burfield, *Medieval Military Medicine*, pp. 75–8.
7. Patricia Skinner, *Living with Disfigurement in Early Medieval Europe* (New York, Palgrave MacMillan, 2017), p. 1, regarding disfigurements, especially facial.
8. Garrison, *Notes on the History of Military Medicine*, pp. 115–16.
9. Riley (trans.), *Memorials of London and London Life*, p. 432.
10. Eyre-Todd (trans.), *The Bruce*, p. 107.
11. Southey (trans.), *Amadís of Gaul*, Vol. II, p. 244.
12. Benjamin Williams (ed.), *Henrici Quinti Angliæ Regis, Gesta* (London, Sumptibus Societatis, 1850), p. 48. This anonymous chronicle was written around 1418. See also, Ian Mortimer, *1415 Henry V's Year of Glory*, p. 332. Henry V made it clear that pages and grooms were not to become involved in questions regarding captured prisoners, weapons and the like, under the threat of having their left ear cut off.
13. Rosenman (trans.), *The Surgery of Master Jehan Yperman*, p. 88. Yperman went further by advising that no part of the body that had been separated from the main could be put back into place and survive.
14. Ibid. Yperman notes that any misalignment of the ear caused during this process could later make the surgeon a laughing-stock.
15. Ibid. In modern times, a running suture is sometimes referred to as the 'baseball suture', resembling the stitches on an American baseball. See also, ibid., p. 50, regarding waxed silk thread being used for sutures.
16. Ibid. Regularly used in shipbuilding, oakum was also favoured by surgeons and physicians for wound care. See also, Rosenman (trans.), *The Surgery of*

Master Henri de Mondeville, Volume II, pp. 731, 814, for de Mondeville's use of oakum.

17. Johnson (trans.), *The workes of that famous chirurgion Ambrose Parey*, p. 295.
18. Ibid.
19. Louis Tanon, *Registre criminal de la justice de St. Martin des Champs à Paris au XIV siècle: publié pour la première fois, d'après le manuscrit des archives nationales, précède d'une étude sur la juridiction des religieux de St. Martin (1060-1674)* (Paris, Léon Willem, 1877), p. CI. This form of punishment was very common, primarily in the fourteenth century. See also, Judges (ed.), *The Elizabethan Underworld*, Introduction p. xxxiv, for this punitive action in Tudor times.
20. Tanon, *Registre criminal*, pp. C and CI, 'Le 12 août 1355, '*Thassin-aus-oz*, de Bazeville, *eut l'oreille coupée*, sous l'échelle de Saint-Martin, pour avoir volé deux draps'. 'Thassin-aus-oz, from Bazeville, had his ear cut off, underneath the ladder of Saint-Martin, for stealing two sheets.'
21. Rawcliffe, *Leprosy in Medieval England*, p. 138.
22. Johnson (trans.), *The workes of that famous chirurgion Ambrose Parey*, p. 295.
23. Ibid., p. 581.
24. Ibid.
25. Ibid.
26. A. N. Williams and J. Williams, '"Proper to the duty of a chirurgeon": Ambroise Paré and sixteenth century paediatric surgery', *Journal of the Royal Society of Medicine*, Volume 97, September 2004, p. 449.
27. Willard (trans.) and Cannon Willard (ed.), *The Book of Deeds of Arms and of Chivalry*, p. 116.
28. Bern, Burgerbibliothek, Mss.h.h.I.16: Diebold Schilling, *Spiezer Chronik*, p. 637. See also, BnF Français 2643, f. 387r, for similar.
29. Johnson (trans.), *The workes of that famous chirurgion Ambrose Parey*, pp. 149, 313. See also, Emily Cockayne, 'Experiences of the Deaf in Early Modern England', *The Historical Journal*, vol. 46, no. 3, 2003, p. 495. This was a problem that would carry on into the centuries to come; K. Conroy and V. Malik, 'Hearing loss in the trenches – a hidden morbidity of World War I', *The Journal of Laryngology & Otology*, 132[11], 2018, p. 953, and Wilfrid Wilson Gibson, *Battle and Other Poems* (New York, The MacMillan Company, 1916), p. 15. The poem *Deaf* by the First World War poet, Wilfrid Wilson Gibson, captures the sad thoughts of so many down the centuries who, because of the guns of war, lost their ability to hear.

30. K. Oshima, S. Suchert, N. H. Blevins and S. Heller, 'Curing hearing loss: Patient expectations, health care practitioners and basic science', *J Commun Disord*, 2010 Jul-Aug; 43[4], p. 311. Even with cochlear implants and hearing aids there is no known cure for hearing loss, although work with stem cells, gene therapy, etc. is ongoing.
31. Rosenman (trans.), *The Surgery of Master Jehan Yperman*, p. 157.
32. Rosenman (trans.), *The Surgery of Lanfranchi of Milan*, p. 167. See also, Rosenman (trans.), *The Surgery of Master Jehan Yperman*, p. 157. Despite completely discounting these cures, Yperman did suggest that there was no harm in a surgeon trying them.
33. Power (trans.), *De arte phisicali et de cirurgia of Master John Arderne*, p. 6.
34. Rosenman (trans.), *The Surgery of Master Jehan Yperman*, p. 157, fn. 133.
35. Ibid., p. 84.
36. Michael Drayton, *The Battaile of Agincourt* (London, Charles Whittingham & Co., 1893), p. 70, for a further, poetic example.
37. Southey (trans.), *Amadís of Gaul*, Vol. I, p. 160.
38. Rosenman (trans.), *The Major Surgery of Guy de Chauliac*, p. 331; Colton (trans.), *John of Mirfield*, p. 62, and Johnson (trans.), *The workes of that famous chirurgion Ambrose Paréy*, p. 577. See also, Rosenman (trans.), *The Surgery of Lanfranchi of Milan*, p. 89 for another example.
39. Rosenman (trans.), *The Surgery of Henri de Mondeville*, Vol. I, p. 463. It was not always possible to reattach the 'dangling' portion of a nose, as de Mondeville describes. So much depended on the quality of the blood supply it received, along with age of the wound.
40. Ibid., Vol. I, p. 465. Mondeville recommended breathing tubes in his surgery, but he also recognized that many of his patients struggled to tolerate them, plus these tubes tended to become contaminated quite quickly with pus and mucus. To eliminate the need for them, he recommended making holes in the bandages where the patient's nostrils were located.
41. Rosenman (trans.), *The Major Surgery of Guy de Chauliac*, p. 331. See also, Rosenman (trans.), *The Surgery of Master Jehan Yperman*, pp. 83–4; Rosenman (trans.), *The Surgery of Henri de Mondeville*, Vol. I, pp. 463–5, and Rawcliffe, *Medicine & Society*, pp. 72, 74. In 1404 a man named Richard Cheddar had his nose nearly severed. It was treated by an unknown English surgeon who was able to successfully repair it.
42. Rosenman (trans.), *The Major Surgery of Guy de Chauliac*, pp. 229, 331. For patients with facial injuries, de Chauliac was a strong proponent of a heavy linen skull cap, with or without a brim. It provided a robust platform for bandages to be attached to.

43. Johnson (trans.), *The workes of that famous chirurgion Ambrose Paréy*, p. 578.
44. Ibid.
45. Ibid., p. 577.
46. Ibid., p. 579.
47. Ibid.
48. Rosenthal (trans.), *Tirant lo Blanc*, p. 77.
49. Ohler, *Krieg und Frieden im Mittelalter*, p. 261, 'Mit ungelöschtem Kalk oder feinem Kohlestaub blendete man Krieger . . .', 'Soldiers were blinded with quicklime or fine coal dust . . .'. See also, Metzler, *A Social History of Disability in the Middle Ages*, p. 55, for a late fifteenth-century civilian incident of lime causing damage to the eyes.
50. Willard (trans.) and Cannon Willard (ed.), *The Book of Deeds of Arms and of Chivalry*, p. 109. See also, Bourchier (trans.) and Macaulay (ed.), *The Chronicles of Froissart*, p. 50, 58, 92.
51. Colton (trans.), *John of Mirfield*, p. 67.
52. Plaine (ed.), *Monuments du procès de canonisation du bienheureux Charles de Blois*, pp. 366–7. See also, ibid., p. 370, here the details are related again, '. . . quedam spina intravit occulum cuiusdam vocati Johannis Hervei, qui cum isto tunc equitabat, directe in pupilla dicti occuli . . .', '. . . a thorn struck the eye of a certain man called John Hervey, who rode with him (Yvon de la Jailla), it went directly into the pupil of the said eye . . .'.
53. Ibid., p. 370, '. . . quia spina erat in loco tam periculoso, quod non potuisset sanari nisi miraculose'.
54. Ibid., pp. 369–70.
55. L. M. Eldredge, 'A thirteenth-century ophthalmologist, Benvenutus Grassus: his treatise and its survival', *J R Soc Med.* 1998 Jan; 91[1], p. 47. See also, Benjamin Z. Kedar, 'Benvenutus Grapheus of Jerusalem, an Oculist in the Era of the Crusades', *KOROT, The Israel Journal of the History of Medicine and Science*, Vol. 11, 1995, p. 14. Kedar notes that Benvenutus Grapheus may have lived in the 'twelfth or thirteenth century'.
56. Rosenman (trans.), *The Surgery of Master Jehan Yperman*, p.130 fn. 98, Yperman appears to have been the first surgeon to include Benvenutus Grapheus' work, and since he refers to him as Master, it may be that he knew him. See also, Eldredge, 'A thirteenth-century ophthalmologist, Benvenutus Grassus: his treatise and its survival', p. 48.
57. Rosenman (trans.), *The Surgery of Master Jehan Yperman*, p. 129, and Nicaise, *La Grande Chirurgie de Guy de Chauliac*, p. 271, 'vertu donnée de

Dieu'. See also, Power (trans.), *De Arte Phisicali et de Cirurgia of Master John Arderne*, p. 5, Arderne called the treatment 'Virtus a deo data' or 'God's Virtue'.

58. Rosenman (trans.), *The Surgery of Master Jehan Yperman*, p. 129, and Rosenman (trans.), *The Major Surgery of Guy de Chauliac*, p. 330.
59. Rosenman (trans.), *The Surgery of Master Jehan Yperman*, p. 129.
60. Johnson (trans.), *The workes of that famous chirurgion Ambrose Parey*, p. 291.
61. Rosenman (trans.), *The Major Surgery of Guy de Chauliac*, p. 330, fn. 423. See also, Nicaise, *La Grande Chirurgie de Guy de Chauliac*, Introduction, p. xxxviii. According to Nicaise, de Chauliac cites Ali ibn Isa al-Kahhal more than 60 times under a few names, including 'Jesu Ali (ou Ali ben issa, Issa ben Ali), que Guy cite plus de 60 fois, sous le nom de Jésus, Jésu Hali, Jésus, fils de Haly . . .'.
62. Rosenman (trans.), *The Major Surgery of Guy de Chauliac*, p. 330, fn. 426. Rosenman notes that Ali ibn Isa al-Kahhal insisted on the use of milk from a nursing mother who had a baby girl. See also, Johnson (trans.), *The workes of that famous chirurgion Ambrose Parey*, p. 291.
63. Sigerist, *Hieronymus Brunschwig and His Work*, p. 23. Brunschwig often sent his patients directly to the stonemasons to perform the removal of such fragments.
64. Johnson (trans.), *The workes of that famous chirurgion Ambrose Parey*, p. 774, '. . . powder of unquenched lime to blinde their eie . . .'.
65. Rosenman (trans.), *The Surgery of Master Jehan Yperman*, p. 89. Yperman makes specific mention of this fact in his surgery, noting that facial injuries from such weapons were common in battles across Europe.
66. Sir Herbert Maxwell (trans.), *The Chronicle of Lanercost - 1272-1346* (Glasgow, James Maclehose and Sons, 1913), p. 270, the Battle of Dupplin Moor took place during the Second War of Scottish Independence. See also, Ian Mortimer, *The Perfect King, The Life of Edward III, Father of the English Nation* (London, Vintage Books, 2008), p. 98.
67. Maxwell (trans.), *The Chronicle of Lanercost - 1272-1346*, p. 279.
68. Rosenman (trans.), *The Major Surgery of Guy de Chauliac*, p. 329.
69. Johnson (trans.), *The workes of that famous chirurgion Ambrose Parey*, p. 576.
70. Sir Herbert Maxwell (trans.), *Scalacronica, The Reigns of Edward I, Edward II and Edward III, as recorded by Sir Thomas Gray* (Glasgow, James MacLehose & Sons, 1907), p. 58. Roger de Horsley was the keeper of Berwick and Bamburgh castles at various stages and did not die until c. 1340. See also, Metzler, *A Social History of Disability in the Middle Ages*, p. 37.

71. Bourchier (trans.) and Macaulay (ed.), *The Chronicles of Froissart*, p. 97. See also, Mortimer, *The Time Traveller's Guide to Medieval England*, p. 36.
72. Sumption, *The Hundred Years War - Trial by Battle*, p. 183, William Montagu. See also, Jonathon Sumption, *The Hundred Years War - Volume II, Trial by Fire* (Philadelphia, University of Pennsylvania Press, 1999), p. 519, Jean de Chalon IV.
73. Garrison, *Notes on the History of Military Medicine*, p. 115.
74. Johnson (trans.), *The workes of that famous chirurgion Ambrose Parėy*, pp. 576–7. Paré included diagrams of both versions of his artificial eye.
75. Southey (trans.), *Amadís of Gaul*, Vol. II, p. 150.
76. Rickert (trans.), *Early English Romances in Verse, Romances of Friendship*, p. 142. See also, Eyre-Todd (trans.), *The Bruce*, p. 107, 'He met the first so eagerly that with the sharp edge of his sword he hewed the arm from the body'.
77. Strachey (ed.), *Le Morte d'Arthur*, p. 37. See also, ibid., pp. 96, 284.
78. Tobias Smollett (trans.), *The Adventures of Don Quixote de la Mancha by Miguel de Cervantes* (New York, Farrar, Straus, Giroux, 1986), p. 3. See also, Motteux (trans.), *Adventures of Don Quixote de la Mancha* (London, Frederick Warne and Co., 1800), Prefactory Memoir, p. vii, '. . . he was wounded in the left hand by a blow from a scimitar, or, as some assert, by a gunshot . . .'.
79. Motteux (trans.), *Adventures of Don Quixote de la Mancha*, Prefatory Memoir, p. vii.
80. Garrison, *An Introduction to the History of Medicine*, p. 172. See also, Siraisi, *Medieval & Early Renaissance Medicine*, p. 192.
81. Johnson (trans.), *The workes of that famous chirurgion Ambrose Parėy*, p. 307.
82. Packard, *Life and Times of Ambroise Pare*, pp. 25, 46, 120.
83. Johnson (trans.), *The workes of that famous chirurgion Ambrose Parėy*, p. 782. See also, Paget (trans.), *Ambroise Paré and His Times*, p. 93, and Siegfried Sassoon, *The War Poems of Siegfried Sassoon* (ReadaClassic, 2011), p. 56, for a similar sentiment in Sassoon's poem of the First World War, *The One-Legged Man*.
84. Southey (trans.), *Palmerin of England*, Vol. II, p. 279. See also, Walter Scheps (trans.), 'The Acts and Deeds of William Wallace', *Medieval Outlaws, Ten Tales in Modern English* (Stroud, Sutton Publishing, 1998), p. 269, from the poem of the second half of the fifteenth century *The Acts and Deeds of Sir William Wallace*, written by Blind Harry (sometimes Henry the Minstrel), 'From an Englishman he struck off his right hand . . . then from the stump

the blood spurted out rapidly and splattered into Wallace's face so that it obscured a good part of his sight'.

85. Burfield, *Medieval Military Medicine*, p. 54.
86. Johnson (trans.), *The workes of that famous chirurgion Ambrose Parèy*, p. 341.
87. Siraisi, *Medieval & Early Renaissance Medicine*, pp. 192–3.
88. Rosenman (trans.), *The Surgery of Henri de Mondeville*, Vol. I, p. 69, fn. 28, Vol. II, pp. 731, 734.
89. Rosenman (trans.), *The Major Surgery of Guy de Chauliac*, p. 477, and Johnson (trans.), *The workes of that famous chirurgion Ambrose Parèy*, p. 341. See also, Warren R. Dawson, *A Leechbook or Collections of Medical Recipes of the Fifteenth Century* (London, MacMillan and Co. Limited, 1934), p. 181, number 560, from a fifteenth-century English Leechbook, 'For a man's leg or arm that is cut off. Make oil seething and put the stump of the leg therein, all seething as it is'.
90. Johnson (trans.), *The workes of that famous chirurgion Ambrose Parèy*, pp. 341–2. See also, Packard, *Life and Times of Ambroise Pare*, p. 47.
91. Siraisi, *Medieval and Renaissance Medicine*, pp. 192–3. See also, Malgaigne, *Surgery and Ambroise Paré*, p. 353.
92. Johnson (trans.), *The workes of that famous chirurgion Ambrose Parèy*, p. 339, '. . . he was much troubled and wearied with the heavy and unprofitable burden of the rest of his Leg . . .'.
93. Ibid.
94. A. Kaur and Y. Guan, 'Phantom limb pain: A literature review', *Chin J Traumatol* 2018 Dec; 21 [6], pp. 366, 368.
95. Johnson (trans.), *The workes of that famous chirurgion Ambrose Parèy*, p. 339.
96. P. Hernigou , 'Crutch art painting in the Middle Ages as orthopaedic heritage (part II: the peg leg, the bent-knee peg and the beggar)', *Int Orthop.* 2014 Jul; 38 [7], p. 1535. See also, Knox and Leslie (trans.), *The Miracles of King Henry VI*, p. 197, no. 149, 'John Curyer, who had been seven years lame, so that he walked upon a wooden prop for support . . .'.
97. Johnson (trans.), *The workes of that famous chirurgion Ambrose Parèy*, p. 771. See also, ibid., p. 588. One of Paré's wooden peg-legged prostheses, which is illustrated in his text, is called 'Jambe de bois poor les vulgaires' or 'A wooden leg for poor men'.
98. Johnson (trans.), *The workes of that famous chirurgion Ambrose Parèy*, pp. 585–8. See also, Burfield, *Medieval Military Medicine*, p. 87, for examples of iron hands and fingers from the earlier centuries of the Middle Ages.

99. K. J. Zuo and J. L. Olson, 'The evolution of functional hand replacement: From iron prostheses to hand transplantation', *Plast Surg (Oakv)* 2014 Spring; 22 [1], pp. 44–5.
100. Ibid., p. 45.
101. Judges (ed.), *The Elizabethan Underworld*, p. 67, from *A Caveat or Warning for Common Cursitors, Vulgarly Called Vagabonds*.
102. E. Cunha and A. M. Silva, 'War lesions from the famous Portuguese Medieval battle of Aljubarrota', *Int. J. Osteoarchaeology*, 7: 1997, p. 597. See also, Hébert, 'L'armée provençale en 1374', p. 23. The troop review of soldiers from the Provençal army in 1374, studied by Michel Hébert, found that about 28 per cent of the men had at least one scar, most of which were to their hands and faces.
103. Metzler, *A Social History of Disability in the Middle Ages*, pp. 37–8. See also, Thordeman, Nörlund and Ingelmark, *Armour from the Battle of Wisby*, p. 196.
104. Burfield, *Medieval Military Medicine*, pp. 89, 106, 173 n120. Despite not fighting, these individuals could still find themselves in harm's way if things went wrong.
105. G. W. Coopland (trans.), *The Tree of Battles of Honoré Bonet* (Liverpool, Liverpool University Press, 1949), p. 168, Chapter LXX. See also, ibid., pp. 18, 189; J.H. Stevenson (ed.), *Gilbert of the Haye's Prose Manuscript (A.D. 1456), Volume I, The Buke of the Law of Armys or Buke of Bataillis* (Edinburgh, William Blackwood and Sons, 1901), p. 195, for translation of Bonet into Scots almost 100 years later.
106. Willard (trans.) and Cannon Willard (ed.), *The Book of Deeds of Arms and of Chivalry*, p. 177.
107. Wylie and Waugh, *The Reign of Henry the Fifth*, Vol. II, pp. 353–4. See also, ibid., p. 354, fn. 1, 'Veillesse et fieblesse'.
108. Annie Abram, *English Life and Manners in the Later Middle Ages* (George Routledge & Sons Limited, London), 1913, p. 96. 'The long wars in which England was engaged also tended to swell the numbers of the unemployed; many soldiers returned from them unfit or unwilling to work.' See also Johannes Fabricius, *Syphilis in Shakespeare's England* (London, Jessica Kingsley Publishers Ltd, 1994), p. 85, for more on the increase of demobilized soldiers and sailors in England at the end of the late medieval period and in the sixteenth century.
109. Rotha Mary Clay, *The Mediaeval Hospitals of England* (London, Methuen & Co., 1909), p. 99.
110. *Calendar of the Patent Rolls, Preserved in the Public Record Office, Henry IV. Vol. III. A.D. 1405-1408* (London, printed for His Majesty's Stationery Office by Mackie and Co Ltd., 1907), p. 290.

111. *Calendar of the Patent Rolls, Preserved in the Public Record Office, Henry IV. Vol. II. A.D. 1401-1405*, p. 410. See also ibid., p. 41, and Grose, *Military Antiquities Respecting a History of the English Army*, Vol. II, pp. 83–4.
112. *Calendar of the Close Rolls, Preserved in the Public Record Office, Edward II: Volume 2, 1313-1318* (London, printed for Her Majesty's Stationery Office by Eyre and Spottiswoode, 1893), p. 335. See also, ibid., p. 192, previously, in August of 1314 Edward II had sent William, son of Thomas le Charetter of Grove, who had his hand cut off by, '. . . the Scotch rebels . . .', to St John's to be looked after for the balance of his life., and Burfield, *Medieval Military History*, p. 90.
113. *Calendar of the Close Rolls, Preserved in the Public Record Office, Edward III. A.D. 1327-1330*, p. 227.
114. Shulamith Shahar, *Growing Old in the Middle Ages - 'Winter clothes us in shadow and pain'* (London, Routledge, 1997), pp. 123–4.
115. Mallett, *Mercenaries and Their Masters*, pp. 138–9. Like some soldiers, da Spagna decided he would rather continue fighting with just one arm than take the pension.
116. James Gairdner and R. H. Brodie (ed.), *Letters and Papers, Foreign and Domestic, Henry VIII, Volume 21 Part 1, January-August 1546* (London, His Majesty's Stationery Office, 1908), p. 583, 'Gonsalo de Villa Panda, Spaniard, maimed in both legs in the wars in Scotland, and recommended hither by Signor Gamboa, 24 March, 4*l*'.
117. Metzler, *A Social History of Disability in the Middle Ages*, p. 138. Dr Metzler notes the rarity of a '. . . military invalid being provided for'.
118. David Knowles and R. Neville Hadcock, *Medieval Religious Houses - England and Wales* (London, Longmans, Green and Co, 1953), p. 319. See also, ibid., p. 313. Founded in 1433, at Thatcham in Berkshire, St George's was a hospital that took in pilgrims, travellers and '. . . lame soldiers returning homewards . . .'.
119. Metzler, *A Social History of Disability in the Middle Ages*, pp. 147–8. See also, Clay, *The Mediaeval Hospitals of England*, p. 9.
120. Knowles and Hadcock, *Medieval Religious Houses*, p. 319.
121. Metzler, *A Social History of Disability in the Middle Ages*, p. 40. See also, Abram, *English Life and Manners in the Later Middle Ages*, p. 97.
122. Henri Duplès-Agier, *Registre Criminel du Chatelet de Paris du 6 Septembre 1389 au 18 Mai 1392, Tome Premier* (Paris, Ch. Lahure, 1861), pp. 373–4.
123. Ibid., p. 374, '. . . il ne povoit plus ouvrer dudit mestier, s'est mis à porter le panier à la porte de Paris', '. . . he could no longer work in the said trade [baking and pastry making], so he became a porter at the gate of Paris'.

124. Thomas H. Ohlgren (ed.), *Medieval Outlaws, Ten Tales in Modern English* (Stroud, Sutton Publishing, 1998), pp. xviii and xix, regarding the crimes of returning soldiers. In England, during 1305, Edward I set up a type of court called 'Trailbaston', which '. . . appointed special judges . . . partly to investigate and to suppress increases in crimes of violence due to the lawlessness of returning soldiery from the foreign wars . . .'. See also, Carter Revard, 'The Outlaw's Song of Trailbaston', *Medieval Outlaws, Ten Tales in Modern English* (Stroud, Sutton Publishing, 1998), p. 103; Bronislaw Geremek, *The Margins of Society in Late Medieval Paris, translated by Jean Birrell* (Cambridge, Cambridge University Press, 1987), pp. 126–7, regarding similar problems in France; Bronislaw Geremek, *Truands et misérables dans l'Europe moderne: (1350-1600)* (Gallimard, Paris, 1980), p. 49, and Metzler, *A Social History of Disability in the Middle Ages*, pp. 162–3, for more on the general increase in crime rates during the late medieval period.
125. Henry Ellis, *Original letters, illustrative of English history; including numerous royal letters; from autographs in the British Museum, and one or two other collections, Second Series, Volume 1* (London, Harding and Lepard, 1827), p. 95, for more information on the battles fought by Thomas Hostell (Hostel). See also, www.medievalsoldier.org/database, this database of English officers and men-at-arms from late medieval England, created by the University of Southampton, includes just one entry for a Thomas Hostell. Sincere thanks to Anne Curry, Emeritus Professor of Medieval History at the University of Southampton and co-director of the medieval soldier database, who very kindly confirmed that this Thomas Hostell is almost certainly the same individual who petitioned the crown for assistance. Professor Curry also notes that to date, nothing is known about Thomas Hostell's campaigns under Henry IV, as suggested in his letter. See also, Curry, *The Battle of Agincourt - Sources and Interpretations*, pp. 435, 449.
126. Sir Harris Nicolas, *History of the Battle of Agincourt, and of the expedition of Henry the Fifth into France in 1415; to which is added the Roll of men-at-arms in the English army* (London, Johnson & Co., 1833), p. 173. See also, Ellis, *Original letters, illustrative of English history*, p. 95.
127. Nicolas, *History of the Battle of Agincourt*, p. 173. Almasse, i.e. alms.
128. Ibid. Among the many hardships that had befallen Thomas Hostell, he claims that he was never paid for his service as a soldier '. . . and being for his said services never yet recompensed nor rewarded . . .'. See also, Ellis, *Original letters, illustrative of English history; Volume 1*, p. 96; Arthur Goldhammer (trans.), *The Poor in the Middle Ages: An Essay in Social History by Michel Mollat* (New Haven, Yale University Press, 1978), pp. 241–2. The knightly classes also suffered during this period. Many ended up in poverty because of

the great economic hardships brought on by prolonged wars, ransom payments and the continual appearances of bubonic plague, and Rochus von Liliencron (ed.), *Deutsches Leben in Volkslied um 1530* (Darmstadt, Wissenschaftliche Buchgesellschaft, 1966), pp. 336–7, for a work from around 1530 entitled 'Ein new lied, von dem landsknecht auf der stelzen' or 'A new song, by the mercenary on stilts'. A mercenary describes his military life. He begins quite positively, but later despairs over what will end up happening to him if he loses an arm or a leg, 'Und wird mir dann geschoßen ein flügel von meinem . . . Und wird mir dann geschoßen ein schenkel von meinem lieb'.

129. Judges (ed.), *The Elizabethan Underworld*, Introduction, p. xiv.
130. Edward Vernon Utterson, *Select Pieces of Early Poetry: Re-Published Principally from Early Printed Copies in the Black Letter, Volume II* (London, William Pickering, Chancery Lane, 1825), p. B2, 'The particular hospital alluded to by Copland may well have been that of St Bartholomew; as he speaks of St Bartholomew's church and of the shepe cotes in its immediate neighbourhood'.
131. Judges (ed.), *The Elizabethan Underworld*, Introduction, p. 5.
132. Ibid., p. 8.
133. George Walter (ed.), *The Penguin Book of First World War Poetry* (London, Penguin Books, 2006), p. 254. Ivor Gurney was a prolific writer who was eventually institutionalized due to his poor mental health, brought on by the horrors of the First World War.

Chapter 7: Two Plagues

1. MacCracken (ed.), *The Minor Poems of John Lydgate*, p. 241, see verse thirteen.
2. May McKisack, *The Fourteenth Century, 1307-1399* (Oxford, Clarendon Press, 1959), pp. 43, 49, 329.
3. Joseph Michon (ed.), *Documents inédits sur la grande peste de 1348 (Consultation de la Faculte de Paris, consultation d'un praticien de Montpellier, description de Guillaume de Machaut)* (Paris, J. -B. Baillière et fils, 1860), p. 26, 'Toute la terre était en guerre', 'The whole world was at war'.
4. Ibid., pp. 26–9. See also, Eric Christiansen, *The Northern Crusades* (London, Penguin Books, 1997), pp. 160–2, for more on the Lithuanian Crusade, and Griffiths, 'The Interaction of War and Plague in the Later Middle Ages', pp. 127–8.
5. Philip Ziegler, *The Black Death* (Harmondsworth, Penguin Books Ltd., 1969), p. 35. See also, William Chester Jordan, *The Great Famine, Northern*

Europe in the Early Fourteenth Century (Princeton, Princeton University Press, 1996), p. 186, and Ann G. Carmichael, 'Plague Persistence in Western Europe: A Hypothesis', *Pandemic Disease in the Medieval World, Rethinking the Black Death* (Kalamazoo, Arc Medieval Press, 2015), pp. 173, 182.

6. Maria A. Spyrou, Rezeda I. Tukhbatova, Michal Feldman, Joanna Drath, Sacha Kacki, Julia Beltrán de Heredia, Susanne Arnold, Airat G., Sitdikov, Dominique Castex, Joachim Wahl, Ilgizar R. Gazimzyanov, Danis K. Nurgaliev, Alexander Herbig, Kirsten I. Bos, and Johannes Krause, 'Historical Y. pestis Genomes Reveal the European Black Death as the Source of Ancient and Modern Plague Pandemics', *Cell Host and Microbe*, Volume 19, Issue 6, 2016, p. 874. See also, John Aberth, *The Black Death, The Great Mortality of 1348-1350, A Brief History with Documents* (Boston, Bedford/St. Martin's, 2005), pp. 1–2.
7. Monica H. Green, 'Taking "Pandemic" Seriously: Making the Black Death Global', *Pandemic Disease in the Medieval World, Rethinking the Black Death* (Kalamazoo, Arc Medieval Press, 2015), pp. 32–4.
8. Ziegler, *The Black Death*, p. 113. See also, Robert S. Gottfried, *The Black Death, Natural and Human Disaster in Medieval Europe* (New York, The Free Press, 1983), p. 42, and Hannah Barker, 'Laying the Corpses to Rest: Grain, Embargoes, and *Yersinia pestis* in the Black Sea, 1346–48', *Speculum, A Journal of Mediaeval Studies*, Volume 96, Number 1, January 2021, pp. 125–6. New research argues that the plague reached the Mediterranean aboard grain ships coming from the Black Sea after peace had been reached in that region and the embargo on grain was lifted in 1347.
9. Aberth, *The Black Death*, p. 1.
10. Ziegler, *The Black Death*, p. 40.
11. Ibid., pp. 40, 43. See also, J. J. de Smet (ed.), *Recueil Chroniques de Flandre, Publié sous la Direction de la Commission Royale D'Histoire, Tome III* (Brussels, M. Hayez, 1856), pp. 14–15. A contemporary letter from a musician called Louis Heyligen describes the progress of the plague from Genoa to Marseilles in late 1347 and early 1348; Sumption, *The Hundred Years War - Volume II*, pp. 6–7, and Gottfried, *The Black Death*, pp. 43, 49.
12. Aberth, *The Black Death*, p. 3. See also, Monica H. Green, 'Editor's Introduction to Pandemic Disease in the Medieval World: Rethinking the Black Death', *Pandemic Disease in the Medieval World, Rethinking the Black Death* (Kalamazoo, Arc Medieval Press, 2015); p. 9, John B. Henneman Jr., 'The Black Death and Royal Taxation in France, 1347–1351', *Speculum, A Journal of Mediaeval Studies*, Vol. XLIII, No. 3, July 1968, p. 413, for French examples.

13. Jean Birdsall (trans.) and Richard A. Newhall (ed.), *Chronicle of Jean de Venette* (New York, Columbia University Press, 1953), p. 49. See also, Thompson (ed.), *Chronicon Galfridi le Baker de Swynebroke*, pp. 99–100. Geoffery le Baker described the plague similarly, 'Uno die letissimi, in crastino defuncti reperiebantur. Torserunt illos apostemata e l diversis partibus corporis subito irrumpencia . . .', 'One day a person could be completely happy but by the next they were dead. Victims of the plague had pustules that burst from various parts of their bodies . . .'; and Tait (ed.), *Chronica Johannis de Reading*, p. 108, '. . . expulsis ulceribus in inguine et sub alis, quae morientes triduo cruciabant', or '. . . painful pustules appeared in the groin and under the arms, before they died three days later'.
14. Aberth, *The Black Death*, p. 23. See also, Ziegler, *The Black Death*, p. 28.
15. Green, 'Taking "Pandemic" Seriously: Making the Black Death Global', p. 32. Septicaemic plague was transmitted through the bloodstream, but by means of an opening in the skin rather than a parasite. Pneumonic plague was transferred by the inhalation of respiratory fluids, and a gastrointestinal or ingested version of the plague is now known to have also existed. See also, Aberth, *The Black Death*, pp. 23–4, and Ziegler, *The Black Death*, pp. 28–9.
16. Rosenman (trans.), *The Major Surgery of Guy de Chauliac*, p. 249, fn. 332. See also, Monica H. Green, 'Preface - The Black Death and Ebola: On the Value of Comparison', *Pandemic Disease in the Medieval World, Rethinking the Black Death* (Kalamazoo, Arc Medieval Press, 2015), p. xiii.
17. Ziegler, *The Black Death*, pp. 106–07, for a map of the progression and devastation of the plague in Europe.
18. Ibid., p. 239, 'To maintain that one European in three died during the period of the Black Death can never be proved but, equally, cannot be wildly far from the truth'.
19. Green, 'Preface – The Black Death and Ebola', p. xi. See also, Green, 'Editor's Introduction to Pandemic Disease in the Medieval World', p. 9, and Ole J. Benedictow, *The Black Death, 1346-1353, The Complete History* (Woodbridge, The Boydell Press, 2004), p. 383.
20. Michon (ed.), *Documents inédits sur la grande peste de 1348*, p. 89, 'Car les batailles et les Guerres, Furent si grans par toutes terres'. From the contemporary poem of the Black Death by Guillaume de Machaut, *Le Jugement dou roy de Navarre*, or *The Judgement of the King of Navarre*.
21. Nicaise, *La grande chirurgie de Guy de Chauliac*, pp. 170–1, '. . . entant que les gens mouroient sans seruiteurs et estoyent enseuelis sans Prestres. Le père ne visitoit pas son fils, ne le fils son père . . . Parquoy elle fut inutile, et honteuse pour les Médecins: d'autant qu'ils n'osoient visiter les malades . . .',

'. . . all the while people died and were buried without priests. The father did not visit his son, nor did the son his father . . . Shamefully, because of the nature of the situation, doctors did not dare visit the sick . . .'.

22. Tait (ed.), *Chronica Johannis de Reading*, p. 106, '. . . vix relinquens vitales mortuorum corpora honeste sepelire, sed fossas altas et latas fodientes, corpora junctim sepeliebant . . .', or '. . . there were hardly enough living to bury the dead in a decent manner, so wide trenches were dug, and the bodies were buried together . . .'.
23. Henneman Jr., 'The Black Death and Royal Taxation in France', p. 414. See also, *Calendar of the Fine Rolls, Preserved in the Public Record Office*, Vol. VI. Edward III. A.D. 1347–1356 (London, Published by His Majesty's Stationery Office, 1921), pp. 199, 214, and Mortimer, *The Perfect King*, p. 257.
24. Michon (ed.), *Documents inédits sur la grande peste de 1348*, p. 88, 'Les estoilles, le ciel, la terre, En significence de guerre, De doleurs et de pestilances'.
25. Christiansen, *The Northern Crusades*, p. 162.
26. Ibid., p. 194. See also, Michael C. Paul, 'Archbishop Vasilii Kalika of Novgorod, the Fortress of Orekhov and the Defence of Orthodoxy', *The Clash of Cultures on the Medieval Baltic Frontier* (Abingdon, Routledge, 2016), p. 268, fn. 57.
27. Mortimer, *The Perfect King*, p. 258. See also, Sumption, *The Hundred Years War - Volume II*, p. 8. At times the truce was used as a stall tactic to buy time to raise enough funds so that the fighting could continue.
28. Sumption, *The Hundred Years War - Volume II*, pp. 45, 47. See also, Mortimer, *The Perfect King*, p. 270; Kenneth Fowler, *The King's Lieutenant: Henry of Grosmont, First Duke of Lancaster, 1310-1361* (New York, Barnes & Noble Inc., 1969), p. 84, and Tait (ed.), *Chronica Johannis de Reading*, p. 111.
29. Ziegler, *The Black Death*, pp. 122–3. See also, Sharon N. DeWitte, 'The Anthropology of Plague: Insights from Bioarcheological Analyses of Epidemic Cemeteries', *Pandemic Disease in the Medieval World: Rethinking the Black Death* (Kalamazoo, Arc Medieval Press, 2015), p. 104.
30. G. H. Martin (ed. & trans.), *Knighton's Chronicle, 1337 – 1396* (Oxford, Clarendon Press, 1995), p. 101.
31. Ibid., p. 103. Knighton quotes a figure of 5,000 dead among the Scottish army. See also, ibid., pp. 59, 83, 155. The number 5,000 is one Knighton uses regularly in his chronicle, generally to describe large numbers of foot soldiers, sheep, crossbowmen, etc., making it difficult to know just how many Scottish soldiers perished due to the plague.
32. Ibid.

33. Cayetano Rosell (ed.), 'Corónica del Muy Alto et Muy Católico Rey Don Alfonso el Onceno, Deste Nombre, Que Venció la Batalla del Rio Salado, et Ganó a las Algeciras', *Crónicas de Los Reyes de Castilla desde Don Alfonso el Sabio, Hasta los Católicos Don Fernando y Doña Isabel, Tomo Primero* (Madrid, Rivadeneyra, 1875), p. 391, '. . . et Caballeros que estaban con el Rey Don Alfonso en el dicho real sobre Gibraltar, le fué dicho et aconsejado que so partiese de la cerca, por quanto morían muchas compañas de aquella pestilencia, et estaba el su cuerpo en grand peligro . . .'.
34. Ibid. See also, J. H. Mann, *A History of Gibraltar and its Sieges* (London, Provost & Co., 1873), pp. 168–9, and Gottfried, *The Black Death*, p. 51.
35. W. J. Simpson, *A Treatise on Plague dealing with the Historical, Epidemiological, Clinical Therapeutic and Preventative aspects of the Disease* (Cambridge, at the University Press, 1905), pp. 26–31. See also, Rosemary Horrox (ed. & trans.), *The Black Death* (Manchester, Manchester University Press, 1994), pp. 85–91; Brian S. Pullan, *Rich and poor in Renaissance Venice; the social institutions of a Catholic state, to 1620* (Cambridge, Mass., Harvard University Press, 1971), p. 219, for the example of Venice, which suffered twenty-two outbreaks of plague between 1361 and 1528, and DeWitte, 'The Anthropology of Plague', pp. 102, 116. The plague of 1361 is sometimes referred to as the 'Pestilence of Children', because so many sadly perished during that outbreak.
36. Aberth, *The Black Death*, p. 1. The term 'Black Death' was not used to describe the plague until a few hundred years after its appearance in the mid-fourteenth century.
37. Luciano Cordiero (ed.), *Cronica de El-Rei D. João I por Fernão Lopes, Vol. III* (Lisbon, Escriptorio, 1897), p. 58.
38. Griffiths, 'The Interaction of War and Plague in the Later Middle Ages', p. 130. See also, Margaret L. King and Diana Robin (ed. & trans.), *Isotta Nogarola, Complete Writings, Letterbook, Dialogue on Adam and Eve, Orations* (Chicago, University of Chicago Press, 2004), p. 66.
39. Johnson (trans.), *The workes of that famous chirurgion Ambrose Paréy*, p. 769, '. . . the plague begun much in our camp . . .'. See also, Packard, *Life and Times of Ambroise Pare*, p. 39, for clarification on the date of the siege as 1542, rather than 1543 as Paré claims.
40. *Calendar of the Close Rolls, Preserved in the Public Record Office, Edward III Vol. IX A.D. 1349-1354* (London, printed for Her Majesty's Stationery Office, Mackie and Co., Ltd., 1906), p. 258.
41. Holy Bible, Containing the Old and New Testaments (Philadelphia, American Baptist Publication Society, 1913), Old Testament, p, 943, Ezekiel 6:11, 'For they shall fall by sword, by famine and by pestilence', and Ibid.,

New Testament, p. 297, Revelations 6:2-8, for the Four Horsemen of the Apocalypse; Pestilence, War, Famine and Death.

42. David K. Coley, *Death and the Pearl Maiden, Plague, Poetry, England* (Columbus, The Ohio State University Press, 2019), p. 167, regarding the lack of direct references to the plague in fourteenth-century English literature.
43. Angel Flores (ed.), *An Anthology of Medieval Lyrics* (New York, Modern Library through Random House, 1962), pp. 355–6, translated by William M. Davis. The three wolves are also referred to as 'the three-pronged one' in the poem. See also, Goldhammer (trans.), *The Poor in the Middle Ages*, p. 206.
44. Cotton, 'Benedetto Reguardati of Nursia (1398-1469)', p. 180. See also, Griffiths, 'The Interaction of War and Plague in the Later Middle Ages', pp. 128–9; Birdsall (trans.) and Newhall (ed.), *Chronicle of Jean de Venette*, p. 5, and Coley, *Death and the Pearl Maiden*, p. 134.
45. Griffiths, 'The Interaction of War and Plague in the Later Middle Ages', pp. 134–5.
46. Seward, *The Hundred Years War*, pp. 73–4. See also, Francis Aidan Gasquet, *The Black Death of 1348 and 1349* (London, George Bell and Sons, 1908), p. 243.
47. *Calendar of the Close Rolls, Edward III Vol. IX A.D. 1349-1354*, p. 258. In Newcastle upon Tyne in the north-east, '. . . the men now in the town, who used to live of their merchandise, are so impoverished by the said pestilence and other adversities in these times of war that they hardly have wherewith to live . . .'; ibid., p. 620, for Dunwich on the Suffolk coast, '. . . has been so wasted and depressed by the late mortal pestilence; and by the king's adversaries of France plundering and slaying the fishermen at sea that they cannot pay . . .', and *Calendar of the Close Rolls, Preserved in the Public Record Office, Edward III Vol. X A.D. 1354-1360* (London, printed for Her Majesty's Stationery Office, Mackie and Co., Ltd., 1908), pp. 268–9, for similar in Seaford in the county of Hampshire. See also, Griffiths, 'The Interaction of War and Plague in the Later Middle Ages', p. 129.
48. Ziegler, *The Black Death*, pp. 173–4. See also, Gasquet, *The Black Death of 1348 and 1349*, p. 152.
49. Colin Platt, *King Death, The Black Death and its aftermath in late-medieval England* (Toronto, University of Toronto Press, 1997), pp. 27–8. See also, Ziegler, *The Black Death*, p. 174, and Gasquet, *The Black Death of 1348 and 1349*, pp. 152–3, 235.
50. Platt, *King Death, The Black Death and its aftermath in late-medieval England*, p. 30. See also, Ziegler, *The Black Death*, p. 174, and Griffiths, 'The Interaction of War and Plague in the Later Middle Ages', p. 129, for

another example of the impact of war and plague in England, being the county of Cheshire in the west of the country.

51. P. S. Lewis, *Later Mediaeval France, The Polity* (London, MacMillan and Co. Ltd., 1968), p. 53, for more general comment on the poor state of France due to war and plague. See also, Sumption, *The Hundred Years War - Volume II*, pp. 9–10, and Gottfried, *The Black Death*, p. 50.
52. C. T. Allmand, 'The War and the Non-Combatant', *The Hundred Years War* (London, The MacMillan Press Ltd, 1971), p. 165.
53. Sumption, *The Hundred Years War - Trial by Battle*, pp. 506–07, 510, 512. See also, Ziegler, *The Black Death*, p. 64.
54. R. Delente, 'L'habitat à Caen aux XIVe et XVe siècles [L'exemple des propriétés de l'abbaye d'Ardenne dans le quartier Saint-Sauveur - rue Écuyère]', *Ann Normandie* 50, 2000, p. 395, 'De fait, on peut considerer que les propriétés ont alores perdu la moitié de le valeur', or 'In fact, we can now consider that properties have lost half their value'. See also, Birdsall (trans.) and Newhall (ed.), *Chronicle of Jean de Venette*, p. 50.
55. Ibid., '*Comme pour cause des Englois nos anemis et pour la mortalité que Dieu a envoyée naguère sur son peuple les mesnages de la ville de Caen et les autres héritages sont apetichiés en revenu et plusieurs demourés gastés et vides places, et plusieurs tournés à non valoir* . . .'. See also, *Calendar of the Close Rolls, Preserved in the Public Record Office, Edward III Vol. X A.D. 1354-1360*, p. 76. The city of Cork in Ireland represents another example of a large community that struggled for many years because of war and the Black Death, as indicated by an entry in the *Calendar of the Close Rolls for 24 May 1354*: '. . . the city is so damaged by a sudden fire and by the late mortal pestilence and by the costs and expenses incurred by the mayor and community upon the war in those parts . . .'.
56. Lauro Martines, *April Blood, Florence and the Plot Against the Medici* (Oxford, Oxford University Press, 2003), p. 186.
57. Thorndike, *University Records and Life in the Middle Ages*, pp. 363–4.
58. J. F. D. Shrewsbury (ed.), *A History of Bubonic Plague in the British Isles* (Cambridge, At the University Press, 1970), p. 146.
59. Rosell (ed.), 'Corónica del Muy Alto et Muy Católico Rey Don Alfonso el Onceno', p. 390.
60. Gottfried, *The Black Death*, pp. 70–1. See also, Aberth, *The Black Death*, pp. 117–20, 138–9, and Ziegler, *The Black Death*, pp. 88–92.
61. Gasquet, *The Black Death of 1348 and 1349*, p. 78, from letters patent of King Magnus Eriksson.
62. Christiansen, *The Northern Crusades*, p. 194.

63. Gasquet, *The Black Death of 1348 and 1349*, p. 79.
64. Ibid.
65. Christiansen, *The Northern Crusades*, p. 194.
66. Nicaise, *La grande chirurgie de Guy de Chauliac*, p. 171. Chauliac says that there was at least a chance with the plagues of old, but nothing worked against this new one, '. . . celles-là esloient remediables en aucune manière, cette-cy en nul'.
67. René de Lespinasse, *Bibliothèque de l'École des Chartes, Tome Deuxième* (Paris, Schneider et Langrand, 1840–1), p. 208. The quotation comes from the prologue of de Covino's 'De Judicio Solis in Conviviis Saturni', 'On the Judgment of the Sun at a Feast of Saturn', '. . . sicut veraciter accidit in Montepessulano, ubi erat major copia medicorum quam alibi, et tamen vix evasit unus ex illis'.
68. Nicaise, *La grande chirurgie de Guy de Chauliac*, p. 171, see note 21 above. See also, Gasquet, *The Black Death of 1348 and 1349*, p. 35.
69. Shrewsbury (ed.), *A History of Bubonic Plague*, p. 146, for Edward IV of England's plague cure, which was very popular during the second half of the fifteenth century.
70. Talbot and Hammond, *The Medical Practitioners in Medieval England*, p. 112. See also, Cornelius Brown, *History of Newark-on-Trent; Being the Life Story of an Ancient Town, Volume I* (Newark, S. Whiles, 1904), pp. 122, 268. Newark was no small town, being about the size of Southampton or Lichfield at the time. Existing evidence points to a significant outbreak of the disease in Newark; and Ziegler, *The Black Death*, p. 184.
71. Rawcliffe, *Leprosy in Medieval England*, p. 238.
72. Power (ed.), *Treatises of Fistula in Ano*, p. 81. See also, Power (trans.), *De Arte Phisicali et de Cirurgia of Master John Arderne*, pp. 38–9.
73. Nicaise, *La grande chirurgie de Guy de Chauliac*, p. 172, 'Et moy pour euiter infamie, n'osay point m'absenter: mais auec continuelle peur me preseruay tant que ie pus . . . Ce neantmoins vers la fin de la mortalité, ie tombay en fiéure continue, auec vn aposteme à l'haine: et maladiay prés de six semaines, et fus en si grand danger que tous mes compagnons croyoient que ie mourusse: mais l'aposteme estant meury . . . i'en eschappay au vouloir de Dieu.'
74. Ibid., 'Pour la preseruation il n'y auoit rien de meilleur, que de fuir la région auant que d'estre infect, et se purger auec pilules aloëtiques: et diminuer le sang par phlebotomie, amander l'air par feu: et conforter le cœur de theriaque . . .'
75. Ibid., 'Pour la curatiue on faisoit des saignées et evacuations, des electuaires et syrops cordials. Et les apostemes extérieurs estoient meuris auec des figues

et oignons cuits, pilez et meslez auec du leuain et du beurre, puis estoient ouuerts, et traitez de la cure des vlceres.'

76. Haeser und Middeldorpf, *Buch der Bündth-Ertznei*, pp. 158–63. These make up the final part of von Pfolspeundt's surgery.
77. Ibid., p. 159, 'Item man sal sich vor dem damp ader adem des kranckenn hütten'.
78. Ibid., p. 162, 'Nim ffygen, wacholderber, rauten, lorbernn, welsche nuss, betonie, angelica, encian, unnd stos es undereinander, unnd vormenge es mith honnige. unnd is do von des morgens und, obenclens, als vil als ein welsche nuss gross. das sselbige ist sunclerlich guth vor die vorgiffte lusst der pestelentz genuttze'.
79. Ibid., p. 161, 'Knobloch geschelth in reinborgen schmer, weiffsen cleyen gestoffsenn, ein kuchen dar aus gemacht, und uff einem herde gebacken. szo heis der mensch erleiden kan, dor auff gebundenn'.
80. Malgaigne, *Surgery and Ambroise Paré*, pp. 330, 406. See also, Packard, *Life and Times of Ambroise Pare*, pp. 6–7.
81. Johnson (trans.), *The workes of that famous chirurgion Ambrose Parey*, pp. 535–75.
82. Ibid., p. 539.
83. Ibid., p. 551.
84. Ibid., pp. 552–3.
85. Ibid., p. 555. Mithridate is similar to theriac, being that it was made from a large number of ingredients, at least one of which was considered poisonous. See also, Judges (ed.), *The Elizabethan Underworld*, p. 501, n. 5.
86. Ibid., p. 545.
87. Solomon Claiborne Martin (trans.), *Hieronymus Fracastor's Syphilis, from the Original Latin; A Translation in Prose of Fracastor's Immortal Poem* (St Louis, The Philmar Company, 1911), p. 55.
88. Lawrence Stone, *Family, Sex and Marriage in England 1500-1800* (London, Weidenfeld and Nicolson, 1977), p. 599. See also, Brown, *The Pox*, p. 8; Fabricius, *Syphilis in Shakespeare's England*, Preface, p. xi, and Burfield, *Medieval Military Medicine*, pp. 100–03, for more on the disease in earlier centuries.
89. Hans Zinsser, *Rats, Lice and History, Being a Study in Biography, which, after Twelve Preliminary Chapters Indispensable for the Preparation of the Lay Reader, Deals with the Life History of Typhus Fever* (London, George Routledge & Sons Ltd., 1935), p. 69. See also, Brown, *The Pox*, p. 8.
90. Power (trans.), *De Arte Phisicali et de Cirurgia of Master John Arderne*, p. 28, 'For the disease which [is called] chaudpisse. [Parsley and boil it] in water [until] it is turned [into a mucilage] let it be well shaken with oil of roses or violets and then add [to it] the milk of a nursing woman, in which

[liquor] camphor is dissolved and inject with a syringe'. See also, Brown, *The Pox*, p. 8.

91. Friedrich W. D. Brie (ed.), *The Brut, or The chronicles of England, Edited from MS. Rawl. B 171, Bodleian Library, &c. Part 1-2* (London, published for the Early English Text Society by Kegan Paul, Trench, Trübner & Co., Limited, 1906), p. 604. See also, Shrewsbury (ed.), *A History of Bubonic Plague*, p. 147.
92. Peter Lewis Allen, *The Wages of Sin – Sex and Disease, Past and Present* (Chicago, The University of Chicago Press, 2000), p. 42. See also, Brown, *The Pox*, Illustration Number 16, between pp. 118 and 119, an American poster from the Second World War entitled, 'She May Look Clean - But', features a large image of a young woman's face being looked at by three small cartoon servicemen, while underneath it reads, 'Pick-Ups, "Good Time" Girls, Prostitutes Spread Syphilis and Gonorrhoea - You can't beat the Axis if you get VD'.
93. Judit Forrai, 'History of Different Therapeutics of Venereal Disease Before the Discovery of Penicillin', *Syphilis – Recognition, Description and Diagnosis* (Rijeka, Croatia, Intech, 2011), p. 40. See also, Fabricius, *Syphilis in Shakespeare's England*, pp. 5, 82, 147, and Zinsser, *Rats, Lice & History*, p .73.
94. L. Smith, 'The French pox', *J Fam Plann Reprod Health Care* 2006 Oct; 32 [4], p. 266. See also, Martin (trans.), *Hieronymus Fracastor's Syphilis*, pp. 35, 41 and 57. Fracastor does include other, less fictional elements in his poem as well, such as how the infection was contracted, its symptoms, and its treatment in the early sixteenth century.
95. John Comrie, *History of Scottish Medicine to 1860, For The Wellcome Historical Medical Museum* (London, Baillière, Tindall & Cox, 1927), Vol. I, p. 45.
96. Brown, *The Pox*, pp. 9–10. See also, M. Tampa, I. Sarbu, C. Matei, V. Benea and S. R. Georgescu, 'Brief history of syphilis', *Journal of Medicine and Life*, 2014 Mar 15; 7 [1], p. 5, and Daniel Turner, *De Morbo Gallico: A Treatise of the French Disease, Publish'd above 200 Years past, By Sir Ulrich Hutten, Kt. of Almayn in Germany. Translated soon after into English by a Canon of Marten-Abbye* (London, Printed for John Clarke at the Bible under the Royal Exchange, 1730), p. 1.
97. L. Smith, 'The French Pox', p. 265. See also, Forrai, 'History of Different Therapeutics of Venereal Disease Before the Discovery of Penicillin', p. 42; E. Tognotti, 'The Rise and Fall of Syphilis in Renaissance Europe', *J Med Humanit* 30, 2009, p. 100, and Zinsser, *Rats, Lice and History*, pp. 70–3.
98. Tampa et al., 'Brief history of syphilis', pp. 5–6. See also, Waldron, *Palaeopathology*, p. 104; Forrai, 'History of Different Therapeutics of

Venereal Disease Before the Discovery of Penicillin', pp. 42–3; Brown, *The Pox*, pp. 6–7; E. Tognotti,'The Rise and Fall of Syphilis in Renaissance Europe', p. 100, and Kerttu Manjander, Saskia Pfrengle, Arthur Kocher, Judith Neukamm, Louis du Plessis, Marta Pla-Díaz, Natasha Arora, Gülfirde Akgül, Kati Salo, Rachel Schats, Sarah Inskip, Markku Oinonen, Heiki Valk, Martin Malve, Aivar Kriiska, Päivi Onkamo, Fernando González-Candelas, Denise Kühnert, Johannes Krause and Verena J. Schuenemann, 'Ancient Bacterial Genomes Reveal a High Diversity of *Treponema pallidum* Strains in Early Modern Europe', *Current Biology*, Volume 30, Issue 19, Oct. 05, 2020, pp. 3796–8.

99. Forrai, 'History of Different Therapeutics of Venereal Disease Before the Discovery of Penicillin', p. 43.
100. Fabricius, *Syphilis in Shakespeare's England*, p. 5. See also, L. Smith, 'The French pox', p. 265; Brown, *The Pox*, p. 3, and Waldron, *Palaeopathology*, p. 102.
101. Iwan Bloch, 'History of Syphilis', *A System of Syphilis, In Six Volumes, Vol. 1* (London, Hodder & Stoughton, 1908), pp. 10–11. See also, Lesa Beth Randall, *Representations of syphilis in sixteenth-century French literature (PhD Dissertation)* (Tucson, University of Arizona, 1999), p. 26, regarding the deceptive nature of syphilis, and Waldron, *Palaeopathology*, p. 103.
102. Fabricius, *Syphilis in Shakespeare's England*, p. 6.
103. Bloch, 'History of Syphilis', p. 11. The time between the first and second stages of the disease appears to have been much shorter with this more virulent form.
104. George Gaskoin (trans.), *The Medical Works of Francisco Lopez de Villalobos, The Celebrated Court Physician of Spain* (London, John Churchill and Sons, 1870), p. 106.
105. Johnson (trans.), *The workes of that famous chirurgion Ambrose Paréy*, p. 579.
106. Alfred Fournier (trans.), *Jean de Vigo, Le Mal Français 1514* (Paris, G. Masson, 1872), p. 79, from Part II, Des Ulcerations Nasales Du Mal Francais, 'Aussi laissent-elles souvent à leur suite des déformations très-affligeantes pour les malades', 'They frequently leave behind deformations that are very distressing for the affected'. See also, Brown, *The Pox*, p. 46.
107. Waldron, *Palaeopathology*, p. 103. See also, Fabricius, *Syphilis in Shakespeare's England*, p. 6; Bloch, 'History of Syphilis', p. 11, '. . . the undoubted frequency of a fatal ending', and Cathryn Corns and John Hughes-Wilson, *Blindfold and Alone, British Military Executions in the Great War* (London, Cassell & Co., 2001). Before the First World War in Britain, it is estimated that 10 per cent of asylum inhabitants were suffering from tertiary syphilis.

108. Judges (ed.), *The Elizabethan Underworld*, p. 5. The pox sufferers and soldiers were often one and the same.
109. Haeser und Middeldorpf, *Buch der Bündth-Ertznei*, Vorwort, p. xxvii, 'Am unzweifelhaftesten deuten auf syphilitische ubel die affectionen . . .', 'The most unquestionable indications of evil syphilitic diseases . . .'. See also, ibid., p. 124.
110. Forrai, 'History of Different Therapeutics of Venereal Disease Before the Discovery of Penicillin', p. 41, for a 1483 example from Denmark. See also, Fabricius, *Syphilis in Shakespeare's England*, p. 58, for examples of the illness in 1494 in England and Ireland.
111. Brown, *The Pox*, pp. 2–3.
112. Ibid., pp. 1–2. See also, Irina Savinetskaya, *The Politics and Poetics of Morbus Gallicus in the German Lands (1495 – 1520) (Thesis)* (Budapest, Central European University, Budapest, 2016), pp. 29–30.
113. Brown, *The Pox*, p. 9. See also, K. Jillings, 'Plague, pox and the physician in Aberdeen, 1495–1516', *J R Coll Physicians Edinb* 2010; 40, p. 71, and C. H. Fuchs, *Die ältesten Schriftsteller über die Lustseuche in Deutschland, von 1495 bis 1510 Nebst mehreren Anecdotis späterer Zeit, gesammelt und mit literarhistorischen Notizen und einer kurzen Darstellung der epidemischen Syphilis in Deutschland* (Göttingen, Dieterichschen, 1843), p. 57, from *Libellus Joephi Grünbeckii de mentulagra alias morbo Gallico*. The Bavarian Joseph Grünpeck (c.1473–c.1532) noted among Charles VIII's men were '. . . et alios, quos belli occasio in copias conscripserat, transfudit', '. . . others whom the occasion of the war had conscripted into the army'.
114. Fuchs, *Die ältesten Schriftsteller über die Lustseuche in Deutschland*, p. 9, 'venenum contagiosum'. See also Zinsser, *Rats, Lice, and History*, pp. 73–4; Fabricius, *Syphilis in Shakespeare's England*, pp. 5–6; Tampa et al., 'Brief history of syphilis', p. 7, and Brown, *The Pox*, p. 9
115. Fuchs, *Die ältesten Schriftsteller über die Lustseuche in Deutschland*, p. 377, 'Davon ist solche kranckheit vonn den teutschen knechten, die man nachvolgents Landesknecht . . .'.
116. Fabricius, *Syphilis in Shakespeare's England*, p. 59.
117. Tampa et al., 'Brief history of syphilis', p. 7; Fabricius, *Syphilis in Shakespeare's England*, p. 82.
118. Burfield, *Medieval Military Medicine*, pp. 100–01, for historical examples of soldiers and STIs.
119. Sassoon, *The War Poems of Siegfried Sassoon*, p. 37 and George J. Firmage, *E.E. Cummings, Complete Poems, 1904-1962* (New York, Liveright, 1991), p. 272.

120. P. M. Gonon, *Séjours de Charles VIII et Loy XII, a Lyon sur le Rosne. Jouxte la copie des Faicts, Gestes et Victoires des Roys Charles VIII et Loys XII* (Lyon, Charvin et Nigon, 1841), pp. 28–30.
121. Iwan Bloch, *Der Ursprung der Syphilis: eine medizinische und kulturgeschichtliche Untersuchung, Erste Abteilung* (Jena, Gustav Fischer, 1901), p. 263, 'Es heisst nun in der ersten Verordnung, derjenigen des Pariser Parlamentes vom 6. März 1497, dass seit zwei Jahren in Frankreich eine Krankheit „Grosse veröle' genannt, herrsche . . .', 'The first decree, that of the Paris parliament of 6 March 1497, notes that for two years the disease called the 'Great Syphilis' had already prevailed in France'. See also Gaskoin (trans.), *The Medical Works of Francisco Lopez de Villalobos*, p. 219.
122. Karl Sudhoff, *Aus der Frühgeschichte der Syphilis; Handschriften- und Inkunabelstudien, epidemiologische Untersuchung und kritische Gänge*, Leipzig, Johann Ambrosius Barth, 1912, p. 13, the original manuscript (cod. germ. 244) where this account was discovered belonged to a convent called Altenhohenau in Bavaria.
123. Ibid., p. 16, '. . . der seit 5 Jahren sein Bett nicht mehr verlassen hate . . .', '. . . he who had not left his bed for 5 years . . .'.
124. Ibid., once he had been completely healed the account notes, '. . . all sein groß locher vnd schaden gehayllt vnd sein smerczen . . .', or 'all the big holes and damage to his body were healed, as was the pain . . .'.
125. Ibid.
126. Holy Bible, p, 72 (New Testament), Mark 15:15, 'And Pilate, wishing to satisfy the multitude, released to them Barabbas, and delivered up Jesus, after scourging him, to be crucified.'
127. Sudhoff, *Aus der Frühgeschichte der Syphilis*, p. 16, 'Darnach hat dy muter gotes den ritter auff gehaben von der erden vnd er hat empfunden gesuntheit an allem seinem leib', 'Afterwards, the mother of God raised the knight from the ground, and he felt health throughout his body'.
128. Ibid., '. . . der Ritter erwachte vor dem Bette knieend und weinte vor Freude', '. . . the knight awoke to find himself kneeling by his bedside, weeping joyously'.
129. Ibid., 'Aber dy Hecken vnd masen hat er etwen lang zeyt gehab', 'But he had these spots and masses for a while'.
130. Claudia Stein, *Negotiating the French Pox in Early Modern Germany* (Farnham, Surrey, Ashgate Publishing Limited, 2009), p. 1 and Bloch, *Der Ursprung der Syphilis*, pp. 273–4. The Nürnbergen Reimchronik von 1580 notes that Landsknechts brought it from France.
131. Fabricius, *Syphilis in Shakespeare's England*, p. 57.

132. Brown, *The Pox*, p. 9. See also, Bloch, *Der Ursprung der Syphilis*, pp, 270–5; Fabricius, *Syphilis in Shakespeare's England*, pp. 58–9, and G. E. Gall, S. Lautenschlager and H. C. Bagheri, 'Quarantine as a public health measure against an emerging infectious disease: syphilis in Zurich at the dawn of the modern era (1496-1585)', *GMS Hyg Infect Control* 2016 Jun 6; 11: Doc 13, p. 2.
133. Jillings, K., 'Plague, pox and the physician in Aberdeen, 1495–1516', p. 71.
134. Comrie, *History of Scottish Medicine to 1860*, pp. 45, 47.
135. Bloch, *Der Ursprung der Syphilis*, p. 273, 'Die Lustseuche scheint erst 1498 durch Kriegsleute nach diesem Teile Nordwestdeutschlands gebracht worden zu sein', 'The plague seems to have been brought to parts of what is now north-west Germany by soldiers in 1498'. See also, ibid., p. 275, 'Prag. — Die Syphilis zeigte sich in Prag erst 1499. 1500 wurde ein Hospital für sie eingerichtet', 'Prague – Syphilis only appeared in Prague in 1499. In 1500 a hospital was set up to treat the sick', and Brown, *The Pox*, p. 9.
136. Fabricius, *Syphilis in Shakespeare's England*, pp. 24–5. See also, Allen, *The Wages of Sin*, p. 45.
137. Craig R. Thompson (trans.), *The Colloquies of Erasmus* (Chicago, The University of Chicago Press, 1965), pp. 428–9, from the colloquy entitled '*The Ignoble Knight or Faked Nobility*'.
138. Brown, *The Pox*, p. 9.
139. Tampa et al., 'Brief History of Syphilis', p. 8.
140. John Hale, *The Civilization of Europe in the Renaissance* (New York, Simon & Schuster, 1993), p. 556. See also, J. R. Hale, 'The Soldier in Germanic Graphic Art of the Renaissance', *The Journal of Interdisciplinary History*, vol. 17, no. 1, 1986, pp. 103–04, and Brown, *The Pox*, p. 9.
141. Hale, 'The Soldier in Germanic Graphic Art of the Renaissance', p. 103, See also Ernst and Johanna Lehner, *Picture Book of Devils, Demons and Witchcraft* (New York, Dover Publications Inc., 1971), p. 107.
142. Hale, 'The Soldier in Germanic Graphic Art of the Renaissance', p. 103.
143. Martin (trans.), *Hieronymus Fracastor's Syphilis*, p. 9.
144. Auguste Alexandre Veinant (ed.), *Les sept marchans de Naples, c'est assavoir l'adventurier. le religieux. l'escolier. l'aveugle. le vilageois. le marchant et le bragart* (Paris, Silvestre, 1838), p. 17, 'L'édition en caractères gothiques sur laquelle a été justifiée la présente copie doit, bein que sans date, avoir paru vers 1530'. See also, Randall, *Representations of syphilis in sixteenth-century French literature*, p. 133. Among more well-known works, Randall's thesis brings to light an obscure set of French poems related to syphilis from the early sixteenth century that are worthy of a much wider audience.

145. Randall, *Representations of syphilis in sixteenth-century French literature*, p. 144.
146. Veinant (ed.), *Les sept marchans de Naples*, p. 2.
147. Ibid., p. 3, 'Comme difforme et pouentable monstre'.
148. Nathan Bailey (trans.) and Rev. E. Johnson (ed.), *The colloquies of Desiderius Erasmus concerning men, manners and things, In Three Volumes, Vol. I*, (London, Gibbings & Company, Limited, 1900), p. 284.
149. Randall, *Representations of syphilis in sixteenth-century French literature*, p. 38.
150. Fournier (trans.), *Jean de Vigo*, p. 30, '. . . l'essential pour nous, c'est de savoir traiter er guérir cette maladie'.
151. Brown, *The Pox*, pp. 11–12. See also, Allen, *The Wages of Sin*, p. 43, and Randall, *Representations of syphilis in sixteenth-century French literature*, p. 26.
152. Allen, *The Wages of Sin*, pp. 42–3. See also, Brown, *The Pox*, p. 18. In the following century, London's St Bartholomew's Hospital struggled to cope with the number of syphilitic patients at its doors. These too were segregated from the other patients and given separate bedding, clothing, and nursing staff. The problem became so great that, here too, patients were sent to accommodations that had once housed lepers.
153. Comrie, *History of Scottish Medicine to 1860*, p. 47.
154. Ibid., pp. 45, 47.
155. Ibid., p. 47.
156. Ibid. See also, Fabricius, *Syphilis in Shakespeare's England*, p. 61. Henry VII of England tried closing the brothels or 'stews' in London, but sex workers just plied their trade elsewhere; and Allen, *The Wages of Sin*, p. 42.
157. Fabricius, *Syphilis in Shakespeare's England*, pp. 25–6. Fabricius notes, 'Everyone knew how the disease began, but nobody knew how it would end'.
158. Gaskoin, *The Medical Works of Francisco Lopez de Villalobos*, pp. 223–4. See also, Randall, *Representations of syphilis in sixteenth-century French literature*, p. 161.
159. Fournier (trans.), *Jean de Vigo*, pp. 61–2, one of de Vigo's mercurial ointments was made with four ounces of quicksilver, a pound of pork fat, one ounce each of chamomile oil, mastic, and pine resin, among other constituents. Once mixed, the patient was to sit in front of a fire while the doctor spread the ointment onto their skin using the palm of their hand and plenty of friction. The skin was then covered with hot compresses, which were kept in place using bandages. See also, Martin (trans.), *Hieronymus Fracastor's Syphilis*, p. 42; F. William Cock, 'An Early Prescription In English', *The British Medical Journal*, vol. 1, no. 3307, 1924, p. 869, for a mercury-based ointment before 1497, and Randall, *Representations of syphilis in sixteenth-century French literature*, p. 161.

160. Gruner (trans.), *The Canon of Medicine of Avicenna*, p. 378.
161. Rosenman (trans.), *The Chirurgia of Roger Frugard*, p. 51. See also, Rosenman (trans.), *The Surgery of Roland of Parma*, p. 44, for similar.
162. Rosenman (trans.), *The Surgery of Master Jehan Yperman*, pp. 102, 103, 208. See also, Rosenman (trans.), *The Major Surgery of Guy de Chauliac*, p. 485. Chauliac notes that the great French physician and professor of medicine at Montpellier, Bernard de Gordon, favoured this remedy too.
163. Fournier (trans.), *Jean de Vigo*, p. 58, 'Ceux qui condamnent le mercure dans le traitement du mal français sont les premiers à le prescrire contre la *scabie*, le phlegme salé, le serpigo, le impétigo, etc.'.
164. Randall, *Representations of syphilis in sixteenth-century French literature*, p. 300.
165. Ibid, pp. 52, 161–2.
166. Fabricius, *Syphilis in Shakespeare's England*, pp. 33–4. See also, Gaskoin, *The Medical Works of Francisco Lopez de Villalobos*, pp. 168–70.
167. Waldron, *Palaeopathology*, pp. 102–03. See also, Fabricius, *Syphilis in Shakespeare's England*, pp. 37–8, and Randall, *Representations of syphilis in sixteenth-century French literature*, p. 104.
168. Waldron, *Palaeopathology*, p. 102. See also, World Health Organization, *Mercury and Health*, 31 March 2017 (on-line article).
169. Martin (trans.), *Hieronymus Fracastor's Syphilis*, p. 42.
170. François Féry-Hue, « De la verolle ». Poèmes inédits sur le péril vénérien (fin du XVe - début du XVIe siècle) In: *Romania*, tome 110 n°439-440, 1989, p. 548, from a manuscript in the Bibliothèque Municipale de Soissons, MS 203, f. 39v. See also, ibid., p. 551, for another harrowing appraisal of such remedies in a poem by Eustorg de Beaulieu (c. 1495–1552), written no later than 1537, entitled *Rondeau d'ung paovre verolli*, or *About a poor syphilitic*, 'I am from my head to my feet Naked, near a big fire and greased Scalded, boiled and fired Without mercy and worth less than a beast'; and Randall, *Representations of syphilis in sixteenth-century French literature*, p. 312, where I discovered this resource.
171. Brown, *The Pox*, p. 21. See also, Fabricius, *Syphilis in Shakespeare's England*, p. 38.
172. Brown, *The Pox*, p. 21. See also, Johnson (trans.), *The workes of that famous chirurgion Ambrose Parëy*, pp. 469.
173. Johnson (trans.), *The workes of that famous chirurgion Ambrose Parëy*, pp. 468–70.
174. Ibid., p. 468, 'Guaiacum hath not sufficient strength to extinguish the venom of the venereous virulencie . . .'. See also, ibid., p. 470.
175. Brown, *The Pox*, p. 35.

176. Turner, *De Morbo Gallico*, p. 12.
177. Brown, *The Pox*, p. 35. See also, W. Buchan, *Observations Concerning the Prevention and Cure of the Venereal Disease. Intended to guard the ignorant and unwary against the baneful effects of that insidious malady* (London, T. Chapman, 1796), p. 245, regarding the decline of guaiacum.
178. Brown, *The Pox*, pp. 61, 99. See also, Buchan, *Observations Concerning the Prevention and Cure of the Venereal Disease*, p. 241.
179. Waldron, *Palaeopathology*, p. 102. See also, Buchan, *Observations Concerning the Prevention and Cure of the Venereal Disease*, pp. 242–7.
180. Brown, *The Pox*, pp. 186–9.
181. A. Grzybowski and K. Pawlikowska-Łagód, 'Some lesser-known facts on the early history of syphilis in Europe', *Clin Dermatol* 2024 Mar-Apr; 42 [2], pp. 128, 132. A recent Polish study has put the fatality numbers for syphilis at around five million.
182. DeWitte, 'The Anthropology of Plague', p. 97. See also, Green, 'Editor's Introduction to Pandemic Disease in the Medieval World', p. 9.
183. Veinant (ed.), *Les sept marchans de Naples*, p. 15,
    Pleurs et en larmes,
    Je laisse les armes
    Et les durs assaubc.
    Pourtant soyez fermes
    Entre vous, gensdarmes,
    D'eviter telz maulx . . .
    En lieu de picque je porte une potence
    Et tiens le champ au devant d'ung moustier,
    En demandant une maille ou denier
    Pour aulmosne, au peuple charitable.

Chapter 8: Damaged Psyches

1. Michon (ed.), *Documents inédits sur la grande peste de 1348*, p. 87, ll, pp. 109–10, 'Et pour ce que merencolie, Esteint toute pensée lie', from Guillaume de Machaut's *Le Jugement dou roy de Navarre*, or *The Judgement of the King of Navarre*.
2. Alexandra Onuf and Nicholas Ealy, 'Introduction', *Violence, Trauma and Memory – Responses to War in the Late Medieval and Early Modern World* (Lanham, Lexington Books, 2022), pp. 3–5. See also, Wendy J. Turner and Christina Lee, 'Conceptualizing Trauma for the Middle Ages', *Trauma in Medieval Society* (Leiden, Brill, 2018), p. 8; Richard Morgan Loomis (trans.), *Dafydd ap Gwilym - The Poems* (Binghamton, Centre for Medieval & Early

Renaissance Studies, 1982), p. 56, 'battle-grief' from *Englynion to Ifor Hael*, a poem by Dafydd ap Gwilym, and Scoble (ed.), *The Memoirs of Philip de Commines*, Vol. I, p. 321, 'melancholy'.

3. Thompson (ed.), *Chronicon Galfridi le Baker de Swynebroke*, p. 152, 'Tunc vexilla titubarunt, vexillarii corruerunt, hii sua viscera fusa calcarunt, alii dentes evomuerunt, multi terre fixi fuerunt, nonnulli stantes brachia precisa perdiderunt'.
4. Bessel van der Kolk, *The Body Keeps Score – Mind, Brain and Body in the Transformation of Trauma* (London, Penguin Books, 2014), pp. 45–7. See also, Peter Bernstein, *Trauma: Healing the Hidden Epidemic* (Petaluma, The Bernstein Institute for Integrative Psychotherapy & Trauma Treatment, 2013), pp. 1–2, 21–9, 72–3; and Judith Lewis Herman, *Trauma and Recovery* (London, Pandora, 2015), p. 34.
5. Adair, 'The Newsletter of Gerhard von Wesel, 17 April 1471', p. 69. See also, Rossell Hope Robbins (ed.), *Historical Poems of the XIVth and XVth Centuries* (New York, Columbia University Press, 1959), p. 227; the contemporary poem *The Battle of Barnet* emphasises the horror of the day, 'Uppon Ester day befelle a pyteous case, Many a man hys lyfe lost in the mornyng.'
6. Bernstein, *Trauma: Healing the Hidden Epidemic*, p. 73.
7. Kaeuper and Kennedy, *The Book of Chivalry of Geoffroi de Charny*, p. 111, Section 19. See also, ibid., p. 177, Section 40.
8. Wilson, *The Book of Geoffroi de Charny*, p. 113, and Vegetius, *De Re Militari*, p. 84.
9. Institute of Medicine of the National Academies, *Treatment for Posttraumatic Stress Disorder in Military and Veteran Populations: Initial Assessment* (Washington D.C., The National Academies Press, 2012), pp. 25–6. See also, M. A. Crocq and L. Crocq, 'From shell shock and war neurosis to posttraumatic stress disorder: a history of psychotraumatology', *Dialogues Clin Neurosci.* 2000 Mar; 2 [1], p. 47.
10. Richard A. Gabriel, *Military Psychiatry: A Comparative Perspective* (Westport, Greenwood Press, 1986), p. 181.
11. Ibid., pp. 181, 188. See also, Bernstein, *Trauma: Healing the Hidden Epidemic*, pp. 72–3.
12. Paulus Grosjean (ed.), *Henrici VI Angliae Regis Miracula Postuma, Ex codice Musei Britannici regio 13. C VIII* (Brussels, Société des Bollandistes, 1935), Liber I, p. 48, 'Unde ille nimirum animo turbatus est, eoque intimius contristatus quo se viderat longius a patria segregatum'. See also, Knox and Leslie (trans.), *The Miracles of King Henry VI*, pp. 58–9.
13. Grosjean (ed.), *Henrici VI Angliae Regis Miracula Postuma*, Liber I, p. 48, '. . . ad tantam devenit impotenciam ut mensis unius et dimidii spacio nullum

prorsus . . .', '. . . he became so helpless that in the space of a month and a half he could do no work at all . . .'. See also, Y. Sun, Y. Qu and J. Zhu, 'The Relationship Between Inflammation and Post-traumatic Stress Disorder', *Front Psychiatry* 2021 Aug 11; 12: 707543, p. 2, for similar symptoms in modern soldiers.

14. Grosjean (ed.), *Henrici VI Angliae Regis Miracula Postuma*, Liber I, p. 48, '. . . cum quippe nec ipsi quotquot accesserant medici hanc illi promittere quovis- modo valuissent', '. . . since indeed even they themselves, the many doctors who had come, were in no way able to help him with this'.
15. Bourchier (trans.) and Macaulay (ed.), *The Chronicles of Froissart*, p. 334.
16. Ibid., p. 335.
17. Bernstein, *Trauma: Healing the Hidden Epidemic*, pp. 8–9.
18. Bourchier (trans.) and Macaulay (ed.), *The Chronicles of Froissart*, p. 316, for an example of de Béarn's war experiences.
19. Ibid., p. 334.
20. Herman, *Trauma and Recovery*, p. 37. See also, Van der Kolk, *The Body Keeps Score*, pp. 134–5, 187–8.
21. Charles Hamilton Sorley, *Marlborough and Other Poems* (Cambridge, Cambridge University Press, 1919), p. 78.
22. Sassoon, *The War Poems of Siegfried Sassoon*, p. 61.
23. E. A. Gebresenbet, Z. Zegeye and T. D. Biratu, 'Prevalence and associated factors of depression and posttraumatic stress disorder among trauma patients: multi-centered cross-sectional study', *Front Psychiatry* 2025 Mar 7;16, p. 2. See also, Bernstein, *Trauma: Healing the Hidden Epidemic*, p. 9.
24. François Morand, *Chronique de Jean Fèvre, seigneur de Saint-Remy, Transcrite d'un manuscrit appartenant a la Bibliothèque de Boulogne-Sur Mer* (Paris, Librairie Renouard, 1876), p. 260, '. . . que deschausser gens mors et désarmer. Soubz lesquelz trouvèrent pluiseurs prisonniers en vie, entre lesquelz le duc d'Orléans en fut ung . . .', '. . . the dead were to be stripped of their shoes and arms. Under them they found several prisoners alive, the Duke of Orleans being one of them . . .'. See also, Pierre Champion, *Vie de Charles d'Orléans (1394-1465)* (Paris, Honoré Champion, 1911), p. 158 fn. 5.
25. Enid McLeod, *Charles of Orleans, Prince and Poet* (London, Chatto & Windus, 1969), p. 129.
26. Livingston and DeVries (ed.), *The Battle of Crécy*, p. 49. See also, ibid., p. 13.
27. Champion, *Vie de Charles d'Orléans (1394-1465)*, p. 359, 'Louis d'Orléans meurt assassiné en 1407 . . .'.
28. Ibid., p. 59, 'Le 4 décembre 1408 Madame Valentine, duchesse d'Orléans, mourut, à son château de Blois . . .'.

29. Ibid., p. 61, fn 1, '. . . que sa femme Isabelle mourut des suites de son accouchement, le 13 septembre 1409 . . .'.
30. Charles-Louis Morand-Métivier, '"Je hé guerre, point ne la doit prisier": Emotions, War, and Trauma in the Poetry of Charles of Orléans', *Violence, Trauma, and Memory – Responses to War in the Late Medieval and Early Modern World* (London, Lexington Books, 2022), pp. 50–1, 60. See also. McLeod, *Charles of Orleans, Prince and Poet*, pp. 180–1, 306.
31. Flores (ed.), *An Anthology of Medieval Lyrics*, p. 180, translated by Muriel Kittel. See also, Morand-Métivier, '"Je hé guerre, point ne la doit prisier"', pp. 52–60, for more examples.
32. Coopland (trans.), *The Tree of Battles of Honoré Bonet*, pp. 18, 159, 189.
33. Ibid., p. 182.
34. Willard (trans.) and Cannon Willard (ed.), *The Book of Deeds of Arms and of Chivalry*, pp. 174–5. See also, Joanne Carnandet (ed.), *Acta Sanctorum, January* [1] (Paris, Victor Palmé, 1863), p. 76, #29. Among the miracles of St Odilo Abbot of Cluny, from centuries earlier, is a similar example, 'Praeterea miles quidam tam mentis inops erat effectus, ut postposita penitus omni cura privata vel publica, per devia solivagus et nudus erraret, inconditas voces emitteret, et tamquam deamoniacum se per inordinati gestus insaniam exhiberet', 'Moreover, a certain soldier was so unfit of mind that he ignored entirely all private or public concerns. He wandered around naked and lonely, uttering incoherent voices, and exhibiting his insanity with strange gestures, as if possessed by a demon', and Corns and Hughes-Wilson, *Blindfold and Alone - British Military Executions in the Great War*, pp. 325–36, for an example from the First World War, Second Lt Eric Skeffington Poole.
35. Coopland (trans.), *The Tree of Battles of Honoré Bonet*, pp. 182–3, Bonet said, '. . . if he killed a thousand he would never be punished for it'. See also, Willard (trans.) and Cannon Willard (ed.), *The Book of Deeds of Arms and of Chivalry*, pp. 174-5. De Pizan uses a figure of one hundred.
36. *Calendar of the Patent Rolls, Preserved in the Public Record Office, Edward I. A.D. 1301-1307*, printed for Her Majesty's Stationery Office (London, Eyre and Spottiswoode, 1898), p. 416, see Winchester, Feb. 20.
37. Wendy J. Turner, *Care and Custody of the Mentally Ill, Incompetent, and Disabled in Medieval England* (Turnhout, Brepolis Publishers, 2013), p. 123.
38. *Calendar of the Patent Rolls, Preserved in the Public Record Office, Edward I. A.D. 1301-1307*, p. 416, Dorchester, Feb. 1. A knight called James de Astlee seems to have been similarly pardoned.
39. Charity Cannon Willard (ed.), *The Writings of Christine de Pizan* (New York, Persea Books, 1994), p. 338.

40. Gebresenbet et al, 'Prevalence and associated factors of depression and posttraumatic stress disorder among trauma patients: multi-centered cross-sectional study', p. 3. PTSD symptoms can develop with the loss of a loved one in terrible circumstances, even if it is not witnessed. See also, H. J. Hewitt, *The Organisation of War under Edward III, 1338-62* (Manchester, Manchester University Press, 1966), p. vii, and C. T. Allmand, *Society at War, The Experience of England and France During the Hundred Years War* (Edinburgh, Oliver & Boyd, 1973), pp. 131–2.
41. Juliet Barker, *Conquest - The English Kingdom of France 1417-1450* (Cambridge, Mass., Harvard University Press, 2012), p. 4.
42. Willard (ed.), *The Writings of Christine de Pizan*, p. 344, n. 1. See also, ibid., p. 343; de Pizan apologises to Marie de Berry for taking as long as she did to write the letter, but she too was struggling.
43. Allmand, 'The War and the Non-Combatant', p. 173.
44. Turner and Lee, 'Conceptualizing Trauma for the Middle Ages', p. 9.
45. Allmand, 'The War and the Non-Combatant, p. 171. See also, Sumption, *The Hundred Years War - Volume II*, pp. 360–1; Shahar, *Growing Old in the Middle Ages*, p. 123, and Bourchier (trans.) and Macaulay (ed.), *The Chronicles of Froissart*, pp. 142–3, '. . . they wasted all the country without any cause, and robbed without sparing all that ever they could get, and violated and defiled women, old and young, without pity . . .'.
46. J. C. Laidlaw (ed.), *The Poetical Works of Alain Chartier* (Cambridge University Press, 1974), p. 32–6.
47. Nicolas, *History of the Battle of Agincourt*, p. 64, 'Upon the day on which the truce was made (Harfleur), Michael de la Pole, Earl of Suffolk, died of the disease which had proved fatal to the Bishop of Norwich . . .'. See also, ibid., pp. 59–60, which provides the identity of the illness which killed both Michael de la Pole, Senior and the Bishop of Norwich, as dysentery.
48. Joseph Hunter, *Agincourt. A Contribution Towards an Authentic List of the Commanders of the English Host in King Henry the Fifth's Expedition to France, in the Third Year of His Reign* (London, John Russell Smith, 1850), p. 28.
49. Ibid., '. . . for he had 3 daughters . . .'.
50. Flores (ed.), *An Anthology of Medieval Lyrics*, pp. 343–4, translated by William M. Davis.
51. The British Library Board, Royal MS 19 B XIII, *f.* 7r, *Roman de la Rose*, see miniature top right. See also, Burfield, *Medieval Military Medicine*, pp. 124, 187, n. 101, for similar examples from earlier centuries.
52. Janet Cowen (ed.), *Sir Thomas Malory, Le Morte D'Arthur, In Two Volumes* (Hammondsworth, Penguin Books Ltd., 1969), Vol. I, pp. 173–4. See also,

Strachey (ed.), *Le Morte d'Arthur*, p. 102. In the version printed by William Caxton, the rape scene, from which this epigraph is taken, is omitted.

53. Bern, Burgerbibliothek, Mss.h.h.I.3: Diebold Schilling, *Amtliche Berner Chronik*, vol. 3, p. 259, for a scene from the Burgundian Wars of the 1470s in which a Burgundian soldier is about to bring his foot down on the stomach of a heavily pregnant woman laying helplessly on the floor, just as two young children are stripped, hung and stabbed by another.
54. Birdsall (trans.) and Newhall (ed.), *Chronicle of Jean de Venette*, pp. 84–5, for villagers sleeping in a fortified church, in constant fear of attacks by English soldiers. See also, Douët-D'Arcq, *Choice de Pièces Inédites Relatives au Règne De Charles VI, Tome Second*, pp. 124–5, from a French record dated 25 March 1417, involving a poor farm labourer named Guillemin Hure in Northern France: 'En laquelle carrière ou caverne et à l'entrée d'icelle, le dit suppliant avoit faicte une manière de logis pour retraire soy, sa femme et enfant, avec un petit de mesnage qu'il avoit, pour la doubte des gens d'armes qui couroient ou pays', 'In which a cave, near the entrance, the supplicant had made a kind of dwelling to retreat with his wife and child, along with a small stock of supplies that he had, because they feared the soldiers who were running around the country'.
55. Caryn A. Reeder, 'Wartime Rape, the Romans, and the First Jewish Revolt', *Journal for the Study of Judaism in the Persian, Hellenistic, and Roman Period*, vol. 48, no. 3, 2017, pp. 363–5, 383. See also, W. A. Tol, V. Stavrou and M. C. Greene *et al*, 'Sexual and gender-based violence in areas of armed conflict: a systematic review of mental health and psychosocial support interventions', *Confl Health* 7, 16 (2013), pp. 7–8.
56. Tol, *et al*, 'Sexual and gender-based violence in areas of armed conflict', p. 8. See also, Claudia Card, 'Rape as a Weapon of War', *Hypatia*, vol. 11, no. 4, 1996, pp. 6–7
57. Johnes (trans.), *The Chronicles of Enguerrand de Monstrelet*, Vol. I, pp. 303–04.
58. Ibid., p. 303. See also, Charles Samaran (trans. and ed.), *Thomas Basin, Histoire de Charles VII, Tome 1er, 1407-1444* (Paris, Société d'édition 'Les Belles lettres', 1933), p. 213, for an equally dreadful but slightly different account of this part of the sack of Soissons.
59. Anne Curry, 'The Theory and Practice of Female Immunity in the Medieval West', *Sexual Violence in Conflict Zones, From the Ancient World to the Era of Human Rights* (Philadelphia, University of Pennsylvania Press, 2011), p. 176.
60. Kaeuper and Kennedy, *The Book of Chivalry of Geoffroi de Charny*, p. 95, Section 12. See also, Wilson, *The Book of Geoffroi de Charny*, p. 124. His

father wrote, 'Love and honour, too, all ladies and damsels, I pray you; and be sure you always speak well of them, for it's thanks to them that one attains true worth'.

61. Twiss (ed.), *Monumenta Juridica, Vol. I*, p. 453, Item 3 from the *Ordinances of War Made by King Richard II, at Durham, AD 1385*, relates, '. . . ne nulle femme, ne de prendre prisoner, sil ne port armes, ne denforcer nulle femme sur peine destre penduz', '. . . not to take any woman prisoner, unless she bears arms and not to ravish any woman on pain of being hanged'.
62. Kingsford (ed.), *The First English Life of King Henry the Fifth*, p. 34. See also, Twiss (ed.), *Monumenta Juridica, Vol. I*, p. 460. In his ordinances decreed at Mantes in 1419, Henry V noted that, upon pain of death, his men were not to rape or threaten a woman.
63. Barbara Donagan, 'Law, War, and Women in Seventeenth-Century England', *Sexual Violence in Conflict Zones, From the Ancient World to the Era of Human Rights* (Philadelphia, University of Pennsylvania Press, 2011), p. 191. See also, Neil Murphy, 'Violence, Colonization and Henry VIII's Conquest of France, 1544–1546', *Past & Present*, Volume 233, Issue 1, November 2016, p. 25.
64. Geremek, *The Margins of Society*, pp. 114–15. See also, Murphy, 'Violence, Colonization and Henry VIII's Conquest of France, 1544–1546', p. 25. Soldiers frequently believed that rape and booty were their right as victors of battles and sieges.
65. Ohler, *Krieg und Frieden im Mittelalter*, p. 274, 'Vergewaltigung kam im Krieg häufiger vor, als die Quellen festhalten, vielleicht deshalb, weil christliche Autoren den sexuellen Bereich weitgehend ausblenden'.
66. Kathryn Gravdal, *Ravishing Maidens, Writing Rape in Medieval French Literature and Law* (Philadelphia, University of Pennsylvania Press, 1991), pp. 128, 137. Gravdal suggests the possibility that the soldier could not be found in order to stand trial in this case. See also, Duplès-Agier, *Registre Criminel du Chatelet de Paris du 6 Septembre 1389 au 18 Mai 1392,* pp. 42–7, for a similar case in which an 18-year-old girl was supplied to a soldier named Jean Braque for sex. Here again, the woman who arranged it, in this case Katherine du Roquier, was burnt to death for her involvement, while the soldier went unpunished.
67. Douët-D'Arcq, *Choice de Pièces Inédites Relatives au Règne De Charles VI, Tome Second*, p. 92, 'Et adont anglois print sa dicte femme devant son dit mary, et coucha avec ques elle et la congnut charnelment contre son gré . . .', 'And the Englishman took the man's wife, right in front of him, and slept with her and knew her carnally against her will . . .'.

68. Ibid., pp. 92–3.
69. Siméon Luce, *Histoire de Bertrand du Guesclin et de son époque, la jeunesse de Bertrand (1320-1364)* (Paris, Librairie Hachette et Cie., 1876), p. 72, fn. 4, Luce cites this example from Bibliothèque Nationale Francais (BnF), mss. lat. no., 5381, t. I, f. 124, 'Ipsa, existens conjugata, rapta fuerat per aliquos de Magna Societate, super quo in tantum turbata fuit et etiam metu ne maritus suus propter hoc istam in odio haberet . . .'.
70. Ibid., '. . . quod ipsa demens et demoniaca fuit effecta'.
71. M. de Barante, *Historie des Ducs de Bourgogne de la Maison de Valois, 1364 – 1477, Tome IX* (Paris, Librairie le Normant, 1854), pp. 406–07, 'Sans cesse des soldats étaient logés chez les habitans, et les maltraitaient sans nul contrôle ni recours . . . Il n'y avait donc sortes de fantaisies auxquelles il ne se livrât : corrompant avec.de l'argent les jeunes filles de tout état, ou les enlevant à leurs parens, leur faisant violence, forçant la clôture des couvens, déshonorant les familles des nobles comme celles des bourgeois', 'Soldiers regularly stayed in the homes of the inhabitants, mistreating them without any control or recourse . . . There were no types of fantasies in which he [Hagenbach] did not indulge. He corrupted young girls of all ranks using money, or by taking them from their parents and violating them. He did the same to nuns, as well as to the daughters of nobles and the bourgeoise.'
72. Ibid., p. 407, 'Il lui arriva un jour de donner une fête, et tout d'un coup, après avoir renvoyé les maris, il fit mettre les femmes toutes nues, en leur couvrant seulement la tête'.
73. Diane Lupig, 'Investigation and Prosecution of Sexual and Gender-Based Crimes before the International Criminal Court', *American University Journal of Gender, Social Policy & the Law* 17, no. 2 (2009), p. 436.
74. Herman, *Trauma and Recovery*, p. 51.
75. Ibid., p. 68. See also, Rape Crisis Scotland, *Information for survivors of sexual violence. Guilt, shame and blame* (Glasgow, Rape Crisis Scotland Helpline, 2024), online pamphlet www. rape crisis scotland. org. uk /resources/Guilt-blame-and-shame.pdf.org.uk), pp. 3–8.
76. C. Espí Forcén and F. Espí Forcén, 'Demonic possessions and mental illness: discussion of selected cases in late medieval hagiographical literature', *Early Sci Med.* 2014;19 [3], p. 262. During the late Middle Ages, 'madness' was thought to be caused by an imbalance of the humours, which could lead to things such as depression, anxiety and mania.
77. Tol, et al, 'Sexual and gender-based violence in areas of armed conflict', p. 8. See also, Herman, *Trauma and Recovery*, p. 58.

78. Rosalind Brown-Grant (trans.), *The Book of the City of Ladies* (Bury St Edmunds, Penguin Books, 1999), p. 147. In *The Book of the City of Ladies*, which was completed in 1405, Christine de Pizan makes it clear just how normalized rape had seemingly become among some men: 'It therefore angers and upsets me when men claim that women want to be raped and that, even though a woman may verbally rebuff a man, she won't in fact mind it if he does force himself upon her. I can scarcely believe that it could give women any pleasure to be treated in such a vile way . . . On the contrary, they think that it is the worst thing that could possibly happen to them.' See also, Luce, *Histoire de Bertrand du Guesclin et de son époque*, p. 72. In the nineteenth century, Luce noted that the incidents of sexual violence against women that led to psychological damage were very common during the Hundred Years War, especially those caused by members of the Great Company. 'Dans les cas de folie furieuse, qui vont devenir si fréquents, surtout chez les femmes à la suite des rapts et des viols commis par les brigands des compagnies . . .'.
79. MacKaye (trans.), *The Canterbury Tales*, p. 205.
80. Wilfred Owen, *Poems*, London, Penguin Classics, 2017, p. 30.
81. Burfield, *Medieval Military Medicine*, pp. 20–2.
82. John O'Rourke, *Suicide Now the Primary Cause of Death among Active Duty US Soldiers*, Boston University, 15 July 2024, online article: www.bu.edu/articles/2024/suicide-now-the-primary-cause-of-death-among-active-duty-us-soldiers/. See also, D. L. Nordstrom, 'Ukraine set to act on high suicide burden', *Injury prevention: Journal of the International Society for Child and Adolescent Injury Prevention* vol. 13,4 (2007), pp. 224–5.
83. Institute of Medicine of the National Academies, *Treatment for Posttraumatic Stress Disorder in Military and Veteran Populations*, p. 36. See also, Bernstein, *Trauma: Healing the Hidden Epidemic*, p. 73, and Aleksandra Nicole Pfau, *Madness in the Realm: Narratives of Mental Illness in Late Medieval France (Thesis)* (Michigan, University of Michigan, 2008), pp. 196–7.
84. Birdsall (trans.) and Newhall (ed.), *Chronicle of Jean de Venette*, pp. 41, 93. See also, Johnes (trans.), *The Chronicles of Enguerrand de Monstrelet*, Vol. I, p. 49, 189; James Gairdner (ed.), *The Historical Collections of a Citizen of London in the Fifteenth Century* (Westminster, Nichols and Sons, 1876), pp. 18, 20; Schullian (trans.), *Diaria de bello Carolino*, p. 159, and Johnson (trans.), *The workes of that famous chirurgion Ambrose Parėy*, pp. 775–6.
85. Birdsall (trans.) and Newhall (ed.), *Chronicle of Jean de Venette*, p. 75.
86. Alexander Murray, *Suicide in the Middle Ages, Volume 1 The Violent against Themselves* (Oxford, Oxford University Press, 1998), pp. 225–6. See also,

J. Schmitt, 'Le suicide au Moyen Age', *Annales. Histoire, Sciences Sociales*, 31[1], 1976, p. 23, n. 35.

87. Schmitt, 'Le suicide au Moyen Age', p. 24 n. 46, 'Jean Lunneton se pendit « a bien environ demie lieue » de sa maison', 'Jean Lunneton hanged himself "about the distance of half a league" from his house'.
88. Douët-D'Arcq, *Choice de Pièces Inédites Relatives au Règne De Charles VI, Tome Second*, p. 176, '. . . et qui avoit perdu la graigneur partie de ses biens par le fait et occasion des guerres . . .'.
89. Ibid., 'Pour lesquelles choses ou autrement, lui, tempté de l'ennemi, s'en ala, icellui deffunct, pendre à un arbre . . .'.
90. Pfau, *Madness in the Realm*, p. 198.
91. Flores (ed.), *An Anthology of Medieval Lyrics*, p. 178, *Ales vous ant, ales, ales* or *Away With You! Begone! Begone!* , translated by Dwight Durling.
92. Siraisi, *Taddeo Alderotti and his Pupils*, p. 234.
93. Luce, *Histoire de Bertrand du Guesclin et de son époque*, p. 72, 'Les malheureux atteints d'aliénation mentale, s'ils ne font de mal à personne, sont gardés chez leurs parents', 'Those unfortunates suffering from mental health problems, provided they do no harm to anyone, are left with their parents'. See also Rawcliffe, *Medicine & Society*, p. 10.
94. Luce, *Histoire de Bertrand du Guesclin et de son époque*, p. 72, fn. 3, from Archives Nationale (Paris) JJ 115 no. 74, 'Perrine, femme de Pierre Mauravaule, étant tombée malade et « en fernisie tellement que elle avoit très petit sens », leseigneurdu lieu ordonne à son mari de la garder de telle sorte qu'elle ne préjudicie ni à lui seigneur ni à autrui . . .'.
95. Siraisi, *Taddeo Alderotti and his Pupils*, p. 234 fn. 87.
96. Grosjean (ed.), *Henrici VI Angliae Regis Miracula Postuma*, Liber II, pp. 125–7.
97. Ibid., p. 126, 'Quocirca saniores quidam et amiciciores affinium et proximorum, cum nequaqum valuissent ullis eum increpacionibus edomare seu pacare blandiciis, iniecta in eum manu violenta . . . manicis quoque ferreis prepeditum, cippis astringentes, quousque in idem volveretur celum salvo custodire curarunt', 'Some of his more sane and friendly relatives and neighbours, who had not been able to bring him under control with rebukes or flattery, restrained him . . . and bound him with iron manacles, binding him with stocks, and took care to keep him safe until he should return to heaven'. See also, Luce, *Histoire de Bertrand du Guesclin et de son époque*, pp. 72–3, fn. 5, Luce brings together a couple of cases, citing from Bibliotheque Nationale, France (BnF), mss. lat. no., 5381, t. II, f. 268, 'Ligatus cum ligaminibus ferreis per pedes et manus et custoditus in domo sua', 'He was bound up by his hands and feet, using iron fetters and then

kept inside his house', and another from Archives Nationale (Paris) JJ 123, no. 280, 'Jeannin Guillon, laboureur de Rousson, étant devenu fou furieux, sa femme le fait 'enfergier par les mains' et conduire à Saint-Mathurin de Larchant pour y faire sa neuvaine', 'Jeannin Guillon, a farm worker from Rousson, went berserk and his wife had him "imprisoned by the hands" and then taken to Saint-Mathurin de Larchant to make his novena.'

98. Judges (ed.), *The Elizabethan Underworld*, p. 17.
99. Catherine Arnold, *Bedlam, London and Its Mad* (London, Pocket Books, 2008), p. 2.
100. Clay, *The Mediaeval Hospitals of England*, p. 33, 'menti capti'. See also, Arnold, *Bedlam, London and Its Mad*, pp. 18–20, and Michel Foucault, *Madness and Civilization, A History of Insanity in the Age of Reason* (New York, Vintage Books, 1988), p. 9.
101. J. J. López-Ibor, 'The founding of the first psychiatric hospital in the World in Valencia', *Actas Esp Psiquiatr.* 2008 Jan-Feb; 36 [1], p. 4.
102. Ibid., p. 1.
103. Clay, *The Mediaeval Hospitals of England*, pp. 33–4. See also, Foucault, *Madness and Civilization*, pp. 9–10, and Rawcliffe, *Medicine & Society*, pp. 10–11.
104. Foucault, *Madness and Civilization*, p. 9.
105. Morand-Métivier, '"Je hé guerre, point ne la doit prisier", p. 50.
106. Champion, *Vie de Charles d'Orléans*, p. 590. Pierre Champion, who authored an important biography of the Duke of Orléans, observed that Charles refused to be a passive victim of the melancholy that assaulted him, 'Toutefois Charles ne sera pas la victime tranquille de cette Mélancolie qui le combat si fort: il s'efforcera de la chasser, comme on poursuit un chien enragé'. See also, McLeod, *Charles of Orleans, Prince and Poet*, p. 180.
107. Flores (ed.), *An Anthology of Medieval Lyrics*, p. 178, translated by Dwight Durling.
108. A. Pope, 'Exploring the Emotional Landscape of Veterans: An Analysis of Poems About PTSD', *Journal of Veterans Studies*, 2024, 10 [1], pp. 24–5.
109. N. Landis-Shack, A. J. Heinz and M. O. Bonn-Miller, 'Music Therapy for Posttraumatic Stress in Adults: A Theoretical Review', *Psychomusicology*. 2017; 27 [4], pp. 336–7.
110. Ibid., pp. 336–40.
111. Burfield, *Medieval Military Medicine*, p. 128.
112. Nicaise, *Chirurgie de Maitre Henri de Mondeville*, p. 145, '. . . et que le corps engraisse par la joie et maigrit par la tristesse'.
113. Ibid., p. 144, '. . . distraie en jouant de la viole ou du psaltérion à dix corde'.
114. Bovey, *Tacuinum Sanitatis*, pp. 19, 44, 73.

115. Peregrine Horden, 'Commentary on Part III, with a Note on Paracelsus', *Music as Medicine, The History of Music Therapy since Antiquity* (Aldershot, Ashgate Publishing Limited, 2000), p. 152, from his treatise *De religione perpetua.*
116. Claude V. Palisca, *Humanism in Italian Renaissance Musical Thought* (New Haven, Yale University Press, 1985), p. 181.
117. Scoble (ed.), *The Memoirs of Philip de Commines*, Vol. I, p. xiii, de Commines fought at battles such as Montlhéry in 1465.
118. Ibid., Vol. I, pp. 321–2. See also, Putnam, *Charles the Bold, Last Duke of Burgundy*, p. 420, and Bernstein, *Trauma: Healing the Hidden Epidemic*, pp. 72–3.
119. Scoble (ed.), *The Memoirs of Philip de Commines*, Vol. I, p. 321.
120. Willard (ed.), *The Writings of Christine de Pizan*, p. 339.
121. Bernstein, *Trauma: Healing the Hidden Epidemic*, pp. 103–04. See also, Van der Kolk, *The Body Keeps Score*, pp. 207, 210.
122. Scoble (ed.), *The Memoirs of Philip de Commines*, Vol. I, p. 321.
123. Van der Kolk, *The Body Keeps Score*, pp. 210–11. See also, Bernstein, *Trauma: Healing the Hidden Epidemic*, p. 104, and Herman, *Trauma and Recovery*, p. 160.
124. Scoble (ed.), *The Memoirs of Philip de Commines, Vol. I*, pp. 321–2. See also, Bernstein, *Trauma: Healing the Hidden Epidemic*, p. 85, and Van der Kolk, *The Body Keeps Score*, p. 207.
125. Putnam, *Charles the Bold, Last Duke of Burgundy*, p. 426.
126. Vatican City, Biblioteca Apostolica, Vaticana, Palatina lat. 1363, f. 168r. I discovered this manuscript in Siraisi, *Taddeo Alderotti and his Pupils*, p. 234, fn. 85.
127. Robert Burton, *The Anatomy of Melancholy: What it is, with all the kinds causes, symptomes, prognostickes, & severall cures of it. In three Partitions, with their severall Sections, members & subsections; Philosophically, Medicinally, Historically, opened & cut up by Democritus Junior* (Oxford, Henry Cripps, 1628), pp. 12, the third of four unnumbered pages between 208 and 209, 379, Democritus Junior was the pseudonym of Robert Burton.
128. Moffat, *SHARP Practice 6*, pp. 22–3.
129. K. Clement, C. R. Covertson, M. J. Johnson and K. Dearing, 'St. John's wort and the treatment of mild to moderate depression: a systematic review', *Holist Nurs Pract.* 2006 Jul-Aug; 20[4], p. 197.
130. Q. Q. Mao, S. P. Ip, Y. F. Xian, Z. Hu and C. T. Che, 'Anti-depressant-like effect of peony: a mini-review', *Pharm Biol.* 2012 Jan; 50[1], pp. 72–4.
131. Brian Stone (trans.), *Medieval English Verse* (Penguin Books, New York, 1988), p. 144, n. 2.

132. Margaret B. Freeman, *Herbs for the Mediaeval Household for Cooking Healing and Divers Uses* (New York, The Metropolitan Museum of Art, 1943), p. 11.
133. Ibid., p. 24.
134. George T. L. Chapman, Frank McCombie and Anne Wesencraft (ed.), *A New Herball by William Turner, Parts II and III*, Cambridge, Cambridge University Press, 1995), p. 489.
135. Freeman, *Herbs for the Mediaeval Household*, pp. 29–30.
136. MacKaye (trans.), *The Canterbury Tales*, pp. 78–9.
137. L. Zhang, C. Wang, Q. Meng, Q. Tian, Y. Niu and W. Niu, 'Phytochemicals of Euphorbia lathyris L. and Their Antioxidant Activities', *Molecules* 2017 Aug 18; 22[8], p. 1.
138. Freeman, *Herbs for the Mediaeval Household*, Introduction p. x, 41.
139. Jack Hartnell, *Medieval Bodies, Life, Death and Art in the Middle Ages* (London, Wellcome Collection, 2018), p. 37.
140. N. K. Yoshikawa, 'Holy medicine and diseases of the soul: Henry of Lancaster and Le livre de seyntz medicines', *Med Hist.* 2009 Jul; 53[3], pp. 408–09.

Conclusion

1. Johnson (trans.), *The workes of that famous chirurgion Ambrose Paréy*, p. 308.
2. Smith and Gnudi (trans.), *The Pirotechnia of Vannoccio Biringuccio*, pp. 422–35, for more on sixteenth-century weapons.
3. Geoffrey Parker, *The Military Revolution, Military innovation and the rise of the West, 1500-1800*, (Avon, The Bath Press, 1988), pp. 1–2.
4. I. Pells, 'Reassessing Frontline Medical Practitioners of the British Civil Wars in the Context of the Seventeenth-Century Medical World', *The Historical Journal*. 2019; 62[2], pp. 401–02.

BIBLIOGRAPHY

Manuscripts

Bern, Burgerbibliothek, Mss.h.h.I.3: Diebold Schilling, *Amtliche Berner Chronik*, vol. 3.

Bern, Burgerbibliothek, Mss.h.h.I.16: Diebold Schilling, *Spiezer Chronik*.

Bibliothèque nationale de France, Français 2643, Chroniques sire JEHAN FROISSART.

British Library Board, Harley MS 1736, *Tracts on Surgery, etc.*

British Library Board, Royal MS 19 B XIII, *Roman de la Rose*.

British Library Board, Sloane MS 2272, *Anatomia Membrorum*.

Christ Church, Oxford, *De Nobilitatibus Sapientii Et Prudentiis Regum*, MS 92.

Die Große Heidelberger Liederhandschrift (*Codex Manesse*) Cod. Pal. Germ. 848; Universitätsbibliothek, Heidelberg.

Huntington Library, San Marino, California HM 937, *De cas des nobles hommes et femmes*, 1462.

Tschachtlan, Bendicht: [*Berner Chronik*]. Bern, [um 1470]. Zentralbibliothek Zürich, Ms A 120.

Vatican City, Biblioteca Apostolica, Vaticana, Palatina lat. 1363.

Wellcome Collection, *Alchemical and Medical Miscellany*, MS.117.

Wellcome Collection, *An English folding almanac in Latin*, MS.8932.

Wellcome Collection, *Jackson, Jane*, MS.373.

Zürich, Zentralbibliothek, Ms. Rh. hist. 33b: *War technology (Illuminated Manuscript)*.

Studies and Journal Reports

Adair, John, 'The Newsletter of Gerhard von Wesel, 17 April 1471', *Journal of the Society for Army Historical Research*, vol. 46, no. 186, 1968, pp. 65–9.

Barker, Hannah, 'Laying the Corpses to Rest: Grain, Embargoes, and *Yersinia pestis* in the Black Sea, 1346–48', *Speculum*, Volume 96, Number 1, January 2021, pp. 97–126.

Boucherie, A., Jørkov, S. ML and Smith M., 'Wounded to the bone: Digital microscopic analysis of traumas in a medieval mass grave assemblage (Sandbjerget, Denmark, AD 1300-1350)'. *Int J Paleopathol*. 2017, Dec;19: pp. 66–79.

Bullough, Vern L., 'Training of the Nonuniversity-Educated Medical Practitioners in the Later Middle Ages', *Journal of the History of Medicine and Allied Sciences*, vol. 14, no. 4, 1959, pp. 446–58.

Card, Claudia, 'Rape as a Weapon of War', *Hypatia*, vol. 11, no. 4, 1996, pp. 5–18.

Carter, Colonel B. Noland, and DeBakey, Lieutenant Colonel Michael E., 'Current Observations on War Wounds of the Chest', *The Journal of Thoracic Surgery*, August 1944, Vol. 13, No. 4, pp. 271–93.

Clement, K., Covertson, C. R., Johnson, M. J., and Dearing K., 'St. John's wort and the treatment of mild to moderate depression: a systematic review', *Holist Nurs Pract*, 2006 Jul-Aug; 20 4, pp. 197–203.

Cobb, T. K., 'Wrong site surgery – where are we and what is the next step?', *Hand* (N Y). 2012 Jun; 7[2], pp. 229–32.

Cock, F. William, 'An Early Prescription In English', *The British Medical Journal*, vol. 1, no. 3307, 1924, pp. 869–70.

Cockayne, Emily, 'Experiences of the Deaf in Early Modern England', *The Historical Journal*, vol. 46, no. 3, 2003, pp. 493–510.

Colleter, R., Bataille, C.P., Dabernat, H., Pichot, D., Hamon, P,. Duchesne, S., Labaune-Jean, F., Jean, S., Le Cloirec, G., Milano, S., Trost, M., Steinbrenner, S., Marchal, M., Guilbeau-Frugier, C., Telmon, N., Crubézy, É., and Jaouen, K., 'The last battle of Anne of Brittany: Solving mass grave through an interdisciplinary approach (paleopathology, biological anthropology, history, multiple isotopes and radiocarbon dating)', *PLoS One*. 2021 May 5; 16 [5], pp. 1–25.

Conroy, K., and Malik, V., 'Hearing loss in the trenches – a hidden morbidity of World War I', *The Journal of Laryngology & Otology*, 2018. 132[11], pp. 952–5.

Cotton, Juliana Hill, 'Benedetto Reguardati of Nursia (1398-1469)', *Medical History*, Volume XIII 1969, pp. 175–89.

Crocq, M.A., and Crocq, L., 'From shell shock and war neurosis to posttraumatic stress disorder: a history of psychotraumatology', *Dialogues Clin Neuroscim*, 2000 Mar; 2 [1], pp. 47–55.

Cunha, E., and Silva, A.M., 'War lesions from the famous Portuguese Medieval battle of Aljubarrota', *Int. J. Osteoarchaeology*, 7, 1997, pp. 595–9.

Delente R., 'L'habitat à Caen aux XIVe et XVe siècles [L'exemple des propriétés de l'abbaye d'Ardenne dans le quartier Saint-Sauveur - rue Écuyère]', *Ann Normandie* 50, 2000, pp. 387–407.

Demmm Eberhard, 'Censorship', in: 1914-1918-online *International Encyclopedia of the First World War*, ed. by Ute Daniel, Peter Gatrell, Oliver Janz, Heather

Jones, Jennifer Keene, Alan Kramer, and Bill Nasson, issued by Freie Universität Berlin, Berlin 2017-03-29.

Eftekhari, Kian, Choe, Christina H., Vagefi, M. Reza, and Eckstein, Lauren A., 'The last ride of Henry II of France: Orbital injury and a king's demise', *Survey of Opthalmology*, Volume 60, Issue 3, May-June 2015, pp. 274–8.

Eldredge, L. M., 'A thirteenth-century ophthalmologist, Benvenutus Grassus: his treatise and its survival', *J R Soc Med.*, 1998 Jan; 91[1], pp. 47–52.

Féry-Hue, Françoise, '« De la verolle ». Poèmes inédits sur le péril vénérien (fin du XVe - début du XVIe siècle)', *Romania*, tome 110 n°439-440, 1989, pp. 542–52.

Forcén, C. Espí and Forcén, F. Espí, 'Demonic possessions and mental illness: discussion of selected cases in late medieval hagiographical literature', *Early Sci Med.* 2014;19[3], pp. 258–79.

Fruergaard, Simon, Braad Lund, Marie, Schramm, Andreas, Vosegaard, Thomas, and Bilde, Trine.,'The myth of antibiotic spider silk', *iScience*, 2021, pp. 1–17.

Gagliardi, Isabella, 'La disparition progressive des femmes médecins du Moyen Âge, une histoire oubliée', *La Conversation*, 3 January 2023, pp. 1–5.

Gall, G. E., Lautenschlager, S., and Bagheri, H.C., 'Quarantine as a public health measure against an emerging infectious disease: syphilis in Zurich at the dawn of the modern era (1496-1585)', *GMS Hyg Infect Control* 2016 Jun 6; 11: Doc 13, pp. 1–10.

Gask, G. E., 'The Medical Staff of King Edward the Third', *Proceedings of the Royal Society of Medicine*, 1 May 1926, pp. 1–16.

Gask, G. E., 'The Medical Services of Henry the Fifth's Campaign of the Somme in 1415', *Proceedings of the Royal Society of Medicine*, 1 May 1923, pp. 1–10.

Gebresenbet, E.A., Zegeye, S,. and Biratu, T.D., 'Prevalence and associated factors of depression and posttraumatic stress disorder among trauma patients: multi-centered cross-sectional study', *Front Psychiatry*, 2025 Mar 7;16, pp. 1–13.

Goodman, Kevin, 'The Strange Case of Henry V's Wandering Wound', *Ramparts: Magazine of the Friends of Dudley Castle*, Summer 2015, pp. 1–5.

Gottfried, Robert S., 'English Medical Practitioners, 1340-1530', *Bulletin of the History of Medicine*, vol. 58, no. 2, 1984, pp. 164–82.

Greco, Manfredi, Ciriaco, Greto, Antonio, Vonella, Marco, Vitagliano, Tiziana 'The Primacy of the Vianeo Family in the Invention of Nasal Reconstruction Technique', *Annals of Plastic Surgery* June 2010, 64[6], pp. 702–05.

Grzybowski, A., and Pawlikowska-Łagód, K.'Some lesser-known facts on the early history of syphilis in Europe', *Clin Dermatol* 2024 Mar–Apr; 42 [2], pp. 128–32.

Gupta, A. K., 'The Pioneer of Plastic Surgery – 'Sushruta'', *Dev Sanskriti Interdisciplinary International Journal*, Vol. 6, July 2015, pp. 39–43.

Hale, J. R., 'The Soldier in Germanic Graphic Art of the Renaissance', *The Journal of Interdisciplinary History*, vol. 17, no. 1, 1986, pp. 85–114.

Harper, April, 'The Image of the Female in Western Vernacular Literature of the Middle Ages', *Social History of Medicine*. Vol. 24, Issue 1, 2011, pp. 108–24.

Harvey, D., Bardelang, P., Goodacre, S.L., Cockayne, A. and Thomas, N.R., 'Antibiotic Spider Silk: Site-Specific Functionalization of Recombinant Spider Silk Using "Click" Chemistry', *Advanced Materials*, Volume 29, Issue 10, March 2017, pp. 1–5.

Hébert, Michel, 'L'armée provençale en 1374', *Annales du Midi, revue archéologique, historique et philologique de la France méridionale*, Tome 91, N°141, 1979, pp. 5–27.

Henneman, John B. Jr., 'The Black Death and Royal Taxation in France, 1347-1351', *Speculum, A Journal of Mediaeval Studies*, Vol. XLIII, No. 3, July 1968, pp. 405–28.

Hernigou P., 'Crutch art painting in the Middle Ages as orthopaedic heritage (part II: the peg leg, the bent-knee peg and the beggar)', *Int Orthop*. 2014 Jul; 38[7], pp.1535–42.

Holzman, Robert S., 'The Legacy of Atropos, the Fate Who Cut the Thread of Life', *Anesthesiology*, 1998, 89, pp. 241–9.

Hooper, Bari, Rickett, Stephanie, Rogerson, Andrew J. G., and Yaxley, Susan, 'The grave of Sir Hugh de Hastyngs, Elsing', *Norfolk Archaeology*, vol. 39 (1984/86), pp. 88–99.

Jessop, Oliver, 'A New Artefact Typology for the Study of Medieval Arrowheads', *Medieval Archaeology*, Vol. XL (1996), pp. 192–205.

Jillings, K., 'Plague, pox and the physician in Aberdeen, 1495–1516', *J R Coll Physicians Edinb* 2010; 40, pp. 70–6.

Juvin, P, and Desmonts, J.M., 'The ancestors of inhalational anesthesia: the Soporific Sponges (XIth-XVIIth centuries): how a universally recommended medical technique was abruptly discarded', *Anesthesiology* 2000 Jul; 93[1], pp. 265–9.

Kaur A., and Guan, Y., 'Phantom limb pain: A literature review', *Chin J Traumatol* 2018 Dec; 21[6], pp. 366–8.

Kedar, Benjamin Z., 'Benvenutus Grapheus of Jerusalem, an Oculist in the Era of the Crusades', *KOROT, The Israel Journal of the History of Medicine and Science*, Vol. 11, 1995, pp. 14–41.

Kjellström, Anna, 'A Sixteenth-Century Warrior Grave from Uppsala, Sweden: The Battle of Good Friday', *International Journal of Osteoarchaeology*, 15: 2005, pp. 23–50.

Landis-Shack, N., Heinz, A.J., Bonn-Miller. M.O., 'Music Therapy for Posttraumatic Stress in Adults: A Theoretical Review', *Psychomusicology*, 2017; 27 [4], pp. 334–42.

Lang, S.J., 'John Bradmore and his book Philomena', *Soc Hist Med.* 1992 Apr;5[1], pp. 21–30.

López-Ibor, J.J., 'The founding of the first psychiatric hospital in the World in Valencia', *Actas Esp Psiquiatr*. 2008 Jan-Feb; 36 [1]: pp. 1–9.

Lupig, Diane, 'Investigation and Prosecution of Sexual and Gender-Based Crimes before the International Criminal Court', *American University Journal of Gender, Social Policy & the Law* 17, no. 2 (2009), pp. 431–96.

Manjander, Kerttu, Pfrengle, Saskia, Kocher, Arthur, Neukamm, Judith, Plessis, Louis du, Pla- Díaz, Marta, Arora, Natasha, Akgül, Gülfirde, Salo, Kati, Schats, Rachel, Inskip, Sarah, Oinonen, Markku, Valk, Heiki, Malve, Martin, Kriiska, Aivar, Onkamo, Päivi, González-Candelas, Fernando, Kühnert, Denise, Krause, Johannes, Schuenemann, and Verena, J., 'Ancient Bacterial Genomes Reveal a High Diversity of *Treponema pallidum* Strains in Early Modern Europe', *Current Biology*, Volume 30, Issue 19, Oct. 05, 2020, pp. 3788–3803.

Mao, Q. Q., Ip, S. P., Xian, Y. F., Hu, Z., and Che, C. T., 'Anti-depressant-like effect of peony: a mini-review.' *Pharm Biol.* 2012 Jan; 50 [1], pp. 72–7.

Markatos, K., Karamanou, M., Arkoudi, K., and Androutsos, G., 'Henry II of France (1519-1559) and His Death From Meningoencephalitis Following Cranial Trauma', *World Neurosurg*, 2017 Oct; 106, pp. 442–5 .

Markatos, K., Karamanou, M., Tsourouflis, G., Androutsos, G., and Mavrogenis, A.F., 'Ambroise Paré (1510-1590): on the diagnosis and treatment of shoulder dislocations', *Int Orthop*, 2018 Jan; 42 [1], pp. 215–18.

Metzler, Irina, 'Disability in the Middle Ages: Impairment at the Intersection of Historical Inquiry and Disability Studies', *History Compass*, Vol. 9, Issue 11, January 2011, pp. 45–60.

Murphy, Neil, 'Violence, Colonization and Henry VIII's Conquest of France, 1544–1546', *Past & Present*, Volume 233, Issue 1, November 2016, pp. 13–51.

Mustain, James K., 'A Rural Medical Practitioner in Fifteenth-Century England', *Bulletin of the History of Medicine*, vol. 46, no. 5, 1972, pp. 469–76.

Nordstrom, D. L., 'Ukraine set to act on high suicide burden', *Injury Prevention: Journal of the International Society for Child and Adolescent Injury Prevention*, vol. 13,4 (2007): pp. 224–6.

Oshima, K., Suchert, S., Blevins, N. H., and Heller, S., 'Curing hearing loss: Patient expectations, health care practitioners, and basic science', *J Commun Disord.* 2010 Jul-Aug; 43[4], pp. 311–18.

Park, Marian T., Mignucci-Jiménez, Giancarlo, Houlihan, Lena Mary and Preul, Mark C., 'Management of injuries on the 16th-century battlefield: Ambroise Paré's contributions to neurosurgery and functional recovery', *Neurosurgical Focus*, 2022 Sep; 53[3], pp. 1–12.

Pells I., 'Reassessing Frontline Medical Practitioners of the British Civil Wars in the Context of the Seventeenth-Century Medical World', *The Historical Journal* 2019; 62[2], pp. 399–425.

Pope, A., 'Exploring the Emotional Landscape of Veterans: An Analysis of Poems About PTSD', *Journal of Veterans Studies*, 2024 10 [1], pp. 22–6.

Reeder, Caryn A., 'Wartime Rape, the Romans, and the First Jewish Revolt', *Journal for the Study of Judaism in the Persian, Hellenistic, and Roman Period*, vol. 48, no. 3, 2017, pp. 363–85.

Salehi, S., Koeck, K., and Scheibel, T., 'Spider Silk for Tissue Engineering Applications', *Molecules* 2020 Feb 8; 25 [3], 737, pp. 1–20.

Schmitt, J., 'Le suicide au Moyen Age', *Annales. Histoire, Sciences Sociales*, 31[1], pp. 3–28.

Smart, William R.E., 'On The Medical Services of the Navy and Army from the Accession of Henry VIII to the Restoration', *The British Medical Journal*, Feb. 7–28, 1874, in 4 parts.

Smith, L., 'The French pox', *J Fam Plann Reprod Health Care* 2006 Oct; 32 [4], pp. 265–6.

Spyrou, Maria A., Tukhbatova, Rezeda I., Feldman, Michal, Drath, Joanna, Kacki, Sacha, Beltrán de Heredia, Julia, Arnold, Susanne, Sitdikov, Airat G., Castex, Dominique, Wahl, Joachim, Gazimzyanov, Ilgizar R., Nurgaliev, Danis K, Herbig, Alexander, Bos, Kirsten I., and Krause, Johannes, 'Historical Y. pestis Genomes Reveal the European Black Death as the Source of Ancient and Modern Plague Pandemics', *Cell Host and Microbe*, Volume 19, Issue 6, 2016, pp. 874–81.

Sun, Y., Qu, Y., and Zhu, J., 'The Relationship Between Inflammation and Post-traumatic Stress Disorder', Front Psychiatry 2021 Aug 11; 12: 707543, pp. 1–6.

Tampa, M., Sarbu, I., Matei, C., Benea, V., and Georgescu, S. R., 'Brief history of syphilis', *Journal of Medicine and Life*, 2014 Mar 15; 7 [1], pp. 4–10.

Tognotti, E., 'The Rise and Fall of Syphilis in Renaissance Europe', *J Med Humanit* 30 (2009), pp. 99–113.

Tol, W. A., Stavrou, V., and Greene, M. C. *et al.*, 'Sexual and gender-based violence in areas of armed conflict: a systematic review of mental health and psychosocial support interventions', *Confl Health* 7, 16 (2013), pp. 7–16.

Watt, James, 'Surgeons of the *Mary Rose*, The practice of surgery in Tudor England', *The Mariner's Mirror - The International Journal of the Society for Nautical Research*, Vol. 69, No. 1, February 1983, pp. 3–18.

Williams, A. N., and Williams, J, '"Proper to the duty of a chirurgeon": Ambroise Paré and sixteenth century paediatric surgery', *Journal of the Royal Society of Medicine*, Volume 97, September 2004, pp. 446-449

Wolfe, Jared A., Christensen, Daniel L., Mauntel, Timothy C., Owens, Brett D., LeClere, Lance E., and Dickens, Jonathan F., 'A History of Shoulder Instability in the Military: Where We Have Been and What We Have Learned', *Military Medicine*, Volume 183, Issue 5-6, May-June 2018, pp. 158–65.

Yoshikawa, N. K., 'Holy medicine and diseases of the soul: Henry of Lancaster and Le livre de seyntz medicines', *Med Hist.* 2009 Jul;53[3], pp. 397–414.

Zhang, L., Wang, C., Meng, Q, Tian, Q., Niu, Y., and Niu, W. 'Phytochemicals of Euphorbia lathyris L. and Their Antioxidant Activities', *Molecules* (2017), Aug 18; 22 8, pp. 1–12.

Zuo, K. J., and Olson, J. L., 'The evolution of functional hand replacement: From iron prostheses to hand transplantation.', *Plast Surg (Oakv)* 2014 Spring; 22 [1], pp. 44–51.

Primary Source Material

Amman, Jost and Sachs, Hans, *The Book of Trades (Ständebuch)*, New York, Dover Publications, Inc., 1973.

Bailey, Nathan (trans.) and Johnson, Rev. E. (ed.), *The colloquies of Desiderius Erasmus concerning men, manners and things, In Three Volumes, Vol. I*, London, Gibbings and Company, Limited, 1900.

Bain, Joseph (ed.), *Calendar of Documents Relating to Scotland, Preserved in Her Majesty's Public Record Office, London, Volume III, A.D. 1307-1357*, Edinburgh, H.M. General House, 1887.

Balfour-Melville, E. W. M., 'Papers Relating to the Captivity and Release of David II', *Miscellany of the Scottish History Society*, Edinburgh, T. and A. Constable Ltd, 1958.

Bellaguet, M. L., *Chronique du Religieux de Saint-Denys, Contenant le Regne de Charles VI, de 1380 a 1422, Publiée en Latin pour la Premiere Fois et Traduite, Tome Premier*, Paris, Imprimerie de Crapelet, 1839.

Birdsall, Jean (trans.) and Newhall, Richard A. (ed.), *Chronicle of Jean de Venette*, New York, Columbia University Press, 1953.

Bourchier, John (Lord Berners) (trans.) and Macaulay, G. C. (ed.), *The Chronicles of Froissart*, London, MacMillan and Co., Limited, 1904.

Brie, Friedrich W. D. (ed.), *The Brut, or The chronicles of England, Edited from MS. Rawl. B 171, Bodleian Library, &c. Part 1-2*, London, published for the Early English Text Society By Kegan Paul, Trench, Trübner & Co., Limited, 1906.

Brizzolara, Guiseppe (ed.), *La Cronica de Cristoforo da Soldo, Raccolta Storici Italiani dal cinquecento al millecinquecento, Tomo XXI, Parte III*, Bologna, Nicola Zanichelli, 1900.

Broeckx, M. C., *La Chirurgie de Maître Jehan Yperman Chirurgien Belge (XIIIe - XIVe Siècle), Publiée pour la Première fois d'après la copie flamande de Cambridge*, Antwerp, J. de Koninck, 1866.

Brown-Grant, Rosalind (trans.), *The Book of the City of Ladies*, Bury St Edmunds, Penguin Books, 1999.

Burton, Robert, *The Anatomy of Melancholy: What it is, with all the kinds causes, symptomes, prognostickes, & seuerall cures of it. In three Partitions, with their severall Sections, members & subsections; Philosophically, Medicinally, Historically, opened & cut up by Democritus Junior*, Oxford, Henry Cripps, 1628.

Calendar of the Close Rolls, Preserved in the Public Record Office, Edward II: Volume 2, 1313-1318, London, printed for Her Majesty's Stationery Office by Eyre and Spottiswoode, 1893.

Calendar of the Close Rolls, Preserved in the Public Record Office, Edward III. A.D. 1327-1330, London, printed for Her Majesty's Stationery Office, Eyre and Spottiswoode, 1896.

Calendar of the Close Rolls, Preserved in the Public Record Office, Edward III Vol. IX A.D. 1349-1354, London, printed for Her Majesty's Stationery Office, Mackie and Co., Ltd., 1906.

Calendar of the Close Rolls, Preserved in the Public Record Office, Edward III Vol. X A.D. 1354-1360, London, printed for Her Majesty's Stationery Office, Mackie and Co., Ltd., 1908.

Calendar of the Fine Rolls, Preserved in the Public Record Office, Vol. VI. Edward III. A.D. 1347-1356, London, published by His Majesty's Stationery Office, 1921.

Calendar of the Patent Rolls, Preserved in the Public Record Office, Edward I. A.D. 1301-1307, London, printed for Her Majesty's Stationery Office, Eyre and Spottiswoode, 1898.

Calendar of the Patent Rolls, Preserved in the Public Record Office, Henry IV. Vol. II. A.D. 1401-1405, London, printed for His Majesty's Stationery Office by Mackie and Co Ltd., 1905.

Calendar of the Patent Rolls, Preserved in the Public Record Office, Henry IV. Vol. III. A.D. 1405-1408, London, printed for His Majesty's Stationery Office by Mackie and Co Ltd., 1907.

Calendar of the Patent Rolls, Preserved in the Public Record Office, Henry V, Vol. II, A.D. 1416-1422, London, published for His Majesty's Stationery Office by Wyman & Sons, 1911.

Campbell, Eldridge and Colton, James (trans), *The Surgery of Theodoric, c. 1267– Volumes I and II*, New York, Appleton-Century Crofts, Inc., 1955.

Carnandet, Joanne (ed.), *Acta Sanctorum, January 1*, Paris, Victor Palmé, 1863.

Chapman, George T. L., McCombie, Frank, and Wesencraft, Anne (ed.), *A New Herball by William Turner, Parts II and III*, Cambridge, Cambridge University Press, 1995.

Cockayne, Revd Oswald, *Leechdoms, Wortcunning and Starcraft of Early England, Volumes I–III*, London, Longman, Green, Longman, Roberts and Green, 1864–6.

Colton, James B. (trans.), *John of Mirfield (d. 1407) Surgery, A Translation of his Breviarium Bartholomei, part IX*, New York, Hafner Publishing Company, 1969.

Coopland, G. W. (trans.), *The Tree of Battles of Honoré Bonet*, Liverpool, Liverpool University Press, 1949.

Cordiero, Luciano (ed.), *Cronica de El-Rei D. João I por Fernão Lopes, Vol. III*, Lisbon, Escriptorio, 1897.

Cowen, Janet (ed.), *Sir Thomas Malory, Le Morte D'Arthur, In Two Volumes*, Hammondsworth, Penguin Books Ltd., 1969.

Davies, Rev. John Silvester, *An English Chronicle of the Reigns of Richard II., Henry IV., Henry V., and Henry VI. - Written before the year 1471*, London, The Camden Society, 1856.

Dawson, Warren R., *A Leechbook or Collections of Medical Recipes of the Fifteenth Century*, London, MacMillan and Co. Limited, 1934.

Denifle, Henricus, *Chartularium Universitatis Parisiensis - Sub Auspichiis Consili Generalis Facultatum Parisiensium - Tomus II*, Paris, Ex Typis Fratrum Delalain (Delalain Brothers), 1889.

Dillon, Harold Arthur, Viscount and Hope, William St. John (ed.), *Pageant of the Birth Life and Death of Richard Beauchamp Earl of Warwick K.G., 1389-1439*, London, Longmans Green and Co., 1914.

Douët-D'Arcq, Louis Claude, *Choice de Pièces Inédites Relatives au Règne De Charles VI, Tome Second*, Paris, Jules Renouard et Cio, 1864.

Drayton, Michael, *The Battaile of Agincourt*, London, Charles Whittingham & Co., 1893.

Duplès-Agier, Henri, *Registre Criminel du Chatelet de Paris du 6 Septembre 1389 au 18 Mai 1392, Tome Premier*, Paris, Ch. Lahure, 1861.

Ellis, Henry, *Original letters, illustrative of English history; including numerous royal letters; from autographs in the British Museum, and one or two other collections, Second Series, Volume 1*, London, Harding and Lepard, 1827.

Eyre-Todd, George (ed.), *Mediaeval Scottish Poetry*, Glasgow, William Hodge & Co., 1892.

Eyre-Todd, George (trans.), *The Bruce, being the Metrical History of Robert the Bruce King of the Scots, Compiled A.D. 1375, by Master John Barbour Archdeacon of Aberdeen*, London, Gowans & Gray Limited, 1907.

Favre, Camille and Lecestre, Léon (ed.) *Le Jouvencel par Jean de Bueil, Suivi du commentaire de Guillaume Tringant, Tome Sécond*, Paris, Renouard H. Laurens successeur, 1887.

Firmage, George J. (ed.), *E.E. Cummings, Complete Poems, 1904-1962*, New York, Liveright, 1991.

Flavius Vegetius Renatus, *De Re Militari – Concerning Military Affairs*, Leonaur, 2012.

Flores, Angel (ed.), *An Anthology of Medieval Lyrics*, New York, Modern Library through Random House, 1962.

Fournier, Alfred (trans.), *Jean de Vigo, Le Mal Français 1514*, Paris, G. Masson, 1872.

Fuchs, C. H., *Die ältesten Schriftsteller über die Lustseuche in Deutschland, von 1495 bis 1510 Nebst mehreren Anecdotis späterer Zeit, gesammelt und mit literarhistorischen Notizen und einer kurzen Darstellung der epidemischen Syphilis in Deutschland*, Göttingen, Dieterichschen, 1843.

Gairdner, James (ed.), *The Historical Collections of a Citizen of London in the Fifteenth Century*, Westminster, Nichols and Sons, 1876.

Gairdner, James and Brodie, R. H. (ed.), *Letters and Papers, Foreign and Domestic, Henry VIII, Volume 21 Part 1, January-August 1546*, London, His Majesty's Stationery Office, 1908.

Gaskoin, George (trans.), *The Medical Works of Francisco Lopez de Villalobos, The Celebrated Court Physician of Spain*, London, John Churchill and Sons, 1870.

Gibson, Wilfrid Wilson, *Battle and Other Poems*, New York, The MacMillan Company, 1916.

Giles, J. A. (trans.), *Roger of Wendover – Flowers of History, In Two Volumes*, London, Henry G. Bohn, 1849.

Gonon, P. M., *Séjours de Charles VIII et Loy XII, a Lyon sur le Rosne. Jouxte la copie des Faicts, Gestes et Victoires des Roys Charles VIII et Loys XII*, Lyon, Charvin et Nigon, 1841.

Grosjean, Paulus (ed.), *Henrici VI Angliae Regis Miracula Postuma, Ex codice Musei Britannici regio 13. C VIII*, Brussels, Société des Bollandistes, 1935.

Gruner, Oskar Cameron (trans.), *The Canon of Medicine of Avicenna*, New York, AMS Press, 1973.

Haeser, H. und Middeldorpf, A., *Buch der Buch der Bündth-Ertznei von Heinrich von Pfolsprundt, Bruder des deutschen Ordens. 1460*, Berlin, Druck und Verlag von Georg Reimer, 1868.

Hardy, Sir William and Hardy, Edward (trans.), *A Collection of the Chronicles and Ancient Histories of Great Britain, Now Called England - by John de Wavrin, Lord of Forestel - from A.D. 1399 to A.D. 1422*, London, Eyre and Spottiswoode, 1887.

Hilton, Geoffrey (trans.), *The Deeds of Henry V Told by John Streeche*, Kenilworth, Published by the Author, 2014.

Holy Bible, Containing the Old and New Testaments, Philadelphia, American Baptist Publication Society, 1913.

Hughes, Shaun F. D., 'The Saga of Án Bow-Bender', *Medieval Outlaws, Ten Tales in Modern English*, Stroud, Sutton Publishing, 1998.

Hunter, Joseph, *Agincourt. A Contribution Towards an Authentic List of the Commanders of the English Host in King Henry the Fifth's Expedition to France, in the Third Year of His Reign*, London, John Russell Smith, 1850.

James, Thomas Beaumont and Simons, John (ed.), *The Poems of Laurence Minot 1333-1352*, Exeter, University of Exeter, 1989.

Jamison, D. F., *The Life and Times of Bertrand de Guesclin, A History of the Fourteenth Century, In Two Volumes*, Charleston, John Russell, 1864.

Johnes, Thomas (trans.), *The Chronicles of Enguerrand de Monstrelet; containing an account of the cruel civil wars between the houses of Orleans and Burgundy; of the possession of Paris and Normandy by the English; their expulsion thence; and of other memorable events that happened in the kingdom of France, as well as in other countries. Beginning at the year MCCCC., where that of Sir John Froissart finishes, and ending at the year MCCCCLXVII, and continued by others to the year MDXVI, In Two Volumes*, London, Henry G. Bohn, 1853.

Johnson, Tho. (trans.), *The workes of that famous chirurgion Ambrose Paréy - Translated out of Latine and compared with the French*, London, Printed by Richard Cotes and Willi Du-gard, 1649.

Judges, A. V. (ed.), *The Elizabethan Underworld - A Collection of Tudor and Stuart Tracts and Ballads, telling of the lives and misdoings of vagabonds, thieves, rogues and cozeners, and giving some account of the operation of the criminal law*, London, Routledge & Kegan Paul Ltd., 1965.

Kaeuper, Richard W. and Kennedy, Elspeth (trans.), *The Book of Chivalry of Geoffroi de Charny: Text, Context, and Translation*, Philadelphia, University of Pennsylvania Press, 1996.

Kingsford, Charles Lethbridge (ed.), *Chronicles of London*, Oxford, Clarendon Press, 1905.

Kingsford, Charles Lethbridge (ed.), *The First English Life of King Henry the Fifth, written in 1513 by an anonymous Author known commonly as The Translator of Livius*, Oxford, Clarendon Press, 1911.

Knox, Father Ronald and Leslie, Shane (trans.), *The Miracles of King Henry VI - Being an account and Translation of Twenty-three Miracles taken from the Manuscript in the British Museum (Royal 13c.viii)* , Cambridge University Press, Cambridge, 1923.

Laidlaw, J. C. (ed.), *The Poetical Works of Alain Chartier*, Cambridge University Press, 1974.

Lang, Andrew (trans.), *The Miracles of Madame Saint Katherine of Fierbois*, London, David Nutt, 1897.

Lespinasse, René de, *Bibliothèque de l'École des Chartes, Tome Deuxième*, Paris, Schneider et Langrand, 1840–1.

Lewis, Timothy (ed.), *A Welsh Leech Book or Llyfr o Feddyginiaeth*, Liverpool, D. Salisbury Hughes, 1924.

Liliencron, Rochus von (ed.), *Deutsches Leben in Volkslied um 1530*, Darmstadt, Wissenschaftliche Buchgesellschaft, 1966.

Livingston, Michael and DeVries, Kelly (ed.), *The Battle of Crécy - A Casebook*, Liverpool, Liverpool University Press, 2015.

Loomis, Richard Morgan (trans.), *Dafydd ap Gwilym - The Poems*, Binghamton, New York, Centre for Medieval & Early Renaissance Studies, 1982.

Lottin, D., *Recherches Historiques sur la Ville d'Orléans, Tome Premier*, Orléans, D'Alexandre Jacob, 1836.

MacCracken, Henry Noble (ed.), *The Minor Poems of John Lydgate*, London, Kegan Paul, Trench, Trübner & Co., Ltd., 1911.

MacKay, J. G. (ed.), *The Historie and Cronicles of Scotland - from the Slauchter of King James the First to the Ane thousande fyve hundreith thrie scoir fyftein zeir - Written and Collected by Robert Lindsay of Pitscottie, Three Volumes*, Edinburgh, William Blackwood and Sons, 1899.

MacKaye, Percy (trans.), *The Canterbury Tales of Geoffrey Chaucer - A Modern Rendering into Prose of the Prologue and Ten Tales*, New York, Duffield & Company, 1914.

Martin, G. H. (ed. & trans.), *Knighton's Chronicle, 1337 – 1396*, Oxford, Clarendon Press, 1995.

Martin, Solomon Claiborne (trans.), *Hieronymus Fracastor's Syphilis, from the Original Latin; A Translation in Prose of Fracastor's Immortal Poem*, St. Louis, The Philmar Company, 1911.

Maxwell, Sir Herbert (trans.), *Scalacronica, The Reigns of Edward I, Edward II and Edward III, as recorded by Sir Thomas Gray*, Glasgow, James MacLehose & Sons, 1907.

Maxwell, Sir Herbert (trans.), *The Chronicle of Lanercost - 1272-1346*, Glasgow, James Maclehose and Sons, 1913.

Michon, Joseph (ed.), *Documents inédits sur la grande peste de 1348 (Consultation de la Faculte de Paris, consultation d'un praticien de Montpellier, description de Guillaume de Machaut)*, Paris, J. -B. Baillière et fils, 1860.

Morand, François, *Chronique de Jean Fèvre, seigneur de Saint-Remy, Transcrite d'un manuscrit appartenant a la Bibliothèque de Boulogne-Sur-Mer*, Paris, Librairie Renouard, 1876.

Motteux (trans.), *Adventures of Don Quixote de la Mancha*, translated from the Spanish of Miguel de Servantes Saavedra, London, Frederick Warne and Co., 1800.

Müller, Axel E. W., *Gunpowder Technology in the Fifteenth Century, A Study, Edition and Translation of the Firework Book*, Woodbridge, The Boydell Press, 2024.

Nicaise, Edouard, *Chirurgie de Maitre Henri de Mondeville, Chirurgien de Philippe le Bel, Roi de France*, Félix Alcan, Paris, 1893.

Nicaise, Edouard, *La Grande Chirurgie de Guy de Chauliac, Chirurgien, Maistre en Médicine de l'Université de Montpellier, Composée en l'an 1363*, Paris, Félix Alcan, 1890.

Ohlgren, Thomas H. (ed.), *Medieval Outlaws, Ten Tales in Modern English*, Stroud, Sutton Publishing, 1998.

Owen, Wilfred, *Poems*, London, Penguin Classics, 2017.

Paget, Stephen (trans.), 'Journeys in Diverse Places, by Ambroise Paré', *The Harvard Classics, Scientific Papers, Physiology * Medicine * Surgery * Geology, Volume 38*, New York, P.F. Collier & Son, 1910.

Pallister, Janis L. (trans.), *Ambroise Paré on Monsters and Marvels*, Chicago, The University of Chicago Press, 1983.

Paré, Ambroyse, *La Méthode de traicter les playes faictes par hacquebutes et aultres bastons à feu et de celles qui sont faictes par flèches, dardz et semblables, aussy des combustions spécialement faictes par la pouldre à canon composée par Ambroyse Paré*, Paris, V. Gaulterot, 1545.

Payne, John (trans.), *Poems of François Villon*, John W. Luce & Company, Boston, 1917.

Petitot, Claude Bernard, 'S'ensuyt l'estat de la maison du duc Charles de Bourgongne, dict le hardy, composé par le memse auteur l'an 1474', *Collection Complète des Mémoires Relatifs a l'histoire de France, Tome X*, Paris, Foucault Libraire, 1825.

Pifteau, Paul (trans.), *Chirurgie de Guillaume de Sâlicet, Achevée en 1275*, Toulouse, Imprimerie Saint-Cyprien, 1898.

Plaine, François (ed.), *Monuments du procès de canonisation du bienheureux Charles de Blois, duc de Bretagne, 1320-1364*, Saint-Brieuc:, Imprimerie de R. Prud'homme, 1921.

Power, Sir D'Arcy (trans.), *De Arte Phisicali et de Cirurgia of Master John Arderne, Surgeon of Newark Dated 1412*, New York, William Wood & Co., 1922.

Power, D'Arcy (ed.), *Treatises of Fistula in Ano, Hæmorrhoids, and Clysters, by John Arderne, from an early fifteenth-century manuscript translation*, London, Kegan Paul, Trench, Trübner & Co., 1910.

Revard, Carter, 'The Outlaw's Song of Trailbaston', *Medieval Outlaws, Ten Tales in Modern English*, Stroud, Sutton Publishing, 1998.

Rickert, Edith (trans.), *Early English Romances in Verse: Done into Modern English by Edith Rickert: Romances of Friendship*, London, Chatto and Windus, 1908.

Rickert, Edith (trans.), *Early English Romances in Verse: Done into Modern English by Edith Rickert: Romances of Love*, London, Chatto and Windus, 1908.

Riley, Henry Thomas (ed.), *Chronica Monasterii S. Albani, Registra Quorundam Abbatum Monasterii S. Albani, qui Sæculo XVmo. floruere Vol. I., Registrum Abbatiæ Johannis Whethamstede, Abbatis Monasterii Sancti Albani*, London, Longman & Co., and Trübner & Co.,1872.

Riley, Henry Thomas (ed.), *Chronica Monasterii S. Albani. Thomæ Walsingham Quondam, Monachi S. Albani, Historia Anglicana, 2 vols*, London, Longman, Green, Longman, Roberts, and Green, 1863–4.

Riley, Henry Thomas (trans.), *Memorials of London and London Life, in the XIIIth, XIVth and XVth Centuries: Being a Series of Extracts, Local, Social, and Political, from the Early Archives of the City of London A.D. 1276-1419*, London, Longmans, Green, and Co., 1868.

Robbins, Rossell Hope (ed.), *Historical Poems of the XIVth and XVth Centuries*, New York, Columbia University Press, 1959.

Rosell, Cayetano (ed.), 'Corónica del Muy Alto et Muy Católico Rey Don Alfonso el Onceno, Deste Nombre, Que Venció la Batalla del Rio Salado, et Ganó a las Algeciras', *Crónicas de Los Reyes de Castilla desde Don Alfonso el Sabio, Hasta los Católicos Don Fernando y Doña Isabel, Tomo Primero*, Madrid, Rivadeneyra, 1875.

Rosenman, Dr Leonard D. (trans.), *The Chirurgia of Roger Frugard*, Xlibris Corporation, 2002.

Rosenman, Dr Leonard D. (trans.), *The Major Surgery of Guy de Chauliac, An English Translation*, Xlibris Corporation, 2005.

Rosenman, Dr Leonard D. (trans.), *The Surgery of Bruno da Longoburgo – An Italian Surgeon of the Thirteenth Century, by Mario Tabanelli*, Pittsburgh, Dorrance Publishing Co., Inc., 2003.

Rosenman, Dr Leonard D. (trans.), *The Surgery of Henri de Mondeville, In Two Volumes*, Xlibris Corporation, 1996.

Rosenman, Dr Leonard D. (trans.), *The Surgery of Lanfranchi of Milan*, Xlibris Corporation, 2003.

Rosenman, Dr Leonard D. (trans.), *The Surgery of Master Jehan Yperman*, Xlibris Corporation, 2002.

Rosenman, Dr Leonard D. (trans.), *The Surgery of Roland of Parma*, Xlibris Corporation, 2001.

Rosenman, Dr Leonard D. (trans.), *The Surgery of William of Saliceto*, Xlibris Corporation, 1998.

Rosenthal, David H. (trans.), *Tirant Lo Blanc, by Joanot Martorell & Martí Joan de Galba*, Baltimore, The Johns Hopkins University Press, 1996.

Samaran, Charles (ed. and trans.), *Thomas Basin, Histoire de Charles VII, Tome 1er, 1407-1444*, Paris, Société d'édition 'Les Belles lettres', 1933.

Sassoon, Siegfried, *The War Poems of Siegfried Sassoon*, ReadaClassic, 2011.

Scheps, Walter (trans.), 'The Acts and Deeds of William Wallace', *Medieval Outlaws, Ten Tales in Modern English*, Stroud, Sutton Publishing, 1998.

Schullian, Dorothy M. (trans.), *Diaria de bello Carolino (Diary of the Caroline War)* , New York, Frederick Ungar Publishing Co., 1967.

Scoble, Andrew R. (ed.), *The Memoirs of Philip de Commines, Lord of Argenton: Histories of Louis XI. and Charles VIII. Kings of France, and of Charles the Bold, Duke of Burgundy. To which is added, The Scandalous Chronicle or Secret History of Louis XI., by Jean de Troyes - Two Volumes*, London, Henry G. Bohn, 1855–6.

Sharpe, Reginald R. (ed.), *Calendar of Letter-Books Preserved Among the Archives of the Corporation of the City of London at the Guildhall, Letter-Book D., Circa A.D. 1309-1314*, London, John Edward Francis, 1902.

Sitwell, Osbert, *Argonaut and Juggernaut*, London, Chatto & Windus, 1919.

Skeat, Walter William (trans.), *The Vision of Piers Plowman, by William Langland Done Into Modern English*, London, Alexander Moring Ltd., 1905.

Skene, Felix J. H. (ed.), *Liber Pluscardensis, Two Volumes*, Edinburgh, William Paterson, 1877.

Smet, J. J. de (ed.), *Recueil Chroniques de Flandre, Publié sous la Direction de la Commission Royale D'Histoire, Tome III*, Brussels, M. Hayez, 1856.

Smith, Cyril Stanley and Gnudi, Martha Teach (trans.), *The Pirotechnia of Vannoccio Biringuccio, The Classic Sixteenth-Century Treatise on Metals and Metallurgy*, New York, Dover Publications, Inc., 1990.

Smith, Trevor Russell and Livingston, Michael (ed.), *Of Knyghthode and Bataile*, Michigan, Medieval Institute Publications, 2021.

Smollett, Tobias (trans.), *The Adventures of Don Quixote de la Mancha, The Adventures of Don Quixote de la Mancha by Miguel de Cervantes*, New York, Farrar, Straus, Giroux, 1986.

Sorley, Charles Hamilton, *Marlborough and Other Poems*, Cambridge, Cambridge University Press, 1919.

Southey, Robert (trans.), *Amadís of Gaul, by Vasco Lobeira - In Four Volumes*, London, T. N. Longman and O. Rees, 1803.

Southey, Robert (trans.), *Palmerin of England, by Francisco de Moraes - In Four Volumes*, London, Longman, Hurst, Rees, and Orme, 1807.

Stevenson, J. H. (ed.), *Gilbert of the Haye's Prose Manuscript (A.D. 1456), Volume I, The Buke of the Law of Armys or Buke of Bataillis*, Edinburgh, William Blackwood and Sons, 1901.

Stone, Brian (trans.), *Medieval English Verse*, New York, Penguin Books, 1988.

Strachey, Sir Edward (ed.), *Le Morte d'Arthur - Sir Thomas Malory's Book of King Arthur and of his Noble Knights of the Round Table - The Text of Caxton*, London, MacMillan and Co., Limited, 1919.

Strange, Richard, *The Life and Gests of St. Thomas of Hereford – From the Original 1674 Printing*, London, Burns and Oates, 1879.

Tait, James (ed.), *Chronica Johannis de Reading et Anonymi Cantuariensis, 1346-1367*, Manchester, University of Manchester Press, 1914.

Tanon, Louis, *Registre criminal de la justice de St. Martin des Champs à Paris au XIV siècle: publié pour la première fois, d'après le manuscrit des archives nationales, précède d'une étude sur la juridiction des religieux de St. Martin (1060-1674)* , Paris, Léon Willem, 1877.

Thomas, J. W. (trans.), *Medieval German Lyric Verse - In English Translation*, Chapel Hill, The University of North Carolina Press, 1968.

Thompson, Craig R. (trans.), *The Colloquies of Erasmus*, Chicago, The University of Chicago Press, 1965.

Thompson, Edward Maunde (ed.), *Chronicon Galfridi le Baker de Swynebroke*, Oxford, Clarendon Press, 1889.

Thorndike, Lynn, *University Records and Life in the Middle Ages*, New York, Columbia University Press, 1944.

Turner, Daniel, *De Morbo Gallico: A Treatise of the French Disease, Publish'd above 200 Years past, By Sir Ulrich Hutten, Kt. of Almayn in Germany. Translated soon after into English, by a Canon of Marten-Abbye*, London, Printed for John Clarke at the Bible under the Royal Exchange, 1730.

Twiss, Travers (ed.), *Monumenta Juridica, The Black Book of the Admiralty, in 4 Volumes*, London, Longman, 1871–6.

Urquhart, Sir Thomas and Motteux, Peter (trans.), *Rabelais, Gargantua and Pantagruel, Translated Into English, Volume I*, London, David Nutt, 1900.

Utterson, Edward Vernon, *Select Pieces of Early Poetry: Re-Published Principally from Early Printed Copies in the Black Letter, Volumes I and II*, London, William Pickering, Chancery Lane, 1825.

Veinant, Auguste Alexandre (ed.), *Les sept marchans de Naples, c'est assavoir l'adventurier. le religieux. l'escolier. l'aveugle. le vilageois. le marchant et le bragart*, Paris, Silvestre, 1838.

Viriville, Vallet de (ed.), *Chronique de Charles VII, roi de France, Par Jean Chartier, Nouvelle Édition Revue Sur Les Manuscrits, Suivie de divers Fragmens inédits, Trois Tomes*, Paris, P. Jannet, 1858.

Walker, Don, *Disease in London, 1st–19th centuries – An illustrated guide to diagnosis*, London, Museum of London Archaeology, 2012.

Walter, George (ed.), *The Penguin Book of First World War Poetry*, London, Penguin Books, 2006.

Willard, Charity Cannon (ed.), *The Writings of Christine de Pizan*, New York, Persea Books, 1994.

Willard, Sumner (trans.) and Cannon Willard, Charity (ed.), *The Book of Deeds of Arms and of Chivalry, Christine de Pizan*, Pennsylvania, The Pennsylvania University Press, 1999.

Williams, Benjamin (ed.) *Henrici Quinti Angliæ Regis, Gesta*, London, Sumptibus Societatis, 1850.

Young, Sydney, *The Annals of the Barber-Surgeons of London, Compiled from Their Records and Other Sources*, London, Blades, East & Blades, 1890.
Zupitza, Julius (ed.), *The Romance of Guy of Warwick, Part II*, London, N. Trübner & Co., 1887.

Secondary Source Material

Aberth, John, *The Black Death, The Great Mortality of 1348-1350, A Brief History with Documents*, Boston, Bedford/St. Martin's, 2005.
Abram, Annie, *English Life and Manners in the Later Middle Ages*, London, George Routledge & Sons Limited, 1913.
Allbutt, Thomas Clifford, *The Historical Relations of Medicine and Surgery to the End of the Sixteenth Century*, London, MacMillan and Co. Limited, 1905.
Allen, Peter Lewis, *The Wages of Sin – Sex and Disease, Past and Present*, Chicago, The University of Chicago Press, 2000.
Allmand, C. T., *Society at War, The Experience of England and France During the Hundred Years War*, Edinburgh, Oliver & Boyd, 1973.
Allmand, C. T., 'The War and the Non-Combatant', *The Hundred Years War*, London, The MacMillan Press Ltd, 1971.
Arnold, Catherine, *Bedlam, London and Its Mad*, London, Pocket Books, 2008.
Barante, M. de, *Historie des Ducs de Bourgogne de la Maison de Valois, 1364 – 1477, Tome IX*, Paris, Librairie le Normant, 1854.
Barker, Juliet, *Conquest - The English Kingdom of France 1417-1450*, Cambridge, Mass., Harvard University Press, 2012.
BBC, History Cold Case, Series One, Episode Three, *Stirling Man*, Shine TV Limited and Red Planet Pictures, 2011.
Beck, R. Theodore, *The Cutting Edge - Early History of the Surgeons of London*, London, Lund Humphries, 1974.
Benedictow, Ole J., *The Black Death, 1346-1353, The Complete History*, Woodbridge, The Boydell Press, 2004.
Bernstein, Peter, *Trauma: Healing the Hidden Epidemic*, Petaluma, The Bernstein Institute for Integrative Psychotherapy & Trauma Treatment, 2013.
Black, Sue, *Written in Bone, Hidden Stories in What We Leave Behind*, London, Transworld Publishers, 2020.
Bloch, Iwan, *Der Ursprung der Syphilis: eine medizinische und kulturgeschichtliche Untersuchung, Erste Abteilung*, Jena, Gustav Fischer, 1901.
Bloch, Iwan, 'History of Syphilis', *A System of Syphilis, In Six Volumes, Vol. 1*, London, Hodder & Stoughton, 1908.
Bottomley, Frank, *The Castle Explorer's Guide*, New York, Avenel Books, 1979.

Bovey, Alixe, *Tacuinum Sanitatis, An Early Renaissance Guide to Health*, London, Sam Fogg, 2005.

Bradbury, Jim, *The Medieval Archer*, Woodbridge, The Boydell Press, 1985.

Brown, Cornelius, *History of Newark-on-Trent; Being the Life Story of an Ancient Town, Volume I*, Newark, S. Whiles, 1904.

Brown, Kevin, *The Pox – The Life and Near Death of a Very Social Disease*, Stroud, Sutton Publishing, 2006.

Buchan, W., *Observations Concerning the Prevention and Cure of the Venereal Disease. Intended to guard the ignorant and unwary against the baneful effects of that insidious malady*, London, T. Chapman, 1796.

Burfield, Brian, *Medieval Military Medicine - from the Vikings to the High Middle Ages*, Barnsley, Pen & Sword Books, 2022.

Carmichael, Ann G., 'Plague Persistence in Western Europe: A Hypothesis', *Pandemic Disease in the Medieval World, Rethinking the Black Death*, Kalamazoo, Arc Medieval Press, 2015.

Champion, Pierre, *Vie de Charles d'Orléans (1394-1465)*, Paris, Honoré Champion, 1911.

Christiansen, Eric, *The Northern Crusades*, London, Penguin Books, 1997.

Clay, Rotha Mary, *The Mediaeval Hospitals of England*, London, Methuen & Co., 1909.

Cohen, Esther, *The Modulated Scream*, Chicago, The University of Chicago Press, 2009.

Coley, David K., *Death and the Pearl Maiden, Plague, Poetry, England*, Columbus, The Ohio State University Press, 2019.

Comrie, John, *History of Scottish Medicine to 1860, For The Wellcome Historical Medical Museum*, London, Baillière, Tindall & Cox, 1927.

Contamine, Philippe, *War in the Middle Ages (La guerre au moyen âge) - Translated by Michael Jones*, New York, Barnes and Noble Books, 1984.

Corns, Cathryn & Hughes-Wilson, John, *Blindfold and Alone - British Military Executions in the Great War*, London, Cassell Co., 2001.

Coughlan, Jennifer and Holst, Malin, 'Dental health and disease', *Blood Red Roses, The archaeology of a mass grave from the Battle of Towton AD 1461*, Oxford, Oxbow Books, 2000.

Curry, Anne, *The Battle of Agincourt - Sources and Interpretations*, Suffolk, The Boydell Press, 2009.

Curry, Anne, 'The Theory and Practice of Female Immunity in the Medieval West', *Sexual Violence in Conflict Zones, From the Ancient World to the Era of Human Rights*, Philadelphia, University of Pennsylvania Press, 2011.

Davies, Jonathan, *The Medieval Cannon 1326-1494*, Oxford, Osprey Publishing Ltd., 2019.

DeWitte, Sharon N, 'The Anthropology of Plague: Insights from Bioarcheological Analyses of Epidemic Cemeteries', *Pandemic Disease in the Medieval World: Rethinking the Black Death*, Kalamazoo, Arc Medieval Press, 2015.

Donagan, Barbara, 'Law, War, and Women in Seventeenth-Century England', *Sexual Violence in Conflict Zones, From the Ancient World to the Era of Human Rights*, Philadelphia, University of Pennsylvania Press, 2011.

Dormandy, Thomas, *The Worst of Evils, The Fight Against Pain*, New Haven, Yale University Press, 2006.

Dupuytren, Guillaume, *Traité, théorique et pratique, des blessures par armes de guerre, rédigé d'après les leçons cliniques de m. le baron Dupuytren, Tome Premier*, Paris, J.B Baillière, 1834.

Fabricius, Johannes, *Syphilis in Shakespeare's England*, London, Jessica Kingsley Publishers Ltd, 1994.

Finucane, Ronald C., *Miracles and Pilgrims – Popular Beliefs in Medieval England*, New York, St Martin's Press, 1995.

Fonblanque, Edward Barrington de, *Annals of the House of Percy, from the Conquest to the Opening of the Nineteenth Century, In Two Volumes*, London, Richard Clay & Sons, 1887.

Forrai, Judit, 'History of Different Therapeutics of Venereal Disease Before the Discovery of Penicillin', *Syphilis – Recognition, Description and Diagnosis*, Rijeka, Croatia, Intech, 2011.

Foucault, Michel, *Madness and Civilization, A History of Insanity in the Age of Reason*, New York, Vintage Books, 1988.

Fowler, Kenneth, *The King's Lieutenant: Henry of Grosmont, First Duke of Lancaster, 1310-1361*, New York, Barnes & Noble Inc., 1969.

Freeman, Margaret B., *Herbs for the Mediaeval Household for Cooking Healing and Divers Uses*, New York, The Metropolitan Museum of Art, 1943.

Gabriel, Richard, A, *Military Psychiatry: A Comparative Perspective*, Westport, Greenwood Press, 1986.

Garrison, Fielding H., *An Introduction to the History of Medicine*, Philadelphia, W. B. Sauders Company, 1929.

Garrison, Fielding H., *Notes on the History of Military Medicine*, Washington, Association of Military Surgeons, 1922.

Gasquet, Francis Aidan, *The Black Death of 1348 and 1349*, London, George Bell and Sons, 1908.

Geremek, Bronislaw, *The Margins of Society in Late Medieval Paris, translated by Jean Birrell*, Cambridge, Cambridge University Press, 1987.

Geremek, Bronislaw, *Truands et misérables dans l'Europe moderne: (1350-1600)*, Paris, Gallimard, 1980.

Getz, Faye, *Medicine in the English Middle Ages*, Princeton, Princeton University Press, 1998.

Gies, Joseph and Frances, *Life in a Medieval Castle*, New York, Harper & Row Publishers, 1981.

Goldhammer, Arthur (trans.), *The Poor in the Middle Ages: An Essay in Social History by Michel Mollat*, New Haven, Yale University Press, 1978.

Gottfried, Robert S., *The Black Death, Natural and Human Disaster in Medieval Europe*, New York, The Free Press, 1983.

Gravdal, Kathryn, *Ravishing Maidens, Writing Rape in Medieval French Literature and Law*, Philadelphia, University of Pennsylvania Press, 1991.

Gravett, Christopher, *Knights at Tournament*, Oxford, Osprey Publishing Ltd. 1988.

Green, Monica H., 'Editor's Introduction to Pandemic Disease in the Medieval World: Rethinking the Black Death', *Pandemic Disease in the Medieval World, Rethinking the Black Death*, Kalamazoo, Arc Medieval Press, 2015.

Green, Monica H., 'Preface - The Black Death and Ebola: On the Value of Comparison', *Pandemic Disease in the Medieval World, Rethinking the Black Death*, Kalamazoo, Arc Medieval Press, 2015.

Green, Monica H., 'Taking "Pandemic" Seriously: Making the Black Death Global', *Pandemic Disease in the Medieval World, Rethinking the Black Death*, Kalamazoo, Arc Medieval Press, 2015.

Griffiths, Ralph A., 'The Interaction of War and Plague in the Later Middle Ages', *Wales and Medicine, An Historical Survey from Papers Given at the Ninth British Congress on the History of Medicine*, Llandysul, J. D. Lewis and Sons Ltd., 1973.

Grose, Francis, *Military Antiquities Respecting a History of the English Army, from the Conquest to Present Times - Two Volumes*, London, T. Egerton Whitehall & G. Kearsley, 1801.

Hale, John, *The Civilization of Europe in the Renaissance*, New York, Simon & Schuster, 1993.

Hartley, Sir Percival Horton-Smith and Aldridge, Harold Richard, *Johannes de Mirfield of St Bartholomew's, Smithfield - His Life and Works*, Cambridge, Cambridge University Press, 1936.

Hartnell, Jack, *Medieval Bodies, Life, Death and Art in the Middle Ages*, London, Wellcome Collection, 2018.

Heizmann, Colonel Charles L., 'Military Sanitation in the Sixteenth, Seventeenth and Eighteenth Centuries', *The Annals of Medicine, Volume I*, New York, Paul B. Hoeber, 1917.

Herman, Judith Lewis, *Trauma and Recovery*, London, Pandora, 2015.

Hewitt, H. J., *The Organisation of War under Edward III, 1338-62*, Manchester, Manchester University Press, 1966.

Himes, Henry W. L., *Gunpowder and Ammunition Their Order and Progress*, London, Longmans, Green and Co., 1904.

Hindley, Geoffrey, *Medieval Sieges and Siegecraft*, New York, Skyhorse Publishing, 2009.

Hogg, Brigadier O. F. G., *English Artillery, 1326-1716, Being the History of Artillery in this Country Prior to the Formation of the Royal Regiment of Artillery*, London, Royal Artillery Institution, 1963.

Horden, Peregrine, 'Commentary on Part III, with a Note on Paracelsus', *Music as Medicine, The History of Music Therapy since Antiquity*, Aldershot, Ashgate Publishing Limited, 2000.

Horrox, Rosemary (ed. & trans.), *The Black Death*, Manchester, Manchester University Press, 1994.

Huard, Pierre and Grmek, Mirko Dražen, *Mille Ans De Chirurgie, En Occident: V – XV Siècles*, Paris, Les Éditions Roger Dacosta, 1966.

Hurd-Mead, Kate-Campbell, *A History of Women in Medicine from the Earliest Times to the Beginning of the Nineteenth Century*, Haddam, Conn., The Haddam Press, 1938.

Institute of Medicine of the National Academies, *Treatment for Posttraumatic Stress Disorder in Military and Veteran Populations: Initial Assessment*, Washington D.C., The National Academies Press, 2012.

Jones, Terry, *Medieval Lives*, London, BBC Books, 2004.

Jones, Terry, *Terry Jones' Medieval Lives*, BBC Video, 2008.

Jordan, William Chester, *The Great Famine, Northern Europe in the Early Fourteenth Century*, Princeton, Princeton University Press, 1996.

King, Margaret L. and Robin, Diana (ed. & trans.), *Isotta Nogarola, Complete Writings, Letterbook, Dialogue on Adam and Eve, Orations*, Chicago, University of Chicago Press, 2004.

Knowles, David and Hadcock, R. Neville, *Medieval Religious Houses - England and Wales*, London, Longmans, Green and Co, 1953.

Koopmans, Rachel, *Wonderful to Relate, Miracle Stories and Miracle Collecting in High Medieval England*, Philadelphia, University of Pennsylvania Press, 2011.

Lang, Sheila J., *The 'Philomena' of John Bradmore and its Middle English Derivative: A Perspective on Surgery in Late Medieval England (Thesis)* , St Andrews, University of St Andrews, 1998.

Lehner, Ernst and Johanna, *Picture Book of Devils, Demons and Witchcraft*, New York, Dover Publications Inc., 1971.

Lewis, P. S., *Later Mediaeval France, The Polity*, London, MacMillan and Co. Ltd., 1968.

Luce, Siméon, *Histoire de Bertrand du Guesclin et de son époque, la jeunesse de Bertrand (1320-1364)* , Paris, Librairie Hachette et Cie., 1876.

Malgaigne, J. F., *Surgery and Ambroise Paré, translated by Wallace B. Hamby*, Norman, University of Oklahoma Press, 1965.

Mallett, Michael, *Mercenaries and Their Masters - Warfare in Renaissance Italy*, New Jersey, Rowman and Littlefield, 1974.

Mann, J. H., *A History of Gibraltar and its Sieges*, London, Provost & Co., 1873.

Martines, Lauro, *April Blood: Florence and the Plot Against the Medici*, Oxford, Oxford University Press, 2003.

McLeod, Enid, *Charles of Orleans, Prince and Poet*, London, Chatto & Windus, 1969.

McKisack, May, *The Fourteenth Century, 1307-1399*, Oxford, Clarendon Press, 1959.

Meyrick, Samuel Rush, *A critical inquiry into antient armour: as it existed in Europe, but particularly in England, from the Norman conquest to the reign of King Charles II, with a glossary of military terms of the middle ages; In Three Volumes*, London, Robert Jennings, 1824.

Metzler, Irina, *A Social History of Disability in the Middle Ages – Cultural Considerations of Physical Impairment*, New York, Routledge, 2013.

Metzler, Irina, *Disability in Medieval Europe – Thinking about physical impairment during the high Middle Ages, c. 1100–1400*, Abingdon, Routledge, 2006.

Metzler, Irina, 'Indiscriminate Healing Miracles in Decline: How Social Realities Affect Religious Perception', *Contextualizing Miracles in the Christian West, 1100-1500*, Oxford, The Society for the Study of Medieval Languages and Literature, 2014.

Mitchell, Emily Sarah Jocelyn, *War, Wounds, and Medicine: A Re-Examination of the Crew of the Mary Rose (Thesis)*, Southampton, University of Southampton, 2022.

Mitchell, Piers D., 'Anatomy and surgery in Europe and the Middle East during the Middle Ages', *Anatomy and Surgery from Antiquity to the Renaissance*, Amsterdam, Adolf Hakkert, 2016.

Mitchell, Piers D., *Medicine in the Crusades – Warfare, Wounds and the Medieval Surgeon*, Cambridge University Press, 2004.

Moffat, Brian, *SHARP Practice 6, The Sixth Report on Researches into the Medieval Hospital at Soutra Scottish Borders/Lothian, Scotland*, Pathhead, SHARP, 1998.

Moffat, Brian, and other Participants in SHARP, *SHARP Practice 4, Fourth Report on Researches into the Medieval Hospital at Soutra, Lothian/Borders Region Scotland*, Edinburgh, SHARP, 1992.

Morand-Métivier, Charles-Louis, '"Je hé guerre, point ne la doit prisier": Emotions, War, and Trauma in the Poetry of Charles of Orléans', *Violence, Trauma, and Memory – Responses to War in the Late Medieval and Early Modern World*, London, Lexington Books, 2022.

Mortimer, Ian, *1415 Henry V's Year of Glory*, London, Vintage Books, 2010.

Mortimer, Ian, *The Perfect King, The Life of Edward III, Father of the English Nation*, London, Vintage Books, 2008.

Mortimer, Ian, *The Time Traveller's Guide to Medieval England – A Handbook for Visitors to the Fourteenth Century*, London, The Bodley Head, 2008.

Moulin, Daniel de, *A History of Surgery, with emphasis on the Netherlands*, Dordrecht, Martinus Nijoff Publishers, 1988.

Mount, Toni, *Everyday Life in Medieval London, from the Anglo-Saxons to the Tudors*, Stroud, Amberley Publishing, 2014.

Murray, Alexander, *Suicide in the Middle Ages, Volume 1 The Violent against Themselves*, Oxford, Oxford University Press, 1998.

Nicolas, Sir Harris, *History of the Battle of Agincourt, and of the expedition of Henry the Fifth into France in 1415; to which is added the Roll of men-at-arms in the English army*, London, Johnson & Co., 1833.

Nicolas, Sir N. Harris, *The Controversy Between Sir Richard Scrope and Sir Robert Grosvenor in the Court of Chivalry, 1385-1390*, London, Samuel Bentley, Vol. II, 1832.

Norris, John, *Medieval Siege Warfare*, Stroud, Tempus Publishing Limited, 2007.

Novak, Shannon A., 'Battle-related trauma', *Blood Red Roses - The Archaeology of a Mass Grave from the Battle of Towton AD 1461*, Oxford, Oxbow Books, 2000.

Ohler, Norbert, *Krieg und Frieden im Mittelalter*, Hamburg, Nikol Verlagsgesellschaft mbH & Co, 1997.

Onuf, Alexandra and Ealy, Nicholas, 'Introduction', *Violence, Trauma and Memory – Responses to War in the Late Medieval and Early Modern World*, Lanham, Lexington Books, 2022.

Packard, Francis R., *Life and Times of Ambroise Pare [1510-1590]. With a New Translation of his Apology and an Account of his Journeys in Divers Places*, New York, Paul B. Hoeber, 1921.

Paget, Stephen (trans.), *Ambroise Paré and His Times, 1510-1590*, New York, G.P. Putnam's Sons, 1897.

Palisca, Claude V., *Humanism in Italian Renaissance Musical Thought*, New Haven, Yale University Press, 1985.

Park, Katherine, 'Stones, Bones and Hernias', *Medicine from the Black Death to the French Disease*, Aldershot, Ashgate Publishing Limited, 1998.

Parker, Geoffrey, *The Military Revolution, Military innovation and the rise of the West, 1500-1800*, Avon, The Bath Press, 1988.

Partington, J. R., *A History of Greek Fire and Gunpowder*, Baltimore, Johns Hopkins University Press, 1999.

Paul, Michael C., 'Archbishop Vasilii Kalika of Novgorod, the Fortress of Orekhov and the Defence of Orthodoxy', *The Clash of Cultures on the Medieval Baltic Frontier*, Abingdon, Routledge, 2016.

Penman, Michael A., *David II, 1329-71*, Edinburgh, John Donald, 2005.

Pfau, Aleksandra Nicole, *Madness in the Realm: Narratives of Mental Illness in Late Medieval France (Thesis)* , Michigan, University of Michigan, 2008.

Platt, Colin, *King Death, The Black Death and its aftermath in late-medieval England*, Toronto, University of Toronto Press, 1997.

Ponting, Clive, *Gunpowder, An Explosive History: From the Alchemists of China to the Battlefields of Europe*, London, Pimlico, 2006.

Prescott, William H., *History of the Reign of Ferdinand and Isabella, The Catholic of Spain, In Three Volumes*, London, Richard Bentley, 1849.

Pullan, Brian S., *Rich and Poor in Renaissance Venice; the social institutions of a Catholic state, to 1620*, Cambridge, Mass., Harvard University Press, 1971.

Putnam, Ruth, *Charles the Bold, Last Duke of Burgundy, 1433-1477*, London, G. P. Putnam's Sons, 1908.

Randall, Lesa Beth, *Representations of syphilis in sixteenth-century French literature* (*PhD Dissertation)*, Tucson, University of Arizona, 1999.

Rawcliffe, Carole, *Leprosy in Medieval England*, Suffolk, The Boydell Press, 2009.

Rawcliffe, Carole, *Medicine & Society in Later Medieval England*, Stroud, Alan Sutton Publishing Limited, 1995.

Richardson, Thom, 'Armour', *Blood Red Roses - The Archaeology of a Mass Grave from the Battle of Towton AD 1461*, Oxford, Oxbow Books, 2000.

Santoni-Rugiu, Paolo and Sykes, Philip J., *A History of Plastic Surgery*, Berlin, Springer, 2007.

Savinetskaya, Irina, *The Politics and Poetics of Morbus Gallicus in the German Lands (1495 – 1520) (Thesis)*, Budapest, Central European University, Budapest, 2016.

Schipperges, Heinrich, *Die Kranken im Mittelalter*, München, c.H. Beck, 1990.

Scoffern, John, *Projectile Weapons of War and Explosive Compounds*, London, Cooke & Whitley, 1852.

Seward, Desmond, *A Brief History of the Hundred Years War, The English in France, 1337-1453*, London, Robinson, 2003.

Shahar, Shulamith, *Growing Old in the Middle Ages - 'Winter clothes us in shadow and pain'*, London, Routledge, 1997.

Shrewsbury, J. F. D. (ed.), *A History of Bubonic Plague in the British Isles*, Cambridge, At the University Press, 1970.

Sigerist, Henry E., *Hieronymus Brunschwig and his Work*, New York, Ben Abramson Publisher, 1946.

Simpson, W. J., *A Treatise on Plague dealing with the Historical, Epidemiological, Clinical Therapeutic and Preventative aspects of the Disease*, Cambridge, At the University Press, 1905.

Siraisi, Nancy, *Medieval and Early Renaissance Medicine, An Introduction to Knowledge and Practicev*, University of Chicago Press, 1990.

Siraisi, Nancy, *Taddeo Alderotti and his Pupils – Two Generations of Italian Medical Learning*, Princeton University Press, 1981.

Skinner, Patricia, *Living with Disfigurement in Early Medieval Europe*, New York, Palgrave MacMillan, 2017.

Skinner, Patricia, 'Looking for Burn Victims or Survivors in Medieval Europe', *Trauma in Medieval Society*, Leiden, Brill, 2018.

Stein, Claudia, *Negotiating the French Pox in Early Modern Germany*, Farnham, Surrey, Ashgate Publishing Limited, 2009.

Stone, Lawrence, *Family, Sex and Marriage in England 1500-1800*, London, Weidenfeld and Nicolson, 1977.

Stoudt, Debra L., 'Medieval German Women and the Power of Healing', *Women Healers & Physicians, Climbing a Long Hill*, Lexington, The University Press of Kentucky, 1997.

Sudhoff, Karl, *Aus der Frühgeschichte der Syphilis; Handschriften- und Inkunabelstudien, epidemiologische Untersuchung und kritische Gänge*, Leipzig, Johann Ambrosius Barth, 1912.

Sumption, Jonathon, *The Hundred Years War - Trial by Battle*, Philadelphia, University of Pennsylvania Press, 1991.

Sumption, Jonathon, *The Hundred Years War - Volume II, Trial by Fire*, Philadelphia, University of Pennsylvania Press, 1999.

Sumption, Jonathon, *The Hundred Years War - Volume III, Divided Houses*, London, Faber and Faber Ltd., 2009.

Talbot, C. H., *Medicine in Medieval England*, London, Oldbourne Book Co. Ltd, 1967.

Talbot, C. H. and Hammond, E. A., *The Medical Practitioners in Medieval England, A Biographical Register*, London, Wellcome Historical Medical Library, 1965,

Thordeman, Bengt, Nörlund, Poul and Ingelmark, Bo E., *Armour from the Battle of Wisby 1361, Vol. I*, Stockholm, Almqvist & Wiksells Boktryckeri-A.-B., 1939.

Time Team (DVD), *Castle Howard and Other Digs*, Disc 2, Episode 2, *Joust Dig It*, Videotext Communications Ltd., in association with The Picture House Television Co. Ltd., 2003.

Turner, Wendy J., *Care and Custody of the Mentally Ill, Incompetent, and Disabled in Medieval England*, Turnhout, Brepolis Publishers, 2013.

Turner, Wendy J. and Lee, Christina, 'Conceptualizing Trauma for the Middle Ages', *Trauma in Medieval Society*, Leiden, Brill, 2018.

Van der Kolk, Bessel, *The Body Keeps Score – Mind, Brain and Body in the Transformation of Trauma*, London, Penguin Books, 2014.

Vrebos, Dr Jacques, *The Legacy of Jehan Yperman to Plastic Surgery*, Brussels, published by the author, 1997.

Waldron, Tony, *Palaeopathology*, Cambridge, Cambridge University Press, 2009.

Whittock, Martyn, *A Brief History of Life in the Middle Ages*, London, Constable & Robinson Ltd, 2009.

Wilson, Ian, *The Book of Geoffroi de Charny, with the Livre Charny edited and translated by Nigel Bryant*, Woodbridge, The Boydell Press, 2021.

Woodhouse, Frederick Charles, *The Military Religious Orders of the Middle Ages, The Hospitallers, The Templars, The Teutonic Knights, and Others*, London, Society for Promoting Christian Knowledge, 1879.

Wylie, James Hamilton and Waugh, William Templeton, *The Reign of Henry the Fifth, in 3 Volumes*, Cambridge, The University Press, 1914–1919.

Yorke, Philip, *The Royal Tribes of Wales*, Wrexham, John Painter, 1799.

Ziegler, Philip, *The Black Death*, Harmondsworth, Penguin Books Ltd., 1969.

Zinsser, Hans, *Rats, Lice and History, Being a Study in Biography, which, after Twelve Preliminary Chapters Indispensable for the Preparation of the Lay Reader, Deals with the Life History of Typhus Fever*, London, George Routledge & Sons Ltd., 1935.

INDEX